Clinical Management of Swallowing Disorders

Third Edition

Clinical Management of Swallowing Disorders

Third Edition

Thomas Murry, PhD
Ricardo L. Carrau, MD

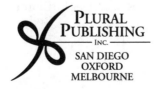

PLURAL
PUBLISHING
INC.
SAN DIEGO
OXFORD
MELBOURNE

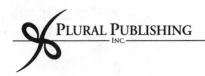

5521 Ruffin Road
San Diego, CA 92123

e-mail: info@pluralpublishing.com
Web site: http://www.pluralpublishing.com

49 Bath Street
Abingdon, Oxfordshire OX14 1EA
United Kingdom

Typeset in 10.5/13 Palatino by Flanagan's Publishing Services, Inc.
Printed in the United States of America by Bang Printing

Cover image courtesy of VEM/Photo Researchers, Inc.

Library of Congress Cataloging-in-Publication Data

Murry, Thomas, 1943-
  Clinical management of swallowing disorders / Thomas Murry and Ricardo L. Carrau.—3rd ed.
    p. ; cm.
  Includes bibliographical references and index.
  ISBN-13: 978-1-59756-425-0 (alk. paper)
  ISBN-10: 1-59756-425-7 (alk. paper)
  1. Deglutition disorders—Handbooks, manuals, etc. I. Carrau, Ricardo L. II. Title.
  [DNLM: 1. Deglutition Disorders—diagnosis. 2. Deglutition Disorders—therapy. WI 250]
  RC815.2.M875 2011
  616.3'1—dc22
                        2011002666

Contents

Preface   ix
Acknowledgments   xiii

I. **Introduction to and Epidemiology of Swallowing Disorders**   1
   Introduction   2
   Need for Early Intervention   4
   Epidemiology   5
   Summary   9
   Study Questions   10
   Discussion Questions   10
   References   10

II. **Anatomy and Function of the Swallowing Mechanism**   13
   Introduction   14
   The Normal Swallow   14
   Sphincters   19
   Cranial Nerves Involved in Swallowing   21
   Central Neural Control   22
   Respiration   23
   Summary   23
   Study Questions   24
   Discussion Question   24
   References   24

III. **The Abnormal Swallow: Conditions and Diseases**   27
   Introduction   28
   Neurological Disorders   33
   Conditions Found in Critical Care Patients   41
   Esophageal Disorders   41
   Infectious Diseases   48
   Medications   49
   Neoplasms   51
   Swallowing Disorders Following Radiation Therapy   52
   Intubation   53
   Autoimmune Diseases   53
   Summary   56
   Study Questions   56
   Discussion Questions   57
   References   57

IV. **Swallowing Disorders Arising From Surgical Treatments**   59
   Introduction   60
   Anterior Cervical Spinal Surgery (ACSS)   60
   Head and Neck Surgery   61

Floor of the Mouth Surgery 63
Partial Glossectomy 63
Palate Surgery 63
Lip Surgery 63
Mandibular Surgery 63
Oropharyngeal Surgery 63
Hypopharyngeal Surgery 64
Skull Base Surgery 64
Tracheotomy 64
Zenker Diverticulum 66
Summary 67
Study Questions 67
Discussion Questions 68
References 68

V. Evaluation of Dysphagia **69**
Introduction 70
Dysphagia Screening 70
Case History and Bedside Swallow Evaluation (BSE) 73
Instrumental Tests of Swallow Function 79
Summary 95
Study Questions 95
Discussion Questions 95
References 96

VI. Nonsurgical Treatment of Swallowing Disorders **99**
Introduction 100
Compensatory Swallowing Therapy 100
Rehabilitative Swallowing Therapy 111
Summary 118
Study Questions 118
Discussion Questions 118
References 118

VII. Prosthetic Management of Swallowing Disorders **121**
Introduction 122
Oral Prosthodontics and Dentures 122
Palate Lowering Prostheses 124
Soft Palate Prostheses 124
Lingual Prostheses 125
Speaking Valves 126
Physical and Environmental Adjustments 128
Summary 128
Study Questions 129
Discussion Question 129
References 129

VIII. Surgical Treatment of Swallowing **131**
Introduction 132
Vocal Fold Medialization 132
Palatopexy 138

Pharyngoesophageal Dilatation   139
Surgical Closure of the Larynx   139
Gastrostomy   139
Tracheotomy   139
Tracheostomy Tubes   141
Swallowing Following Head and Neck Cancer   142
Summary   144
Study Questions   144
Discussion Question   144
References   145

IX. **Pediatric Swallowing and Feeding Disorders**   **147**
Introduction   148
Incidence of Feeding and Swallowing Disorders in the Pediatric Populations   148
Anatomy   151
Physiology   152
Instrumental Examination   155
Radiological Examination   159
FEES and FEESST Examinations   159
Treatment of Feeding and Swallowing Disorders   161
Options and Considerations in Treatment of Feeding Disorders in Infants and Children   167
Additional Factors in Infant Feeding and Swallowing   168
Summary   169
Study Questions   170
Discussion Questions   170
References   170

X. **Nutrition and Diets**   **173**
Introduction   174
Properties of Liquids and Foods   174
Oral Nutrition and Dysphagia Diets   182
Nonoral Diets   184
Malnutrition and Dehydration   188
Nutrition in the Aging Population   189
Summary   190
Study Questions   190
Discussion Question   191
References   191

XI. **Patients With Voice and Swallowing Disorders**   **193**
Introduction   194
Diagnosis   195
Instrumentation   196
Personnel   197
Facilities   198
Case Studies From Voice and Swallowing Centers   198
Summary   206
Study Questions   207
Discussion Question   207
References   207

Glossary   209
Appendix I: Eating Assessment Tool (EAT-10)   221
Appendix II: Reflux Finding Score (RFS)   222
Appendix III: Reflux Symptom Index (RSI)   223
Appendix IV-A: Voice Handicap Index (VHI)   224
Appendix IV-B: Voice Handicap Index-10 (VHI-10)   226
Answers to Study Questions   227
Index   229

Preface

The *Clinical Management of Swallowing Disorders, Third Edition* is a core textbook that addresses the needs of those who will treat swallowing disorders as well as those clinicians who currently treat swallowing disorders in hospitals, rehabilitation centers, nursing homes, and in private outpatient clinics. This textbook addresses the diagnosis and treatment of swallowing disorders in children and adults as a major medical discipline that traverses multiple medical specialties, especially speech-language pathology and otolaryngology. The essential aspects of dysphagia management are presented in a format that both students and clinicians needing a practical update on dysphagia will find useful. Because of our daily clinical involvement treating swallowing disorders in major teaching institutions, we saw a need to revise a text that was well accepted by clinicians, students, and teachers as a practical text that addresses clinical issues at the current level of clinical understanding. With this edition, we hope to improve the standard of care in hospitals and medical centers.

The material contained in the *Clinical Management of Swallowing Disorders, Third Edition* derives from a vast storehouse of recent knowledge and academic pursuits, along with our daily experiences from multispecialty swallowing disorder clinics. Since the second edition, new evidence has demonstrated the importance of early intervention and aggressive treatment of dysphagia. Outcome data is now available to show the importance of proper assessments and treatment to deter and prevent aspiration. The third edition addresses clinical issues in a concise way, provides handy tabular information, and offers practical treatment options for a wide variety of swallowing problems with medical, surgical, and behavioral treatment models. We have tried to distill the complexity of the pathophysiology of dysphagia to a practical level useful to clinicians.

Throughout the book, certain terms are highlighted. These terms, which are germinal to the understanding of swallowing, are briefly explained. However, the reader may want to pursue these in greater depth, thus the reason for highlighting them in the text and in tables. We have tried to maintain the focus on treatment of swallowing disorders and have purposely avoided long discussions on the causes and complications of many conditions that result in dysphagia. Rather, we have focused on the essentials of diagnosis and treatment of swallowing disorders in children and adults.

Although we now work in two separate universities, we continue to share a philosophy that focuses on treatment based on sound research where available, consistent clinical methods, and the review of the outcomes of treatment to enhance our future clinical care.

Chapter 1 presents the clinical arena of dysphagia—who has dysphagia, the indications for intervention, the importance of treating dysphagia, and the relationship of the disorder to associated medical conditions. There are almost no medical conditions or diseases in which swallowing disorders do not occur. Although many swallowing disorders may be temporary, the need to intervene early and address them must be considered in light of the primary disease or disorder. An updated review of the extent of swallowing disorders in hospitals, nursing homes, and otherwise healthy individuals is provided.

Chapter 2 reviews the essential anatomy and function of the swallowing mechanism. We have chosen to present a summary of normal swallowing anatomy along with a concise review of the contributions of the cranial nerves rather than extensive anatomical and neuroanatomical descriptions of swallowing, in keeping with the clinical focus of this text. The contributions of the cranial nerves are presented in tables that the clinician can easily access. In this addition, we have included a review of the sensory information that, in the past, has been given little or no attention in much of the swallowing literature.

Chapter 3 provides a current description of the abnormal swallow and the swallowing disorders that arise from various neurological and head and neck disorders and diseases. Definitions of aspiration and aspiration pneumonia are given. A list of diseases with their major associated swallowing problems is found in this chapter. An array of tables that provide access to diseases and disorders and the swallowing problems associated with these disorders accompanies this chapter. In addition, the effects of medication on swallowing are discussed.

In Chapter 4, we present an expanded overview of swallowing disorders arising from surgical interventions. With the increasing popularity of surgical procedures that were previously considered extensive or dangerous, there is a greater need to understand those procedures and how they will effect swallowing in the short and long terms. The effects of surgery to the head, neck, and upper airway always produce a swallowing disorder, often temporary but in some cases permanent. The authors relate their daily experiences in the team treatment of these disorders. Treatments of long-term swallowing disorders arising from oral cancer or skull base surgical procedures are discussed, with emphasis on safety and recovery from the underlying disease. Indications for either aggressive or conservative surgical treatments are presented in this chapter.

Chapter 5 presents the current methods to evaluate dysphagia. We begin this chapter with an extensive review of the clinical bedside assessment. We have found this to be a starting point for subsequent testing and treatment. Moreover, our experience with the clinical bedside assessment has led us to identifying the appropriate tests to be done subsequent to identifying additional needs early in the treatment process. Although the bedside swallow evaluation is rarely the only evaluation of swallowing, it is an essential first step in the treatment process. Dysphagia screening is also discussed in this chapter. Finally, the most common instrumental tests used by speech-language pathologists and members of the swallowing team are reviewed, with indications for each test. Importance is placed on the criteria for test selection, the needs of the patient, and the expectations in the plan of treatment as a result of new or additional tests.

In Chapter 6, the nonsurgical treatment approaches to swallowing are presented in a modern format. This chapter has been revised extensively based on the plethora of current information. Since the earlier editions of this book, a number of clinicians have shown that many of the procedures are valuable in treatment, especially those that involve laryngeal elevation and upper esophageal sphincter relaxation. As the majority of treatments for swallowing disorders are nonsurgical, this important chapter outlines exercises for improving oral motor strength and bolus propulsion. Techniques are divided in compensatory swallowing therapy and rehabilitative swallowing therapy. Specific instructions for many of the clinical treatments are provided.

Chapter 7 addresses the prosthetic management of swallowing disorders. This includes oral prosthodontics as well as other biomechanical and adaptive devices to aid the patient to swallow safely. New materials that make the prosthetic appliances lighter and easier to use are included.

Chapter 8 provides a description of the newest and most common surgical procedures for treating swallowing disorders that are not amenable to direct or indirect nonsurgical treatments. This chapter has been revised to update the surgical techniques most often used to treat swallowing disorders. The surgical focus is primarily on prevention of aspiration and improving vocal fold closure. This chapter offers the nonsurgical clinician an understanding of the surgical procedures used to manage aspiration, from conservative vocal fold medialization techniques to extensive procedures such as laryngotracheal separation. Although the surgical procedures are briefly described, the importance of decision making by the dysphagia team in planning surgery is emphasized.

Chapter 9 is an entirely new chapter describing the conditions, diseases, and treatments for feeding and swallowing problems in infants and children. Although most infants and children develop and learn to swallow normally, a host of pediatric swallowing and feeding disorders may result from a multitude of medical problems that develop before, during, or after birth. Emphasis in this chapter is placed on the need to manage swallowing problems in the population aggressively, as they can affect growth, mental status, and psychological development even after the swallowing problem is resolved. Congenital and acquired neurological disorders and disorders and diseases that affect the anatomy and physiology of the developing infant are discussed with appropriate treatment options.

Chapter 10 addresses nutrition and diets and their importance in the management of swallowing disorders. A unique aspect of this chapter is the extensive explanation of the properties of liquids and their importance in menu planning. The current knowledge of fluid properties and their effects on swallowing are presented in a manner so that clinicians will understand the application of fluid dynamics to the treatment of swallowing disorders. Malnutrition and dehydration are also discussed in relation to swallowing disorders. An added feature of this chapter is the list of online references for food supplements and instruments to aid in feeding.

Chapter 11 presents our philosophical approach to the organization of a swallowing center. It combines the management of certain voice and swallowing disorders into one center, as the diagnosis and treatment may involve treating both issues concurrently. Cases are presented to show the value of a combined voice and swallowing center. The contributions of the speech-language pathologist and otolaryngologist in the diagnosis and treatment phases are described. The concept of a voice and swallowing center implies efficiency, comprehensiveness, and timeliness in the clinical management process of patients who will benefit from a combined management approach.

An expanded glossary is included to help the beginning swallowing therapist quickly find important terms. The glossary in the third edition has been completely revised and includes explanations of the terms as they relate to swallowing and other disease conditions, not simply definitions. The glossary alone provides the active swallowing clinician with a quick reference to an alphabetically listed wealth of information.

This text evolved from our interest in improving the treatment of swallowing disorders and from our daily involvement in treating those disorders emanating from a variety of medical conditions, diseases, and disorders. We have translated our clinical experiences into a series of chapters that contain information that we draw on daily. The *Clinical Management of Swallowing Disorders, Third Edition* offers the practicing clinician a reference text of the procedures for the diagnosis and management of swallowing disorders.

Acknowledgments

The authors acknowledge the contributions by colleagues in the various disciplines who diagnose and treat swallowing disorders. We have maintained a multidisciplinary approach to the treatment of dysphagia over our careers and we acknowledge all of those individuals who manage swallowing disorders in a multidisciplinary format.

The authors are deeply indebted to Marie-Pierre Murry for her work in reviewing the final version of the text, for preparing the glossary, which includes extended details as they relate to both swallowing and the underlying disease process, and for her unending encouragement while completing the third edition.

Contributions by Sarah Shulman, Yael Herzkof-Oreamuno, Trina Felton, and Ruth Jimenez, graduate students in swallowing disorders courses at Teachers College, Columbia University are gratefully acknowledged.

The authors acknowledge the editorial work of Sandy Doyle of Plural Publishing for her attention to the initial chapters of this manuscript. Her early suggestions and attention were invaluable. The final product is the extensive and detailed work of Caitlin Thompson Mahon, the patient copy editor who kept all of us focused to the finished product.

I

Introduction to and Epidemiology of Swallowing Disorders

CHAPTER OUTLINE

I. INTRODUCTION
    A. Normal Swallowing
    B. Abnormal Swallowing
    C. Impact of Swallowing Disorders on Quality of Life
    D. Other Impacts of Swallowing Disorders on Quality of Life
II. NEED FOR EARLY INTERVENTION
    A. Quality of Life
III. EPIDEMIOLOGY
    A. Cerebrovascular Accidents (CVAs) and Neurological Diseases
    B. Dementia
    C. Elderly Population
    D. Head and Neck Oncology
    E. Hospitalized Patients
    F. Nursing Home Residents
    G. Cardiac-Related Conditions
    H. Other Conditions
IV. SUMMARY
V. STUDY QUESTIONS
VI. DISCUSSION QUESTIONS
VII. REFERENCES

INTRODUCTION

Normal Swallowing

The normal swallow is a rapid and overlapping sequence of neurologically controlled movements involving the muscles of the oral cavity, pharynx, larynx, esophagus, and stomach. When the muscles of these organs or the nerves that govern these organs are disordered, disrupted, damaged, or destroyed, swallowing can no longer be normal. However, because of the neuroplasticity of the swallowing organs and their ability to develop compensatory strategies, certain types of foods and liquids can be swallowed safely by individuals with neurological or muscular damage to the swallowing organs. Although most individuals take normal swallowing for granted, everyone experiences an abnormal swallow at some time in their life, most likely resulting in an episode of a sudden choking sensation. However, in a normal, healthy person, this usually is resolved quickly by a cough or throat clearing.

Abnormal Swallowing

Abnormal swallowing includes difficulty with swallowing or the total inability to swallow, referred to as dysphagia and aphagia, respectively.

> The global definition of **dysphagia** is simply "difficulty in swallowing."

When someone cannot swallow at all, the term **aphagia**, or "inability to swallow anything," is used. The terms dysphagia and aphagia refer to swallowing saliva, liquids, foods, and medications of all consistencies. Dysphagia may also include such problems as foods or liquids "sticking" in the throat or regurgitation of swallowed liquids or foods. Swallowing difficulties may arise from mechanical problems of the swallowing mechanism, neurological disorders, gastrointestinal disorders, or loss of organs due to surgery or traumatic injury. Dysphagia and aphagia may also involve the disruption of the timing of the events needed to swallow normally.

Impact of Swallowing Disorders on Quality of Life

Swallowing disorders, even when subtle, eventually take a toll on quality of life. Because eating is a natural part of social interaction, daily nutrition, and general health, the importance of normal swallowing cannot be overstated. Swallowing affects quality of life in a number of ways, regardless of the severity of the problem.

Aspiration

Aspiration is a condition in which foods or liquids, pills, or oropharyngeal secretions pass into the airway below the level of the true vocal folds. This happens occasionally to most people; but in the absence of injuries to the muscles or nerves of swallowing, most people have the ability to sense the food or liquid in the airway and cough it out. When there is an injury or damage to the swallowing mechanism and aspiration is frequent or extensive, there is a higher risk of lung infections, dehydration, and malnutrition, and the enjoyment of eating diminishes; thus, quality of life also diminishes.

Aspiration Pneumonia

When pulmonary infection results from acute or chronic aspiration of fluids, foods, or oral secretions from the mouth or from fluids arising in the stomach and flowing into the airway, **aspiration pneumonia** develops. This is a potentially life-threatening condition and requires significant medical attention.

Dehydration

Dehydration is the state when there is not enough water in the body to maintain a healthy level of fluids in the body's tissues.

> Even in an otherwise healthy person, lack of adequate water intake can lead to dehydration.

For patients with neurological impairments, who may be at risk for aspiration when swallowing liquids, fluid intake may require constant monitoring.

Other factors such as medications that have dehydrating side effects, as discussed in Chapter 3, may impact one's ability to swallow. For example, when there is not enough natural saliva in the mouth, chewing becomes more difficult, food does not easily form a bolus, and particles may break apart and require multiple swallows.

Malnutrition

Malnutrition is the condition that occurs when your body does not get enough nutrients either due to the inability to ingest food safely, the reluctance to eat or fear of eating/drinking due to past swallowing problems, or the inability to digest or absorb ingested nutrients. Once a person is unable to ingest food safely, his or her ability to maintain health decreases. This is especially important for patients who are recovering from extensive surgeries, strokes, or other debilitating diseases and will require extensive rehabilitation. Once malnutrition develops, its treatment may be as important as any other part of the rehabilitation process. Recovery from malnutrition has been shown to help in the rehabilitation process, including in the treatment of dysphagia, leading to improvement in the patient's quality of life.

Weight Loss

There is a great preoccupation with weight loss in our society. Extensive weight loss, either induced or without reason, requires attention. Significant weight loss is always associated with the loss of muscle mass, which may produce weakness severe enough to change the daily activities of an individual. Weight loss associated with starvation, intentionally or unintentionally, may lead to damage of other vital organs, namely, the heart. When unplanned weight loss develops, a swallowing disorder should be suspected. Weight loss should not be so extensive that it affects quality of life nor should it continue beyond normal weight ranges.

> The impact of weight loss on various medical conditions or postsurgical recovery has been shown to slow or delay recovery.

Temporary nonoral feeding arrangements are now more commonly used to stabilize weight during recovery from severe diseases and disorders and to speed up such recovery.[1,2]

Types of Pneumonia

Not all pneumonia is the result of dysphagia or aphagia. Infections, poor health, and lack of proper posthospital care may lead to other types of pneumonia. Clinicians who treat swallowing disorders must be aware of these, as aspiration may play a part in their cause.

Nosocomial Pneumonia. **Nosocomial pneumonia**, also called hospital-acquired pneumonia, is usually the result of bacterial infections acquired during the first 48 to 72 hours following admission to a hospital. Nosocomial pneumonia is often the cause of death following admission to an intensive care unit. Factors such as old age, aspiration of saliva, fever, and gastric contents rising and falling into the airway (gastric reflux) are common causes of nosocomial pneumonia.

Community-Acquired Pneumonia. Community-acquired pneumonia (CAP) is an infection of the lungs in people who have not been hospitalized. It is a disease that can affect people of all ages and is often the leading cause of death in countries where vaccination against diseases has not been established.

> In CAP, the patient may appear to be swallowing normally but, due to fever or breathing difficulty, the lungs slowly absorb fluids, resulting in infection.

CAP is treated with antibiotics and may require hospitalization. In undeveloped countries, CAP can occur in patients who have recently been hospitalized.[3]

Other Impacts of Swallowing Disorders on Quality of Life

General Health

The inability to swallow correctly may lead to a decline in general health. This may be slow or rapid and is usually, but not always, associated with other diseases. For individuals with systemic diseases such as **Parkinson disease**, diabetes mellitus, and high blood pressure; or disorders such as gastroesophageal reflux; diseases such as **Charcot-Marie-Tooth disease**; or autoimmune disorders, the concomitant dysphagia increases the severity of the primary problem. With the onset of dysphagia, the body is not able to cope as well with the primary disease. Moreover, the primary disease may be exacerbated by the dysphagia.

Psychological Well-Being

Eating is a social function as well as a nutritional necessity. When an illness or disease is further compounded by dysphagia, the natural social functions in which food plays a role are limited. The person with a swallowing disorder can no longer participate seamlessly in the social interactions that surround meals.

Financial Well-Being

The financial impact caused by dysphagia can be significant if there is a need for special foods, supplemental feeding, primary **enteral** or **parenteral nutrition**, dysphagia therapy, special gadgets and appliances to aid in the preparation of meals, or the need for others to assist with feeding. Some or all of these expenses may be paid for by insurance; however, the costs of all dysphagia-related management issues may be substantial and may continue for extended periods of time, straining the financial condition of the patient, his or her family, and the economic welfare of the patient's society.[4] Limitations brought by insurance capitation or personal financial abilities often compromise ideal rehabilitation strategies.

The true financial impact of dysphagia remains unknown, as research has not yet determined the total cost of major events such as aspiration pneumonia and hospital readmissions nor the cost/benefit ratio for the early identification and management of swallowing disorders. Conventional wisdom suggests that early intervention may prevent extensive comorbidities that result from the interaction of swallowing disorders with other diseases or disorders. Clinical research ultimately will lead to the confirmation of methods of dysphagia rehabilitation.

NEED FOR EARLY INTERVENTION

"Not everything that counts can be counted."
Dennis Burket, as quoted in *Kitchen Table Wisdom* by R. N. Remen[5]

Quality of Life

There is only limited, albeit strong and intuitively correct, evidence that the diagnosis and treatment of dysphagia is efficacious from the standpoint of significantly reducing aspiration pneumonia. Most of the evidence that exists is based on studies of stroke patients, although, as pointed out in Chapter 8, there also is evidence derived from research on patients undergoing treatment for cancers of the head and neck. The limited evidence suggests that, in the acute care setting, dysphagia management is accompanied by reduced pneumonia rates. Furthermore, the use of a complete **bedside swallow evaluation (BSE)** appears to be cost-effective.[6] Others have found dysphagia management to be useful in the rehabilitation of swallowing disorders in other populations. Wasserman et al[7] have shown that, with accurate reporting of bedside swallow evaluation information, an early aggressive treatment program is efficacious in reducing the length of hospital stays in patients undergoing major surgery for head and neck cancer. Additionally, development of valid screening procedures, such as the scale developed by Foster and colleagues,[8] may offer a further basis for early treatment of patients with dysphagia. They administered a dysphagia screening instrument to 299 inpatients and found that the scale provided a means for targeting patients for early swallowing assessment and intervention.

McHorney and colleagues[9] presented early versions of two quality of life assessments to determine the need and value of treaing swallowing disorders. The SWAL-QOL is a validated, 44-item tool that assesses quality-of-life concepts. The SWAL-CARE is a 15-item tool that assesses quality of care and patient satisfaction. The scales identify patients with oropharyngeal dysphagia from normal swallowing subjects and are sensitive to differences in dysphagia severity. The SWAL-QOL and SWAL-CARE may help clinicians to identify and focus on patients who are in critical need of treatment and to determine treatment effectiveness. Recently, McHorney and colleagues[10] validated the SWAL-QOL and SWAL-CARE on a group of 386 patients with oropharyngeal dysphagia as it relates to bolus flow. They found that, as the severity of bolus flow increased, there was a decrease in the measures of SWAL-QOL and SWAL-CARE. The two scales were related primarily to oral transit duration and total swallow duration.

> What groups of patients might the SWAL-QOL and SWAL-CARE be most useful for? In what groups might its use be limited?

In general, the lack of control groups, the undefined effects of diseases, and the lack of long-term follow-up data limit the statements that can be made about the true effects of early dysphagia intervention. Nonetheless, the clinical evidence of those treating patients with dysphagia on a day-to-day basis suggests that intervention improves quality of life. The lack of prospective, controlled, randomized research should not suggest that swallowing programs using the BSE or other programs such as the **modified barium swallow** (MBS; see Chapter 5) or the flexible endoscopic evaluation of swallowing (FEES; see Chapter 5) should not be continued. On the contrary, studies such as that by Odderson et al[11] provide strong arguments for continued early intervention in dysphagia. These investigators looked at pneumonia rates before and after initiating a BSE program in a hospital setting.

> Aspiration pneumonia rates in stroke patients were substantially reduced after an early intervention swallowing program was initiated compared to pneumonia rates before the program was started.[11]

Additional research is needed to provide further evidence for BSE programs, as well as for programs that rely on instrumental diagnosis of the swallowing problem. It is important for programs in dysphagia intervention to include a data acquisition format that offers an opportunity to assess their contribution to reduction of hospital stays and readmissions due to swallowing-related problems.

EPIDEMIOLOGY

Dysphagia can be caused by many different disorders, including natural aging, neurological diseases, head injury, degenerative diseases, systemic diseases, autoimmune disorders, neoplasms, and infections. Treatment modalities such as surgery, radiation therapy, and medications can also lead to dysphagia. Chronic reflux laryngitis, often overlooked, may also interfere with normal swallowing. Patients with head or neck cancer have a variable presentation. They often have significant dysphagia at the time of initial presentation, and their swallowing function also often suffers as a result of treatment, although some deficits improve with time. Patients with Parkinson disease suffer from dysphagia that becomes more severe as the disease progresses. Because of these varied and often compounded etiologies, it may not be possible to ascertain the true incidence of any particular category of disorder. In addition to these factors, there is no single test that is 100% accurate for diagnosing dysphagia.

Swallowing disorders may arise as comorbidities of other disorders or as precursors to more significant diseases and disorders. Moreover, the incidence of swallowing disorders may vary depending on the type of diagnostic evaluation. Table 1–1 shows the incidence of oropharyngeal dysphagia in patients who exhibited aspiration during videofluoroscopic examination.[12,13]

More recent data by Daniels and Huckabee[14] suggest that incidence of swallowing disorders following a stroke remains high; however, with the advent of improved assessment techniques, the treatment process following evidence of aspiration is now better understood. If all of the tests for examination

Table 1–1. Incidence of Oropharyngeal Dysphagia in Patients Who Exhibited Aspiration During Videofluoroscopic Examination[12] and Flexible Endoscopic Evaluation of Swallowing.[13]

Cause of Dysphagia	Number (%) of Patients
Head and neck oncologic surgery	59 (36)
Cerebrovascular accident	47 (29)
Cardiac-related event*	294 (22)
Closed head injury	12 (7)
Spinal cord injury	10 (6)
Degenerative neurologic disease**	9 (6)
Adductor vocal fold paralysis	7 (4)
Zenker diverticulum	4 (2)
Generalized weakness	5 (3)
Cerebral palsy	3 (2)
CNS involvement from AIDS	Unknown
Craniotomy (for aneurysm repair)	2 (1)
Undetermined	4 (2)

*Data from Aviv JE, Murry T, Zschommler A, Cohen M, Gartner C. Flexible endoscopic evaluation of swallowing with sensory testing: patient characteristics and analysis of safety in 1340 consecutive examinations. *Ann Otol Rhinol Laryngol.* 2005;114(3):173–176.

**Includes Parkinson disease, motor neuron disease, and multiple sclerosis

Source: Adapted from Rasley A, Logemann JA, Kahrilas P, Rademaker AW, Pauloski BR, Dodds WJ. Prevention of barium aspiration during videofluoroscopic swallowing studies: value of postural change. *Am J Roentgenol.* 1993;160:1005–1009.

of swallowing are considered, the true incidence of swallowing disorders may be substantially higher. When the swallowing disorder accompanies other medical conditions, the primary condition may be affected by the swallowing disorder. Conversely, a swallowing disorder may be the symptom of another neurological disease or condition requiring treatment. Thus, the exact incidence of swallowing disorders remains unknown.

Cerebrovascular Accidents (CVAs) and Neurological Diseases

Stroke is the third leading cause of death in the United States. Approximately 500 000 new cases are reported yearly, and 150 000 individuals die of CVAs every year. Prospective studies have demonstrated an incidence of dysphagia as high as 41.7% in the first month after a CVA.

> The overall rate of aspiration resulting from a CVA is approximately 33.3%. One-half of these patients will aspirate silently (with no obvious clinical symptoms or signs).

As many as 20% die of aspiration pneumonia in the first year after a CVA, and 10% to 15% will die of aspiration pneumonia after the first year following the stroke. In general, the larger the area of ischemia, the more significant the swallowing disorder. Although the site of lesion does not always correlate with the type and severity of the swallowing disorder, brainstem strokes produce dysphagia more frequently than cortical strokes. Table 1–2 shows the epidemiological data recently obtained from the Agency for Healthcare Policy and Research and Quality (AHRQ) for neurological diseases including stroke.[6]

Dementia

Dementia refers to the inability to carry out tasks due to the loss of brain function. The loss of brain function depends on the part of the brain that is damaged. Dysphagia is common in elderly patients with dementia. According to videofluoroscopic reports, normal swallowing function is found in only 7% of patients with dementia. This group of patients is the most difficult to assess with any type of functional study, due to their dementia. The effectiveness of therapeutic maneuvers that require patient cooperation is also low. Nonoral nutrition alternatives must be considered in patients with dementia and dysphagia. Recurrences of aspiration pneumonia, continued weight loss, and/or refusal to eat are the key indications for implementing nonoral nutrition alternatives.

Table 1–2. Epidemiological Data from the Published Literature: Neurological Diseases and the Rate of Dysphagia Within Each

Disease	Prevalence (per 100,000)	Incidence (per 100,000)	Study	Reason	Diagnosed Occurrence of Dysphagia (%)	Study	Reason
Stroke	NA	145	Brown et al[15]	Mayo Clinic	VFSS: 74.6	Daniels et al[25]	Median of VFSS studies
		289	Modan and Wagener[16]	Mayo Clinic seemed low: this provides an upper estimate	BSE: 41.7	DePippo et al[26]	Median of BSE studies
Parkinson disease	106.9	13	Mayeux et al[17]	Only number on general population that included elderly	VFSS: 69.1	Bushmann et al[27]; Fuh et al[28]	Mean of 2 studies in which L-dopa was withheld
Alzheimer disease	259.8	NR	Beard et al[18]	Only published number	VFSS: 84	Horner et al[29]	Only published number
Multiple sclerosis	170.8	NR	Wynn et al[19]	Only number; Mayo Clinic	NR	NA	NA
Motor neuron disease	170.8	6.2	Lilienfeld et al[20]	Only published number	51.2 (method not reported)	Leighton et al[30]	Exam, not survey
Amyotrophic lateral sclerosis	NR	1.8	McGuire et al[21]	Exam, not survey	29 (method not reported)	Litvan et al[31]	Only published number
Progressive supranuclear palsy	1.39	1.1	Golbe et al[22]; Bower et al[23]	Only published number	VFSS: 55.6	Kagel and Leopold[32]	Only published number
Huntington disease	1.9	0.2	Kokmen et al[24]	Only published number	VFSS: 100		

BSE = bedside swallowing evaluation; NA = not applicable; NR = not reported; VFSS = videofluoroscopic swallowing examination

Dementia presents unique problems to the clinician treating dysphagia. Why?

Elderly Population

Seventy to 90% of elderly patients, even those without known neurological disease, have some degree of swallowing dysfunction, if not true dysphagia. Objective functional tests are necessary to rule out specific diseases and to assess the risk of aspiration. As many as 50% of elderly patients have difficulty eating, leading to nutritional deficiencies with associated weight loss, increased risk of falling, poor healing, and increased susceptibility to other illnesses. Weight loss, increased length of meals, depression, and general complaints of fatigue are often observed in this group prior to the diagnosis of a swallowing disorder.

Head and Neck Oncology

The presence of a tumor in the upper aerodigestive tract may affect swallowing by:

1. Mechanical obstruction due to bulk or extraluminal compression;
2. Decreased pliability of the soft tissue due to neoplastic infiltration;
3. Direct invasion leading to paralysis of important pharyngeal or laryngeal muscles;
4. Loss of sensation caused by nerve injury; and
5. Pain.

Treatments for squamous cell carcinoma, namely surgery, radiation, or chemotherapy, produce disabilities that are usually proportional to the volume of the resection and/or the radiation field. Surgery produces division and fibrosis of muscles and anesthetic areas due to the transection or extirpation of afferent neural fibers and/or receptors.

> Radiation therapy leads to **xerostomia** (dryness of the mouth), which, in many cases, is permanent and a main source of swallowing complaints made by patients.

Irradiation also produces fibrosis of the oropharyngeal and laryngeal musculature. Chemotherapy may lead to weakness, nausea, or reduced sensory processes and may add to immediate radiation side effects such as mucositis, the thickening of mucus in the mouth, pharynx, and esophagus.

Swallowing function after radiation treatment appears to be related to both site and stage of disease. In general, patients with so-called anterior tumors, such as on the floor of the mouth or anterior oral tongue, have better posttreatment outcomes regarding swallowing than do patients with posterior tumors, such as on the oropharynx or hypopharynx.

Reconstructive methods also influence the swallowing outcome. Patients who are reconstructed with primary closure have fewer problems swallowing than patients who are reconstructed with bulky insensate flaps.

Hospitalized Patients

The incidence of swallowing disorders in patients admitted to critical care units is increased by the need for endotracheal and nasogastric intubation and tracheotomy, the use of sedatives, impaired consciousness, and the debilitated status of many of the patients requiring critical care.

> Acute care patients should be assessed for swallowing disorders within the first 24 hours of hospitalization.

In many hospitals, a standing order exists for a clinical bedside evaluation (CBE) of the acute patient within 24 hours of admission. Patients requiring mechanical ventilation are at higher risk for aspiration pneumonia. The mortality of nosocomial pneumonia is estimated to be between 20% to 50% for hospitalized patients. Hospital costs due to nosocomial infection may exceed $18,000 per occurrence.

Nursing Home Residents

Studies carried out in nursing homes have demonstrated that 40% to 60% of the residents have clinical evidence of dysphagia. This number appears to be increasing in recent years.

> Smith et al[33] suggest that the high number of nursing home residents with dysphagia is due, at least in part, to discharging patients with swallowing disorders from acute care settings into institutional care.

The prevalence of all types of pneumonia has been estimated to be 2%, although it is unknown how many of these patients developed pneumonia as a result of aspiration. The death rate for patients diagnosed with pneumonia in a nursing home and admitted to acute care centers may exceed 40% of all readmissions.

Cardiac-Related Conditions

The number of patients seen in major medical centers for cardiac-related conditions is always increasing, due to the life-sustaining procedures available in emergency settings and the types of surgical treatment available to patients following cardiac events. In 2004, a large cohort of patients (1,340) with swallowing disorders was examined by Aviv and colleagues[34] in an effort to identify safety and comfort factors related to assessment of swallowing disorders using the flexible endoscopic examination of swallowing with sensory testing (FEESST) procedure in in- and outpatients. The largest patient subgroup, as might be expected, was poststroke patients; however, surprisingly, the second-largest group was patients with cardiac-related events (22.2%). The majority of cardiac-related cases in the acute, inpatient setting were patients who had undergone open-heart surgery (almost 60% of cases), followed by patients who had had heart attacks and those with congestive heart failure and newly diagnosed arrhythmias. The authors found that a large percentage of these patients had significant vagal nerve sensory dysfunctions when tested with FEESST and thus were at risk for **silent aspiration**, that is, aspiration without sensing the need to cough.

Other Conditions

Patients may present to an outpatient facility with numerous problems that include difficulty with swallowing or the inability to swallow. Other swallowing disorders may also be identified when a patient is hospitalized for the care of other conditions. Table 1–3 outlines the most common conditions that may indicate a swallowing disorder is also present. The true incidence of swallowing disorders in patients presenting with these problems is unknown.

Table 1–3. **Conditions That May Lead to or Are Directly Related to Swallowing Disorders**

Type of Condition	Common Examples
Congenital	Dysphagia lusoria
	Tracheoesophageal fistula
	Laryngeal clefts
	Other foregut abnormalities
Inflammatory	Gastroesophageal reflux disease (GERD)
	Laryngopharyngeal reflux (LPR)
Infections	Lyme disease
	Neuropathies/encephalitis
	Chagas disease
Trauma	CNS
	Upper aerodigestive tract
	Blunt traumatic injuries to the oral, laryngeal, and/or esophageal organs
Endocrine	Goiter
	Hypothyroid
	Diabetic neuropathy
Neoplasia	Oral cavity and contents
	Upper aerodigestive tract
	Thyroid
	Central nervous system
Systemic	Autoimmune disorders
	Dermatomyositis
	Scleroderma
	Sjögren disease
	Amyloidosis
	Sarcoidosis
Iatrogenic	Surgery
	Chemotherapy
	Other medications
	Radiation

SUMMARY

Swallowing disorders have a significant effect on a patient's quality of life, including the patient's physical, financial, and psychological well-being.

Dysphagia leads to a number of complicating factors, whether the patient is generally healthy or is recovering from a neurological event, cancer, or other surgery. The inability to swallow leads to weight loss, weakness, and, in severe cases, complicating medical problems.

Although research is somewhat limited, there appears to be a general clinical consensus that early intervention in dysphagia through proper diagnosis and treatment may reduce the comorbidities and thus shorten the length and cost of the hospital stay.

Treatment of swallowing disorders varies according to the underlying pathophysiology and status of the patient. Outpatients with minor problems are generally cooperative and willing to make adjustments in lifestyle and diet to improve their swallowing disorder. Hospitalized patients may be severely deconditioned or their cognitive status may limit their cooperation in the rehabilitation process. The patient with dysphagia presents a unique opportunity for team diagnosis and treatment. The remainder of this text explores the methods and approaches to treating swallowing disorders.

STUDY QUESTIONS

1. Aspiration refers to
   A. Liquid or food caught in the throat
   B. Liquid or food passing into the airway below the vocal folds
   C. Coughing after swallowing liquids or foods
   D. Inability to cough when choking on liquids or foods

2. Malnutrition develops when
   A. A person has not drunk enough water
   B. A person fails to eat a balanced diet
   C. A person does not take in the proper amount of protein calories
   D. A person goes on a crash diet not approved by a physician

3. In today's society, weight loss
   A. Is desirable when people are hospitalized
   B. May have negative effects on hospitalized patients
   C. Is usually recommended for overweight people when they are hospitalized
   D. Improves swallowing ability

4. The bedside swallowing evaluation
   A. Provides the basis for deciding what type of foods to give a patient with a swallowing disorder
   B. Provides the clinician with the patient's underlying swallowing problem
   C. Reduces the need for an instrumental swallowing examination
   D. May be used as a screening tool for identifying patients at risk for a swallowing disorder

5. Silent aspiration
   A. Occurs rarely in patients following strokes
   B. May be reduced using thickened consistencies of food
   C. Cannot be adequately identified during a bedside swallow evaluation
   D. Does not affect patients after their acute recovery period from a CVA

DISCUSSION QUESTIONS

Gather relevant information about the following questions:

A. Why the need to study normal swallowing?

B. What is the importance of understanding the financial impact of swallowing on a patient, a hospital, and a nursing home?

C. What are the limitations of a sole provider of swallowing rehabilitation such as might be found in a nursing home?

D. What are the complications that might exist with a patient with dementia in assessing and treating a swallowing problem?

REFERENCES

1. Mercuri A, Lim Joon D, Wada H, Rolfo A, Khoo V. The effect of an intensive nutritional program on daily set-up variations and radiotherapy planning margins of head and neck cancer patients. *J Med Imaging Rad.* 2009; 53(5):500–505. doi:10.1111/j.1754-9485.2009.02105.

2. Marcason W. What are the primary nutritional issues for a patient with Parkinson's disease? *J Am Diet Assoc.* 2009; 109(7):1316–1319.

3. Dimopoulos G, Matthaiou DK, Karageorgopoulos DE, Grammatikos AP, Athanassa Z, Falagas ME. Short- versus long-course antibacterial therapy for community-acquired pneumonia: a meta-analysis. *Drugs.* 2008;68(13): 1841–1854.

4. Leslie P, Carding PC, Wilson JA.Investigation and management of chronic dysphagia. *Br Med J.* 2003;326:433–436.

5. Remen RN. *Kitchen Table Wisdom.* New York, NY: Penguin; 1996.

6. Agency for Health Care and Policy Research. *Diagnosis and Treatment of Swallowing Disorders (Dysphagia) in Acute Care Stroke Patients.* Summary, Evidence Report/Technology Assessment: No. 8. Rockville, MD: Agency for Health Care Policy and Research; 1999: AHCPR Publication 99-EO24.

7. Wasserman T, Murry T, Johnson JT, Myers EN. Management of swallowing in supraglottic and extended supraglottic laryngectomy patients. *Head Neck.* 2001;23(12): 1043–1048.

8. Foster CB, Gorga D, Padial C, et al. The development and validation of a screening instrument to identify hospitalized medical patients in need of early functional rehabilitation assessment. *Qual Life Res.* 2004;13(6):1099–1108.

9. McHorney CA, Robbins J, Lomax K, et al. The SWAL-QOL and SWAL-CARE outcomes tool for oropharyngeal dysphagia in adults: III. Documentation of reliability and validity. *Dysphagia.* 2002;17(2):97–114.

10. McHorney CA, Martin-Harris B, Robbins J, Rosenbek J. Clinical validity of the SWAL-QOL and SWAL-CARE outcome tools with respect to bolus flow measures. *Dysphagia.* 2006;21(3):141–148

11. Odderson IR, Keaton JC, McKenna BS. Swallow management in patients on an acute stroke pathway: quality is cost effective. *Arch Phys Med Rehabil.* 1995;76(12):1130–1133.

12. Rasley A, Logemann JA, Kahrilas P, Rademaker AW, Pauloski BR, Dodds WJ. Prevention of barium aspiration during videofluoroscopic swallowing studies: value of postural change. *Am J Roentgenol.* 1993;160:1005–1009.

13. Aviv JE, Di Tullio MR, Homma S, et al. Hypopharyngeal perforation near-miss during transesophageal echocardiography. *Laryngoscope.* 2004;114(5):821–826.

14. Daniels SK, Huckabee ML. *Dysphagia Following Stroke.* San Diego, CA: Plural Publishing; 2008:7–15.

15. Brown RD, Whisnant JP, Sicks JD, O'Fallon WM, Wiebers DO. Stroke incidence, prevalence, and survival: secular trends in Rochester, Minnesota, through 1989. *Stroke.* 1996;27(3):373–380.

16. Modan B, Wagener DK. Some epidemiological aspects of stroke: mortality/morbidity trends, age, sex, race, socioeconomic status. *Stroke.* 1992;23(9):1230–1236.

17. Mayeu R, Marder K, Cote, LJ, et al. The frequency of idiopathic Parkinson's disease by age, ethnic group, and sex in northern Manhattan, 1988–1993. *Am J Epidemiol.* 1995;142(8):820–827.

18. Beard CM, Kokmen E, Offord K, Kurland LT. Is the prevalence of dementia changing? *Neurology.* 1991;41(12): 1911–1914.

19. Wynn DR, Rodriguez M, O'Fallon WM, Kurland LT. A reappraisal of the epidemiology of multiple sclerosis in Olmsted County, Minnesota. *Neurology.* 1990;40(5): 780–786.

20. Lilienfeld DE, Sprafka JM, Pham DL, Baxter J. Parkinson's and motoneuron disease morbidity in the Twin Cities metropolitan area: 1979–1984. *Neuroepidemiology.* 1991;10(3):112–116.

21. McGuire V, Longstreth WT Jr, Koepsell TD, van Belle G. Incidence of amyotrophic lateral sclerosis in three counties in western Washington state. *Neurology.* 1996;47(2): 571–573.

22. Golbe LI, Davis PH, Schoenberg BS, Duvoisin RC. Prevalence and natural history of progressive supranuclear palsy. *Neurology.* 1988;38(7):1031–1034.

23. Bower JH, Maraganore DM, McDonnell SK, Rocca WA. Incidence of progressive supranuclear palsy and multiple system atrophy in Olmsted County, Minnesota, 1976 to 1990. *Neurology.* 1997;49(5):1284–1288.

24. Kokmen E, Ozekmekci FS, Beard CM, O'Brien PC, Kurland LT. Incidence and prevalence of Huntington's disease in Olmsted County, Minnesota (1950 through 1989). *Arch Neurol.* 1994;51(7):696–698.

25. Daniels SK, McAdam CP, Brailey K, Foundas AL. Clinical assessment of swallowing and prediction of dysphagia. *Am J Speech-Lang Pathol.* 1997;6:17–24.

26. DePippo KL, Holas MA, Reding MJ. Respiration and relative risk of medical complications following stroke. *Arch Neurol.* 1994;51(10):1051–1053.

27. Bushmann M, Dobmeyer SM, Leeker L, Perlmutter JS. Swallowing abnormalities and their response to treatment in Parkinson's disease. *Neurology.* 1989;39(10):1309–1314.

28. Fuh JL, Lee RC, Wang SJ, et al. Swallowing difficulty in Parkinson's disease. *Clin Neurol Neurosurg.* 1997; 99(2): 106–112.

29. Horner J, Alberts MJ, Dawson DV, Cook GM. Swallowing in Alzheimer's disease. *Alzheimer Dis Assoc Disord.* 1994; 8(3):177–189.

30. Leighton SE, Burton MJ, Lund WS, Cochrane GM. Swallowing in motor neurone disease. *J Roy Soc Med.* 1994; 87(12):801–805.

31. Litvan I, Sastry N, Sonies BC. Characterizing swallowing abnormalities in progressive supranuclear palsy. *Neurology.* 1997;48(6):1654–1662.

32. Kagel MC, Leopold NA. Dysphagia in Huntington's disease: a 16-year retrospective. *Dysphagia.* 1992;7(2):106–114.

33. Smith TL, Sun MM, Pippin J. Research and professional briefs: characterizing process control of fluid viscosities in nursing homes. *J Am Diet Assoc.* 2005:104(6):969–971.

34. Aviv JE, Murry T, Zschommler A, Cohen M, Gartner C. Flexible endoscopic evaluation of swallowing with sensory testing: patient characteristics and analysis of safety in 1340 consecutive examinations. *Ann Otol Rhinol Laryngol.* 2005;114(3):173–176.

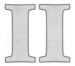

Anatomy and Function of the Swallowing Mechanism

CHAPTER OUTLINE

I. INTRODUCTION

II. THE NORMAL SWALLOW
   A. Oral Preparatory Phase
   B. Oral Phase
   C. Pharyngeal Phase
   D. Esophageal Phase
   E. Phase Relationships

III. SPHINCTERS
   A. Velopharyngeal Sphincter
   B. Laryngeal Sphincter
   C. Upper Esophageal Sphincter
   D. Lower Esophagus

IV. CRANIAL NERVES INVOLVED IN SWALLOWING
   A. Vagus Nerve (CN X)
   B. Trigeminal Nerve (CN V)
   C. Glossopharyngeal Nerve (CN IX)

V. CENTRAL NEURAL CONTROL

VI. RESPIRATION

VII. SUMMARY

VIII. STUDY QUESTIONS

IX. DISCUSSION QUESTION

X. REFERENCES

INTRODUCTION

A thorough understanding of the anatomical and functional aspects of swallowing is critical to understanding the disorders of swallowing and the management of the dysphagic patient. This chapter provides a thorough but not complete review of all anatomical aspects of swallowing. The reader will be directed to specific references to obtain more in-depth information. This chapter represents an approach to understanding the functional events of the normal swallow. A more complete discussion of the anatomy and physiology of the swallowing mechanisms may be found in Daniels and Huckabee,[1] Ludlow,[2] Aviv and Murry,[3] Sasaki and Isaacson.[4] and Perlman and Schulze-Delrieu.[5] The functional anatomy of the swallowing mechanism may be divided into four major components: (1) oral cavity, (2) oropharynx, (3) hypopharynx, and (4) esophagus. Within each component, specific nerves carry out motor and sensory control and regulate the mechanical aspects of swallowing. Table 2–1 outlines these components of the normal swallowing mechanism.[6] The key afferent and efferent neural responsibilities for each of the swallowing mechanisms are shown in Table 2–2.

THE NORMAL SWALLOW

Traditionally, the normal swallow has been described as a series of four phases that relate to the passage of the **bolus** through specific anatomic structures. These phases are the oral preparatory, oral, pharyngeal, and esophageal.

> The phases of swallowing were generally thought to occur sequentially; however, studies have shown that the oral and pharyngeal phases are interdependent.[7]

Martin-Harris and colleagues[7] recently presented evidence obtained from measuring the onset of the swallow and specific respiratory timing patterns associated with swallowing. Using confirmatory

Table 2–1. *Functional Components of the Normal Swallowing Mechanism*

A. Oral Cavity — Responsible for bolus containment and preparation 1. Containment a. Lips: closure after bolus intake b. Cheeks: adequate tension to assist in lip closure 2. Bolus Preparation a. Teeth: mastication b. Tongue: driving force to initially propel the bolus c. Gingival and buccal gutters: channel the bolus d. Soft palate: contact with tongue
B. Oropharynx 1. Oropharyngeal Propulsion Pump a. Soft palate b. Lateral pharyngeal walls c. Base of tongue 2. Velopharyngeal Function a. Soft palate: elevates as tongue propels b. Tongue elevation: necessary for propulsion
C. Hypopharynx 1. Muscular Propulsion a. Pharyngeal constrictors b. Piriform sinuses c. Cricopharyngeal function 2. Larynx a. Closure: glottis, ventricular folds, epiglottis b. Pharyngeal squeeze c. Hyoid elevation
D. Esophagus 1. Upper Esophageal Sphincter Opening 2. Primary Peristaltic Wave 3. Secondary Peristaltic Wave

Source: Adapted from Murry T, Carrau RL. *Clinical Management of Swallowing Disorders.* San Diego, CA: Plural Publishing; 2006:20.

factor analysis, they concluded that there is an overlap between the start of the oral and pharyngeal phases of swallowing. In order to understand bolus preparation and bolus transit, the phases of swallowing will be described sequentially. Nonetheless, the reader should remember that theses phases overlap and normal swallowing involves the integration of phases. Moreover, it is also important to understand the interaction between the organs of swal-

Table 2–2. Contributions of Cranial Nerves to the Oral and Pharyngeal Phases of Deglutition

STRUCTURE	AFFERENT	EFFERENT
LIPS	V2 (maxillary), V3 (lingual)	VII
TONGUE	V3 (lingual)	XII
MANDIBLE	V3 (mandibular)	V (muscles of mastication), VII
PALATE	V, IX, X	IX, X
BUCCAL REGION/CHEEKS		V (muscles of mastication), VII
TONGUE BASE	IX	XII
EPIGLOTTIS (lingual surface)	IX	X
EPIGLOTTIS (laryngeal surface)	X (internal branch of superior laryngeal nerve)	X
LARYNX (to level of true vocal folds)	X (internal branch of superior laryngeal nerve)	X
LARYNX (below true vocal folds)	X (recurrent laryngeal nerve)	X
PHARYNX (naso- and oro-)	IX	X (except for stylopharyngeus, which is innervated by IX)
PHARYNX (hypo-)	X (internal branch of superior laryngeal nerve)	X

Source: Adapted with permission from Aviv J. The normal swallow. In: Carrau RL, Murry T, eds., *Comprehensive Management of Swallowing Disorders.* San Diego, CA: Singular Publishing;1998:24–25, Tables 3–1 and 3–2.

lowing and respiration function prior to, during, and after swallowing. These temporal relationships may affect bolus transit, retention and/or penetration, and aspiration.

The oral preparatory and oral phases of swallowing involve mastication and bolus transfer. For the swallow to be normal, the anatomical structures of the upper aerodigestive system must be intact, and their function in sequence with each other must be appropriately timed. This requires the integrity of both the motor and sensory nervous systems. Clinicians involved with diagnosing and treating swallowing disorders should be familiar with the basic anatomy of the upper aerodigestive system. The anatomy of the larynx is shown in brief in Figure 2–1. An endoscopic view of the hypopharynx with residual bolus remaining is shown in Figure 2–2. The material in the cricopharyngeus area shows the residual

of a bolus that did not completely pass through all of the stages of swallowing.

Oral Preparatory Phase

The oral preparatory and oral phases of swallowing are sometimes considered one phase of swallowing. Traditionally, they are divided. The lips, tongue, mandible, dentition, soft palate, and muscles of the buccal cavity are temporally integrated to grind and position the food. The lips are essential for directing the food back to the tongue and teeth for bolus mastication and transfer.

The oral preparatory phase includes a **transfer phase** during which the tongue arranges the bolus and moves it posteriorly to a position where it can be chewed. In the normal swallow, the transfer stage

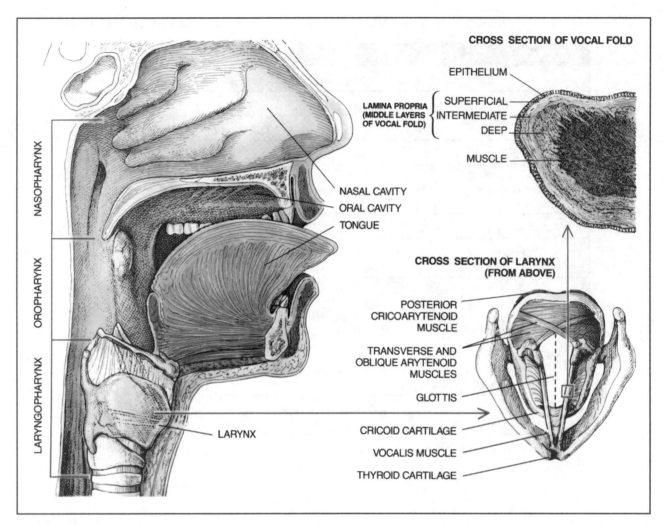

Figure 2–1. An overview of the nasopharynx, oropharynx, and laryngopharynx and the region of the vocal folds. Source: *Reprinted with permission from Sataloff RT. The human voice.* Sci Am. *1992;267:108–115.*

usually results in the food being placed in the region of the molar teeth. At this point, the **reduction phase** takes over and the food is chewed, ground, and mixed with saliva to form the bolus that eventually will be swallowed.

> During the oral preparatory phase, factors such as taste, temperature, and the viscosity and size of bolus are sensed, and appropriate lip, tongue, buccal, and dental manipulations are carried out to prepare the bolus for the next phase.

The trigeminal nerve (cranial nerve [CN] V), through its second and third divisions, provides sensory and motor innervations, respectively, to the muscles of mastication. Sensory information related to taste is mediated by CN VII (anterior two-thirds of the tongue) and CN IX (posterior one-third of the tongue).

Oral Phase

The food bolus is transported via the action of the tongue and its interaction with the palate, teeth, and

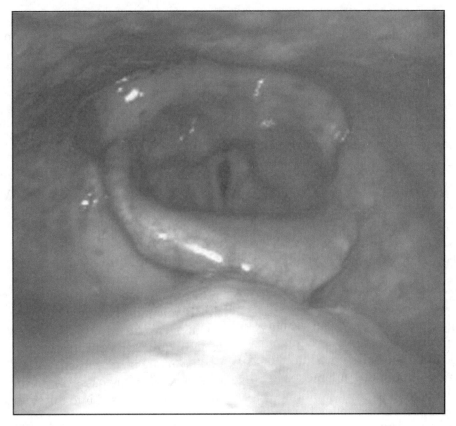

Figure 2–2. *View from flexible endoscope showing the epiglottis and vocal folds shortly after the bolus has passed into the upper esophagus.*

cheeks. The oral phase is primarily a delivery system. Contact of the back of the tongue with the soft palate retains the bolus in the oral cavity, preventing early spillage into the pharynx. Once the bolus is prepared, it is positioned posteriorly on the tongue. The velum then elevates as the lips and buccal muscles contract to build pressure and reduce the volume of the oral cavity. The posterior tongue is depressed, and the anterior and middle portions of the tongue differentially elevate and begin the propulsion of the bolus to the oropharynx.

It should be emphasized that the tongue is the primary manipulator of food during the oral phase.

> Any injury or surgical treatment to the tongue will affect the oral preparatory and oral phases of swallowing.

Injury to the lips may complicate the problems in the oral phase. If lip closure and the maintenance of lip pressure are inadequate, the oral preparatory and oral phases of swallowing will be affected due to lack of bolus containment. If normal bolus transit does not occur, there is a high probability that material will be found in the cricopharyngeus area after the swallow is completed. When the food is properly masticated and formed into a bolus, the entire bolus is propelled into the oropharynx by the tongue. This leads to the next stage of swallowing.

It is clear that with damage to the cranial nerves involved in swallowing, the oral preparatory and oral phases of swallowing become abnormal, which may lead to further abnormalities as the bolus reaches or fails to reach the next phase in a coordinated manner. In the oral phase of swallowing, results from fMRI studies have revealed that the primary motor and sensory areas of the brain, as well as the anterior cingulate cortex and insular cortex, are active in healthy adults.[8]

Pharyngeal Phase

The pharyngeal phase of swallowing begins when the bolus reaches the level of the anterior tonsillar pillars.

> Normal function of the pharyngeal phase is dependent on the consistency of the bolus, the size of the bolus, and whether swallowing is a single or continuous event.

A small well-organized bolus may pass the anterior faucial arches rapidly, whereas a poorly organized bolus will extend from the oral cavity into the oropharynx, requiring continuous interaction of the pharyngeal mechanisms.

The pharyngeal phase of swallowing involves the complex interaction of the tongue, velopharynx, and larynx. As the tongue elevates, velopharyngeal closure begins. This activity triggers the forward motion of the hypolaryngeal mechanism to increase the opening of the upper esophageal sphincter; the larynx also elevates, all of which leads to relaxation of the cricopharyngeus musculature. When these actions occur with appropriate temporal integration, the bolus moves through the pharyngeal segment without penetration/aspiration into the airway. This activity is considered to be involuntary.

Table 2–3, adapted from Simonian and Goldberg,[9] summarizes the signs and possible causes of dysphagia and its treatment according to the phases of swallowing. A detailed description of the treatment options is offered in Chapters 6 and 8.

Esophageal Phase

The **esophageal body** is a muscular tube extending 20 to 25 cm in length from its origin just caudal to the cricopharyngeus muscle to its termination at the gastric cardia. The esophagus shortens by about 10% through longitudinal muscle contractions during swallowing. Although the primary function of the esophageal body is passage of injected material from the pharynx to the stomach, recent studies indicate that the esophagus is not merely a hollow, passive conduit for food transport. Rather, it has several active functions for acid control and mucosal protection.

Peristalsis, or sequential contraction of the esophagus and relaxation of the lower esophageal sphincter, characterizes the esophageal phase of swallowing. The bolus is propelled through the esophagus by contraction above and relaxation below the bolus. This relaxation is referred to as **descending inhibition.**

Primary peristalsis occurs when a swallow induces peristaltic activity, whereas **secondary peristalsis** refers to the initiation of a propagated contraction wave in the absence of a swallow. Initiation of secondary peristaltic contractions is involuntary and normally is not sensed. Ultimately, in a normal swallow, the bolus passes from the proximal to the distal esophagus and into the stomach.

Phase Relationships

It is clear from recent studies that the phases of swallowing involve a type of parallel processing from the cortex to the peripheral nervous system. Problems during any one phase of swallowing may lead to problems at other phases. As will be pointed out in the remainder of this chapter, central nervous system structures control the motor sequencing of the transfer of the bolus from the lips to the stomach. However, these central processes require the coordination of the peripheral nervous system to carry out the functional passage of the bolus to the stomach.

> The phase relationships in swallowing are somewhat variable, affected by the type, size, and consistency of the bolus.

Even in the normal individual, the order of events and especially the timing of those events may not be entirely consistent. Moreover, the timing of events may vary for an individual depending on the con-

Table 2–3. Diagnosis of Dysphagia According to Four Phases of Swallowing

Type	Signs	Possible Causes	Treatment Options
Oral Preparatory	Lip flaccidity Labial leakage	CN V	Place food
Oral	Buccal pocketing	Facial weakness Surgical revision	Oral motor exercises, present food to stronger side
	Labored mastication	Lack of dentition Poor cognition	Modify food texture
	Premature spill	Lingual weakness	Chin tuck position Modify food texture
Pharyngeal	Delayed swallow initiation	Poor oral phase Vagus nerve dysfunction Prolonged intubation	Thermal stimulation Posterior tongue strengthening
	Decreased laryngeal elevation	Tracheotomy Nasogastric tube Suprahyoid muscle	Tracheotomy cuff deflation, d/c NGT Edema
	Multiple swallow pattern	Decreased pharyngeal peristalsis/contraction.	Alternate liquid and solid swallows
	Cough/throat clear immediately after the swallow	Aspiration secondary to decreased epiglottic deflection Poor oral phase Tracheoesophageal fistula (rare)	Supraglottic swallow Modify food texture
	Delayed cough, throat clear	Aspiration after the swallow secondary to pooling in the pharynx	Utilize dry swallow, alternating liquid and more solid swallows
	Change in vocal quality	Penetration to the level of the vocal cords Vocal cord weakness	NPL Modify food texture
Esophageal	Significantly delayed aspiration	Reflux, stricture	Medication Modify foods GI referral

Source: Adapted and revised with permission from Simonian MA, Goldberg AN. Swallowing disorders in the critical care patient. In: Carrau RL, Murry (eds). *Comprehensive Management of Swallowing Disorders.* San Diego, CA: Singular Publishing; 1998:367, Table 52–1.

ditions under which he or she is swallowing (distraction, multiple swallows, rapid swallows, etc). Nonetheless, Martin-Harris and colleagues have suggested an approximate order for the events of the normal swallow to be initiated.[10,11] The course of these events and the variation in timing are variable, but they follow the pattern recently described by Rosenbek and Jones[12] and outlined in Table 2–4.

SPHINCTERS

Swallowing can be visualized as the passage of the bolus through a series of dynamic chambers. These chambers are separated by sphincters (gates) that help prevent spillage of the material before the next chamber is ready to receive it.

Table 2–4. Clinical Results after Cranial Nerve Injury

Cranial Nerve	Clinical Result of Injury
V—Trigeminal nerve (motor)	Slight weakness in mastication
VII—Facial nerve	Slight weakness in bolus control, weak lip closure
IX—Glossopharyngeal nerve (sensory)	Failure to trigger the pharyngeal stage of the swallow, premature spill of material from the mouth into the airway
IX—Glossopharyngeal nerve (motor)	Deficit from loss of function not great secondary to intact function of other elevators of the larynx
X—Superior laryngeal nerve (sensory)	Loss of protective glottic closure and cough reflex protecting airway from material on the supraglottic larynx
X—Vagus nerve (motor)	Inadequate velopharyngeal closure, nasal regurgitation, Incomplete clearing of residue in the hypopharynx, pooling of material above the level of the vocal folds, aspiration once the vocal folds open Inadequate glottic closure during pharyngeal transit
XII—Hypoglossal nerve	Bolus control problems; crippled swallow if bilateral

Source: Adapted and modified with permission from Perlman A, Schulze-Delrieu K. *Deglutition and Its Disorders.* San Diego, CA: Singular Publishing;1997:354.

> Sphincters maintain a watertight closure that aids in building up the pressure in the particular chamber to facilitate the propulsion of the bolus into the next chamber. Damage to any of the sphincters may affect disruption of the normal swallow.

The specific sphincteric actions of the upper aerodigestive tract involved in swallowing are discussed below. Sphincter relaxation in a normal swallow generally precedes the onset of pharyngeal transit (bolus entry into the pharynx) and the initiation of swallow. Manometric studies have proven useful in interpreting the actions of the upper esophageal sphincter in the act of swallowing.[13,14] During a swallow of more than 5 cc of fluid, failure to coordinate the onset of pharyngeal transit (entry of the bolus into the pharynx) with the onset of swallow gestures can result in nasal reflux, aspiration, or regurgitation. In other swallows, however, particularly those associated with mastication, the linguopalatal sphincter may open repeatedly to allow small amounts of the bolus into the oropharynx and valleculae long before swallow sequence is initiated. Opening of the linguopalatal sphincter usually coincides with the onset of **pharyngeal transit** (bolus entry into the pharynx) and the initiation of the swallow.

Velopharyngeal Sphincter

Failure to close the velopharyngeal sphincter results in leakage of the bolus or air into the nasopharynx and a diminished ability to generate appropriate oropharyngeal pressures to propel the bolus through the oropharynx. Recent data by Pauloski and colleagues[15] in a study of manometry and fluoroscopy found that increased tongue base activity resulted in increased pressure on the bolus, resulting in a more efficient swallow that was characterized by shorter transit times and better bolus clearance.

Laryngeal Sphincter

Laryngeal closure occurs in a sequential fashion, with approximation of the true vocal folds (CN X) preceding false vocal fold approximation, and finally approximation of the arytenoids to the petiole of the epiglottis. Failure to close the supraglottic and glottic sphincters during the swallow results in penetration and aspiration and in decreased ability to generate adequate hypopharyngeal pressures to propel the bolus through the pharyngoesophageal segment and into the esophagus.

Upper Esophageal Sphincter

The upper esophageal sphincter (UES) is a tonically contracted group of skeletal muscles separating the pharynx from the esophagus. The major component of the sphincter is the cricopharyngeus muscle. At rest, the sphincter is in a state of **tonic contraction** that minimizes the entrance of air into the gastrointestinal tract during respiration. Equally important is its function to prevent the entry of refluxed material from the esophagus into the pharynx.

The tonically contracted UES relaxes during the pharyngeal peristaltic sequence. The relaxation begins after the onset of swallowing and lasts 0.5 to 1 second. The onset of the pharyngeal peristaltic wave is marked by apposition of the soft palate to the pharyngeal wall, generating a contraction that lasts over 0.1 seconds and generates a pressure greater than 180 mm Hg. Pharyngeal peristalsis transverses the oropharynx and hypopharynx at about 15 cm/sec and reaches the UES in about 0.7 seconds. After the relaxation phase, the sphincter contracts with an increase in force, in which the pressure may exceed twice the pressure of the resting tone for approximately a second prior to returning to baseline.

Poor coordination of the pharyngoesophageal segment may occur due to neurological deficits such as recurrent laryngeal nerve paralysis or brain stem stroke. Inadequate elevation of the hyoid-laryngeal complex and/or weakness of the pharyngeal constrictors also affect the function of the pharyngoesophageal segment as a sphincter.

Lower Esophagus

The lower esophagus is a specialized segment of smooth tubular muscle extending 20 to 25 cm in length from its origin just caudal to the cricopharyngeus muscle to its termination at the gastric cardia. It relaxes to permit the bolus to enter the gastric cavity and contracts to prevent gastroesophageal reflux in its resting state. Gross and histological examinations of the lower esophageal sphincter have failed to identify a specific sphincteric structure. Compared to adjacent structures, the lower esophageal muscle also possess an increased sensitivity to many excitatory agents, suggesting a greater influence on sphincter tone by nerves and hormones.

CRANIAL NERVES INVOLVED IN SWALLOWING

Vagus Nerve (CN X)

The vagus nerve provides motor and sensory innervation to the palate, pharynx, esophagus, stomach, and respiratory tract and is intimately involved in the regulation of blood pressure. Central contributions include motor innervation from the nucleus ambiguus and sensory innervation from the nucleus solitarius.

Recurrent Laryngeal Nerve (RLN)

All of the muscles of the larynx, except the cricothyroid, are innervated by this nerve. It is responsible for glottic closure during swallowing.

Superior Laryngeal Nerve (SLN)

The SLN bifurcates into two major divisions, an internal and an external division. The external division innervates the cricothyroid muscle, which retracts the posterior cricoid facet from the thyroid lamina, tensing the vocal fold and thus lengthening the anterior to posterior dimension of the glottis and changing the vocal pitch.

The internal branch of the SLN provides mucosal touch and proprioceptive sensory input from the supraglottic larynx, cricoarytenoid joints, posterior aspect of the larynx, and the pharyngeal mucosa in the piriform sinuses.

> Loss of sensation due to damage to the SLN results in anesthesia of the supraglottis and piriform sinuses, which leads to aspiration.

Despite secretions into the trachea, patients do not cough when the SLN is not functional. Jafari et al[16] found evidence that damage to the SLN alone without additional lesions in the brain or airway obstructions or diseases can result in aspiration. They suggested that following various conservative laryngeal surgeries, SLN injury was a main factor in dysphagia and aspiration.

Trigeminal Nerve (CN V)

The third division of the trigeminal nerve supplies sensory innervation to the tongue (lingual nerve) and to the inferior alveolus, buccal mucosa, and the lower lip (inferior alveolar nerve). Although sensation of the base of the tongue is supplied through CN IX (glossopharyngeal nerve), innervation of the oral tongue is conferred via the lingual nerve. The trigeminal nerve also supplies motor innervation to the mastication muscles, including those with mandibular and maxillary insertions.

Glossopharyngeal Nerve (CN IX)

This nerve provides sensory innervation to the oropharynx and the base of the tongue and supports taste fibers at the base of tongue. Its motor innervation is to the stylopharyngeus muscle.

CENTRAL NEURAL CONTROL

Normal deglutition, the act of swallowing, is initiated voluntarily. Central neural control of swallowing can be divided into cortical and subcortical components. **Neural control** is composed of a very complex interaction of afferent sensory neurons, motor neurons, and interneurons that control voluntary and involuntary/reflexive actions of swallowing.

Cortical regulation includes centers in both hemispheres of the brain with representation for the pharynx and the esophagus. These cortical areas have interhemispheric connections and projections to the motor nuclei of the brain stem. Bilateral hemispheric stimulation produces a greater response than unilateral impulses, and this response is intensity- and frequency-dependent. Both motor and premotor cortical areas are involved in the initiation of swallowing or at least have the potential to modulate the contraction of the pharyngeal and esopharyngeal musculature. Input from these cortical areas to the pharynx, however, seems greater than input to the esophagus. Similarly, afferent impulses from the pharynx, largely from the superior laryngeal nerve and glossopharyngeal nerve, have greater effects on cortical areas than those from the upper esophagus via the recurrent laryngeal nerve.

The "swallowing center," identified as an area within the reticular system of the brain stem that comprises the nucleus ambiguus (cranial nerves IX, X, and XI) and the nucleus of the tractus solitarius (cranial nerves VII, IX, and X) interact with other nuclei of the cranial nerves (V, IX, X, and XII).

> The collection of brain stem nuclei coordinate the swallow sequence, acting as **"the central pattern generator"** (sequential or rhythmic activities that are initiated by neural elements without external feedback).

Cranial nerve deficits cause changes in function that range from minor to life-threatening. Perlman and Shulze-Delrieu[5] describe the results of cranial nerve injury. Tables 2–2 through 2–4 summarize the findings of deficits to the cranial nerves.

Impulses from afferent fibers arising from pharyngeal receptors respond to touch, pressure, chemical stimuli, and water and provide the means to elicit the pharyngeal swallow. Miller has described this as "the most complex all-or-none reflex in the mammalian central nervous system."[17] Thus, sensory impulses from the pharynx serve to adjust the frequency and intensity of the contraction of the pharyngeal musculature and direct the protective reflexes of the laryngeal sphincter.

Similarly, at the cortical level, impulses from sensory receptors from the oral cavity provide the CNS with information regarding touch, pressure, texture, shape, temperature, chemicals, and taste. Automatic adjustments and voluntary movements are combined to prepare the bolus before swallowing.

RESPIRATION

Once the vocal folds are completely adducted for swallowing, respiration stops. This is known as swallowing **apnea.** The study of apnea events and respirometric activity during the act of swallowing offers additional clues to the understanding of aspiration. Normal deglutition causes an abrupt decrease in airflow, leading to a short interval of apnea, the time of which is dependent on the size of the bolus and whether the swallow is spontaneous or cued. Normal swallowing is always followed by a period of expiration.[18]

Although the act of swallowing is usually described in phases to facilitate understanding of the anatomical structures that are involved in swallowing, there is sufficient evidence to suggest that the involuntary and voluntary phases of swallowing occur simultaneously rather than serially.

> The importance of respiration in managing the action of swallowing has been studied, and it has been shown that rate and time of the stoppage of breathing is well coordinated with the normal swallow.[18]

Shaker and colleagues[19] demonstrated that vocal fold adduction occurs prior to the onset of hyoid bone movement, base of tongue movement, and submental surface myoelectric activity. Onset of vocal fold adduction also preceded the initiation of peristalsis in the nasopharynx and its propagation to the oropharynx. They concluded that it is apparent

that abnormal coordination of the laryngeal motion with bolus transport will lead to disruption in swallowing, and this lack coordination may play a significant role in swallow-induced aspiration. Thus, after each swallow, there is a respiratory cycle "reset"; that is, the swallow causes the normal respiratory pattern to restart with exhalation after each swallow.

In normal swallowing, the onset of the apneic event has been studied by Perlman and colleagues.[20] They demonstrated that respiratory events of swallowing were occurring simultaneously in the oral cavity, base of tongue valleculae, piriform sinuses, upper esophageal sphincter, and esophagus using respirometric data obtained from the onset of respiratory flow decrease to complete apnea combined with videofluoroscopy.

Kelly and colleagues[21] examined normal healthy subjects during sleep and wakefulness and found that although expiration is usually associated with volitional (awake) swallows; reflexive swallows (those during sleep) are more variable and occurred during the expiratory-inspiratory cusp more often than did volitional swallows. Onset of vocal fold adduction also preceded the initiation of peristalsis in the nasopharynx and its propagation to the oropharynx. Thus, it is apparent that abnormal coordination of the laryngeal motion with bolus transport will lead to disruption in swallowing, and this lack of coordination may play a significant role in swallow-induced aspiration.

Once the vocal folds are completely adducted, respiration stops. Thus, the study of respirometric activity during the act of swallowing offers additional clues to the understanding of aspiration. Normal deglutition causes an abrupt decrease in air. It appears that there is an apnea event for the normal swallow but the event may vary depending on the state of the patient, the bolus, and the age of the patient.

SUMMARY

Both the cortical and subcortical pathways are important to the initiation and completion of swallowing. Oral musculature is represented symmetrically between the two hemispheres; laryngeal and esophageal muscles are asymmetrically represented. Most individuals, however, have a dominant swallow hemisphere.

A thorough knowledge of the anatomical structures and physiological functions of the structures involved in swallowing is necessary to understand the complexity of swallowing. The physiology of swallowing includes the interaction of sensory and motor functions and the interaction of the voluntary and involuntary aspects of swallowing. Traditionally, it was thought that swallowing occurred in sequential phases, beginning with chewing. Involuntary phases of swallowing are the responsibility of the brain stem. The recent studies by Miller,[17] Martin-Harris,[11] and Perlman[20] provide evidence of the interaction between the involuntary and voluntary aspects of swallowing. Nonetheless, the interaction between these aspects remains to be fully understood. In addition, recent evidence suggests that the oral and oropharyngeal phases are interdependent. Moreover, evidence from sensory testing suggests that the role of sensation obtained from studies of the superior laryngeal nerve may be more important than originally considered. In future chapters, the role of sensory testing as an integral part of the swallowing evaluation will be presented.

STUDY QUESTIONS

1. The primary afferent control of the tongue, lips, and mandible is via cranial nerve
   A. VII
   B. X
   C. V
   D. XI

2. The oral phase of swallowing liquid varies with
   Age   **T F**
   Type of bolus   **T F**
   Quality of dentition   **T F**
   Discuss why each answer is true or false.

3. Sensory and motor integration of the phases of swallowing suggest that
   A. Each phase of the swallow must be completed before the next one begins
   B. It is impossible to determine when one phase of swallow ends and the next begins
   C. Voluntary and involuntary aspects of swallowing may occur in parallel
   D. Unless the voluntary oral phase of swallowing is completed, the involuntary phases cannot begin

4. The involuntary phases of swallowing are regulated
   A. By unilateral cortical representation
   B. By unilateral brain stem representation
   C. By bilateral brain stem representation
   D. By sensory and motor branches of cranial nerve X

DISCUSSION QUESTION

What additional information of the oropharyngeal swallow does fMRI provide?

REFERENCES

1. Daniels SK, Huckabee MK. *Dysphagia Following Stroke.* San Diego, CA: Plural Publishing; 2008:19–41.
2. Ludlow CL. Recent advances in laryngeal sensorimotor control for voice, speech and swallowing. *Curr Opin Otlaryngol Head Neck Surg.* 2004;12:160–165.
3. Aviv JE, Murry T. *FEESST: Flexible Endoscopic Evaluation of Swallowing with Sensory Testing.* San Diego, CA: Plural Publishing; 2005:8–24.
4. Sasaki CT, Isaacson G. Functional anatomy of the larynx. *Otolaryngol Clin North Am.* 1988;21:595–612.
5. Perlman A, Schulze-Delrieu K. *Deglutition and Its Disorders.* San Diego, CA: Singular Publishing; 1997:354.
6. Murry T, Carrau RL. *Clincal Management of Swallowing Disorders.* San Diego, CA: Plural Publishing; 2006.
7. Martin-Harris B, Michel Y, Castell DO. *Physiologic model of oropharyngeal swallowing revisited.* Paper presented at: AAO-HNS Annual Meeting; September 20, 2004; New York, NY.
8. Humbert I, Robbins J. Normal swallowing and functional magnetic resonance imaging: a systematic review. *Dysphagia.* 2007;22:266–275.
9. Simonian MA, Goldberg AN. Swallowing disorders in the critical care patient. In: Carrau RL, Murry T, eds. *Comprehensive Management of Swallowing Disorders.* San Diego, CA: Singular Publishing; 1999:367–368.

10. Martin-Harris, B. Temporal coordination of pharyngeal and laryngeal dynamics with breathing during swallowing: single liquid swallows. *J Appl Physiol.* 2003;94:1735–1743.

11. Martin-Harris B, Michal Y, Castell DO. Physiologic model of oropharyngeal swallowing revisited. *Otolaryngol Head Neck Surg.* 2005;133:234–240.

12. Rosenbek JC, Jones H. *Dysphagia in Movement Disorders.* San Diego, CA: Plural Publishing; 2009:12.

13. Leonard R, Belafsky PC, Rees CJ. Relationship between fluoroscopic and manometric measures of pharyngeal constriction: the pharyngeal constriction ratio. *Ann Otol Rhinol Laryngol.* 2006;115:897–901.

14. Hila A, Castell JA, Castell DO. Pharyngeal and upper esophageal sphincter manometry in the evaluation of dysphagia. *J Clin Gstroenterol.* 2001;33:355–361.

15. Pauloski BR, Rademaker AW, Lazarus C, Boeckxstaens G, Kahrilas PJ, Logemann JA. Relationship between manometric and videofluoroscopic measures of swallow function in healthy adults and patients treated for head and neck cancer with various modalities. *Dysphagia.* 2009 Jun;24(2):196–203.

16. Jafari S, Prince RA, Kim DY. Paydarfar D. Sensory regulation of swallowing and airway protection: a role for the internal superior laryngeal nerve in humans. *J Physiol.* 2003;550:287–304.

17. Miller, AJ. *The Neuroscientific Principles of Swallowing and Dysphagia.* San Diego, CA: Singular Publishing; 1998.

18. Paydarfar D, Gilbert RJ, Poppel CS, Nassab PF. Respiratory phase resetting and airflow changes induced by swallowing in humans. *J Physiol.* 1995;483(pt 1):273–288.

19. Shaker R, Dodds WJ, Dantas RO, et al. Coordination of deglutitive closure with ororpharyngeal swallowing. *Gastroenterology.* 1990;98:1478–1484.

20. Perlman AL, Ettema SL, Barkmeier J. Respiratory and acoustic signals associated with bolus passage during swallowing. *Dysphagia.* 2000;15(2):89–94.

21. Kelly BN, Huckabee ML, Cooke N, The coordination of respiration and swallowing for volitional and reflexive swallows: a pilot study. *J Med Speech-Lang Path.* 2006; 14(2):67–77.

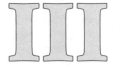

The Abnormal Swallow:
Conditions and Diseases

CHAPTER OUTLINE

I. INTRODUCTION
   A. Penetration
   B. Aspiration
   C. Aspiration Pneumonia
II. NEUROLOGICAL DISORDERS
   A. Amyotrophic Lateral Sclerosis (ALS)
   B. Cerebrovascular Accident
   C. Parkinson Disease
   D. Myasthenia Gravis
   E. Myopathies
   F. Traumatic Brain Injury
III. CONDITIONS FOUND IN CRITICAL CARE
   PATIENTS
IV. ESOPHAGEAL DISORDERS
   A. Esophageal Cancer
   B. Other Esophageal Disorders
V. INFECTIOUS DISEASES
   A. Oral Cavity/Oropharynx
   B. Esophagitis
   C. Deep Neck Infections
   D. Laryngeal Infections
VI. MEDICATIONS
   A. Analgesics
   B. Antibiotics
   C. Antihistamines
   D. Antimuscarines, Anticholinergics, and
      Antispasmodics

     E. Mucolytic Agents
     F. Antihypertensives
     G. Antineoplastic Agents
     H. Vitamins
     I. Neurological Medications
  VII. NEOPLASMS
 VIII. SWALLOWING DISORDERS FOLLOWING
        RADIATION THERAPY
   IX. INTUBATION
    X. AUTOIMMUNE DISEASES
   XI. SUMMARY
  XII. STUDY QUESTIONS
 XIII. DISCUSSION QUESTIONS
 XIV. REFERENCES

INTRODUCTION

Swallowing is a complex activity requiring the interaction of sensory and motor mechanisms. In the previous chapter, the normal swallow was described as three discrete events, **bolus preparation**, **airway protection**, and **bolus propulsion**. Neural impulses from cortical and subcortical pathways integrate motor and sensory data to the muscles of the oral cavity and the pharyngeal and laryngeal structures. The muscles of the oral and pharyngeal regions transfer data to the brain stem, reticular formation, medulla, and frontal cortex via the facial, glossopharyngeal, and vagus nerves.

> A safe, normal swallow entails the timely interaction of the muscles of mastication, which are innervated by the trigeminal nerve, and the pharyngeal and laryngeal muscles, which are controlled by the efferent and afferent fibers of the glossopharyngeal and vagus nerves, respectively.

Additional muscular innervation of the strap muscles of the swallowing mechanism by the ansa hypoglossis and ansa cervicalis aids in the complex motion of swallowing. A more detailed description of the muscular actions and neuromuscular control of these actions can be found in Aviv and Murry.[1] Damage to any of the nerves involved in swallowing or to the corresponding areas of the central nervous system (brain stem, medulla, and cortex) has an effect on normal swallowing. Thus, swallowing involves an intact nervous system, which drives the biomechanical events of the swallow.

Many conditions can disrupt the muscular actions of a normal swallow at any point along the pathway leading to the stomach. In addition, conditions of the bolus in the stomach may affect the transit of the boluses that have not yet arrived in the stomach.

Prior to reaching the stomach, the bolus must pass along a lumen that is shared with the combined respiratory and phonatory pathway. Each swallow involves the interruption of breathing (an apneic event) and the protection of the airway, and then the return of respiration once the bolus is safely beyond the laryngeal inlet. Airway protection during normal swallowing is brought about by the 3-tier closure of the laryngeal sphincter. This is composed of the closure of the true vocal folds, including the arytenoids and the false vocal folds, the aryepiglottic folds, and the epiglottis (ie, supraglottis). The superior and anterior motion of the larynx caused by the contraction of the suprahyoid muscles opens the posterior cricoid space and moves the larynx superiorly to a protected position beneath the base of the tongue. Following the swallow, normal subjects resume respiration activities with exhalation.[2] When airway protection is incomplete or delayed, penetration of the bolus and even aspiration of the bolus may occur. Kendall et al[3] showed that, in most subjects, the arytenoids/epiglottic approximation occurs before the bolus reaches the upper esophageal sphincter, but in some cases it may occur after; however, the delay is never greater than 0.1 second. They also noted no delay of the supraglottic closure in normal elderly patients. More recently, others have found that following radiation therapy to the head or neck regions, these delays may extend beyond normal times. Fibrosis and stenosis of the tongue, pharynx, and esophagus as well as pharyngeal constriction contribute to the delays in oral pharyngeal transit, leading to delays in closure of vocal folds, which may result in penetration and aspiration.[4,5] It is clear that any condition that results in failure of the glottic sphincter to close timely and appropriately may allow the entry of food or liquid into the airway.

Although the neuromuscular pathogenesis is beyond the scope of this book, we will outline the most common conditions associated with a disordered swallow in adults. In this chapter, we introduce the terms of penetration, aspiration, and aspiration pneumonia, as their understanding is important to the remainder of the chapter.

Penetration

Penetration is defined as the entry of bolus contents into the larynx to a level that does not extend beyond the true vocal folds. Figure 3–1 shows an example of penetration obtained during transnasal flexible endoscopy. Note the material below the epiglottis and above the vocal folds.

Aspiration

Aspiration is the entry of material into the airway below the true vocal folds. Aspiration can occur before, during, or after the swallow. **Prandial aspiration** is the result of food or liquid entering the airway. Table 3–1 summarizes and updates Mendelsohn's

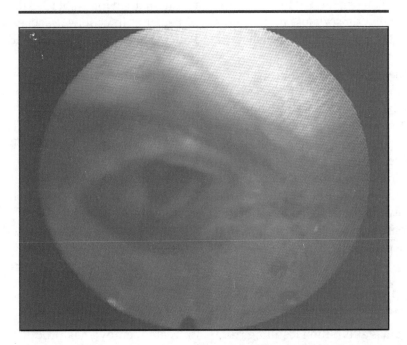

Figure 3–1. *An example of penetration found during flexible endoscopy.*

Table 3–1. Classification of Prandial Aspiration

Aspiration Before the Pharyngeal Stage
- most common type in central neurological diseases
- due to loss of bolus control during oral phase or to delayed pharyngeal swallow
- conservative management: thicken the diet, neck flexation during deglutition, supraglottic swallow, effortful swallow, thermal stimulation
- surgical management: horizontal epiglottoplasty, tongue base flaps, laryngeal suspension

Aspiration During the Pharyngeal Phase
- least common type of aspiration
- due to vocal palsy, paresis, or incoordination
- conservative management: vocal adduction exercises, chin tuck, bolus modification
- surgical management: augment the paralyzed vocal fold

Aspiration After the Pharyngeal Phase
- due to inhalation of uncleared residue at the laryngeal inlet
- conservative management: thinning the diet, alternating liquids, Mendhelson maneuver, head rotation, reduce bolus size
- surgical management: translaryngeal resection of the cricoid lamina, cricopharyngeal myotomy, laryngeal elevation
- medical management: botulinum toxin injection to the superior pharyngeal constrictor muscle

Source: Adapted and expanded from Mendelsohn M. New concepts in dysphagia management. J Otolaryngol. 1993;22(suppl 1):9.

classic review of the nature of prandial aspiration.[6] Figure 3–2 shows a portion of a food bolus below the vocal folds. In this patient, sensory loss to the vagus nerve is apparent, as the bolus is in the airway and the patient did not expel the bolus.

Factors that influence the tolerance to aspiration include amount, frequency, and type of the aspirate, oral hygiene, pulmonary conditions, and immune function of the host. These factors and their interaction with the neuromuscular system of the host are extremely variable. Thus, the definition of what constitutes "significant" aspiration should be individualized. Pulmonary syndromes that are related to aspiration are shown in Table 3–2. They include: (a) chemical pneumonitis, (b) bacterial infection, and (c) acute airway obstruction.[7]

Aspiration Pneumonia

Aspiration pneumonia is a condition resulting from the entrance of foreign materials, usually foods, liq-uids, or vomit, into the bronchi of the lungs with resultant infection. Table 3–3 describes the two types of bacterial infections associated with pneumonia.[7] Patients may present with a wide spectrum of severity of aspiration syndromes prior to aspiration pneumonia. Multiple risk factors for aspiration are listed in Table 3–4.[8] Technically known as bronchopneu-monia, aspiration pneumonia may consist of one of three distinct types:

Anaerobic pneumonia, in its early stages, results in a low grade fever. However, extended periods of aspiration, with fatigue, cough, and unconscious-ness secondary to hypoxia, lead to more severe symptoms.

Lung abscess is an accumulation of pus which has been contained by a surrounding inflammatory process. Radiologically, it appears as a spherical-looking area with an air fluid level often resembling a lung mass.

Empyema is pus in the pleural space. If left untreated, empyemas produce destructive changes resulting in rupture of the pleural walls.

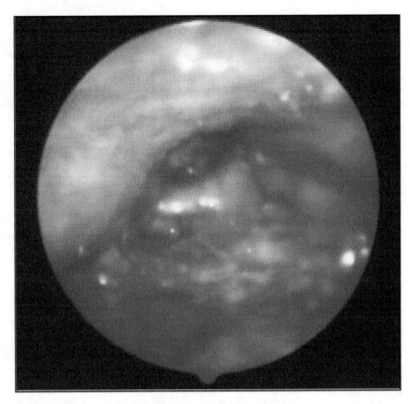

Figure 3–2. *A portion of the food bolus is shown below the vocal folds before the patient expels it.*

Table 3–2. Pulmonary Syndromes Related to Aspiration

1. **Acute respiratory distress syndrome (ARDS):** Interstitial and/or alveolar edema and hemorrhage, as well as perivascular lung edema. It may be caused by aspiration of acid refluxate.

2. **Lipid (lipoid) pneumonia:** Aspiration of oil-based liquids such as mineral oil given as a laxative, oil-based nasal sprays, or contrast material. In unconscious patients, especially those requiring mechanical ventilation, fever, hypoxia, and excessive tracheal secretions may suggest pneumonia. For patients requiring mechanical ventilation, placement in a semirecumbent position and active suction of the hypopharynx may reduce the risk of aspiration.

3. **Aspiration pneumonia:** Aspiration pneumonia is usually polybacterial and is associated with a high morbidity and mortality. It is usually found in dependent pulmonary lobes.

4. **Chronic pneumonia:** Some patients do not develop a radiographic consolidate that could be diagnosed as a pneumonia, but present with purulent, foul-smelling bronchorrhea, low-grade spiking fever, and varying degrees of respiratory compromise. A prominent bronchial pattern may be present in the chest radiogram.

Source: Adapted from Falestiny MN, Yu VL. Chapter 55. In: Carrau RL, Murry T, eds. *Comprehensive Management of Swallowing Disorders.* San Diego, CA: Singular Publishing; 1999:385.

Table 3–3. *Bacteriology of Aspiration Pneumonia*

Community-acquired	Nosocomial-acquired
Anaerobes	**Anaerobes**
Fusobacterium nucleatum	*Fusobacterium nucleatum*
Peptostreptococcus spp	*Peptostreptococcus spp*
Bacteroides melaninogenicus	*Bacteroides spp*
Other *bacteroides spp*	
Aerobes	**Aerobes**
Microaerophilic streptococci	*Staphylococcus aureus*
Streptococcus viridans	*Enterobacteriaceae*
Moraxella catarrhalis	*Escherichia coli*
Eikenella corrodens	*Klebsiella spp*
Streptococcus pneumoniae	*Enterococcus spp*
Haemophilus influenzae	*Citrobacter freundii*
	Acinetobacter lwoffi
	Pseudomonas aeruginosa

Source: Adapted from Falestiny MN, Yu VL. Chapter 55. Carrau RL, Murry T, eds. *Comprehensive Management of Swallowing Disorders.* San Diego, CA: Singular Publishing; 1999:383–388.

Table 3–4. *Aspiration: Risk Factors*

Altered level of consciousness
 Head trauma
 Coma
 Cerebrovascular accident (CVA), acute stage
 Metabolic encephalopathy
 Seizure disorders
 General anesthesia
 Alcohol intoxication
 Altered drug states
 Excessive sedation
 Cardiopulmonary arrest

Gastrointestinal dysfunction
 Scleroderma
 Esophageal stricture
 Gastroesophageal reflux
 Laryngopharyngeal reflux
 Erosive esophagitis
 Zenker diverticulum
 Tracheoesophageal fistula
 Esophageal cancer
 Hiatal hernia
 Pyloric stenosis/gastric outlet obstruction
 Enteral feeding
 Pregnancy
 Anorexia/bulimia

Iatrogenic
 Prolonged mechanical ventilatory support
 Tracheotomy
 Anticholinergic drugs

Miscellaneous
 Obesity
 Neck malignancies
 Medication overdose

Postsurgical
 Skull base
 Head and neck
  Thyroid carcinoma
  Supraglottic laryngectomy
  Major oropharyngeal resection
  Carotid endarterectomy
  Anterior spinal fusion

Source: Adapted and revised from Pou AM, Carrau RL. In: Carrau RL, Murry T, eds. *Comprehensive Management of Swallowing Disorders.* San Diego, CA: Singular Publishing; 1999:155–158.

Aspiration pneumonia may be initially difficult to identify and diagnose even with invasive studies. In stroke patients, the overall debilitation, malnutrition, dehydration, and other systemic problems that accompany the stroke or that precede the stroke increase the risk of aspiration pneumonia after the stroke. Other risk factors often present in patients with a stroke, as well as with head and neck cancer, such as poor oral hygiene with bacterial overgrowth, loss of sensory awareness that may occur after other prolonged illness, or degradation in pulmonary function even after an acute event has been stabilized medically or surgically.

The following conditions include the most important groups of patients that are predisposed to aspiration pneumonia:

Altered mental status: Nearly 70% of patients with altered mental status, regardless of the underlying disease, aspirate, possibly because of the inability to protect the airway and/or the discoordination between breathing and swallowing. Common conditions of altered mental status include diabetic coma, seizure, and medication overdose.

Prolonged mechanical ventilation: Patients requiring prolonged mechanical ventilation and patients with a tracheostomy are especially at risk for aspiration. Aspiration pneumonia can occur after only 2 weeks on mechanical ventilation and nearly 85% of these patients fail flexible endoscopic evaluation of swallowing or swallow testing using fluoroscopy for detection of aspiration.[9]

Gastroesophageal reflux: Acute findings in acid aspiration-induced lung injury include mucosal edema, hemorrhage, and focal ulceration, followed by the development of focal necrosis and diffuse alveolar hyaline membrane formation. Gastroesophageal reflux is discussed in great detail in a later section of this chapter.

Neuromuscular disorders: These patients lose motor and sensory function of the upper aerodigestive tract, leading to a variety of disorders affecting cognition, coordination of reflexive actions, and loss of sphincteric and propulsive mechanisms.

Upper aerodigestive tract tumors: Most of these patients experience some swallowing difficulty, either from the mechanical effects of the tumor, its interference with the sphincteric mechanism of the larynx, or due to the anatomical and functional changes produced by surgery, radiation therapy, and chemotherapy. Their swallowing problems are not limited to the time of treatment or shortly after treatment. Surgery, radiation, and/or chemotherapy can result in long-term changes in bolus propulsion, ability to close the airway, and motility disorders of the esophagus.

The remainder of this chapter reviews the most common conditions and diseases that may require assessment and treatment of a swallowing disorder.

NEUROLOGICAL DISORDERS

Dysphagia caused by neurological injuries and diseases is usually the end result of an impairment of the sensorimotor components of the oral and pharyngeal phases of swallowing. The onset and progression and severity of the disease, as well as the symptoms, may occur suddenly or may result in a slow progressive degeneration of neuromuscular systems.

> Not only swallowing but other neuromuscular systems (phonation, locomotion, etc) may also be affected and reduce the opportunity to effectively treat the swallowing disorder.

A recent review of the advances in sensorimotor control of the swallowing mechanisms suggests that brain stem mechanisms are now thought to control many of the reflexive laryngeal functions associated with swallowing. These functions are thought to control the integration of respiration and swallowing.[10,11] Table 3–5 lists the more common neurological disorders causing dysphagia, as identified by Perlman and Shultze-Delrieu[12] and by Coyle et al.[13]

Evaluation of the cause of unexplained dysphagia should include a careful history, referral for neurological examination, including possible magnetic resonance imaging (MRI) of the brain, blood tests (routine studies plus muscle enzymes, thyroid screening, vitamin B_{12} and antiacetylcholine receptor antibodies), electromyography nerve conduction studies, and, in certain cases, muscle biopsy or cerebrospinal fluid examination. The following pages describe neurogenic conditions that have a significant incidence of swallowing disorders.

Amyotrophic Lateral Sclerosis (ALS)

Amyotrophic lateral sclerosis (ALS) is a progressive disease involving degeneration of the upper and lower motor neurons. It has an incidence around 2 per 100,000. Men are affected slightly more frequently than women, with onset around age 60,

Table 3–5. *Neurologic Disorders Causing Dysphagia*

Cerebrovascular accident (CVA)
Parkinson disease and other movement and neurodegenerative disorders
Amyotrophic lateral sclerosis
Myasthenia gravis
Polymyositis/dermatomyositis
Guillain-Barré syndrome
Dystonia/tardive dyskinesia
Vocal fold paralysis
Progressive muscular dystrophy
Meningitis
Traumatic brain injury
Cerebral palsy
Progressive supranuclear palsy
Olivopontocerebellar atrophy
Huntington disease
Wilson disease
Torticollis
Alzheimer disease and other dementias
Guillain-Barré syndrome and other polyneuropathies
Neoplasms and other structural disorders
Primary brain tumors
Intrinsic and extrinsic brain stem tumors
Base of skull tumors
Syringobulbia
Arnold-Chiari malformation
Neoplastic meningitis
Multiple sclerosis
Postpolio syndrome
Infectious disorders
Chronic infectious meningitis
Syphilis and Lyme disease
Diphtheria
Botulism
Viral encephalitis, including rabies
Myopathy
Polymyositis, dermatomyositis, including body myositis and sarcoidosis
Myotonic and oculopharyngeal muscular dystrophy
Hyper- and hypothyroidism
Cushing syndrome

Source: Adapted from Perlman AL, Schulze-Delrieu K. *Deglutition and Its Disorders.* San Diego, CA: Singular Publishing Group; 1997:322.

although it may present earlier. An updated overview of ALS diagnosis and its effects on swallowing can be found in Siddique and Doonkevert.[14]

> Diagnosis of ALS requires the **presence and progression** of lower motor neuron and upper motor neuron deficiency.

Upper limb muscles are affected more frequently than lower limb muscles, and bulbar muscles may be affected, leading to significant prominent dysarthria and dysphagia. Bulbar involvement in ALS is associated with a worse prognosis because of the higher risk of pulmonary aspiration and malnutrition. It is important to monitor the weight of dysphagic patients with ALS and their nutritional status, and to begin discussions of **percutaneous endoscopic gastrostomy (PEG)** before the patient becomes severely deteriorated.

Lower motor neuron signs result from damage to the motor nuclei in the spinal cord (anterior horn cells) and brain stem motor nuclei. Upper motor neuron symptoms are due to damage to the corticospinal and corticobulbar tracts. Atrophy with or without fasciculations may be observed in the tongue and face. Spasticity or flaccidity may also be detected throughout affected regions. Patients with bulbar involvement are likely to show early lingual and labial weakness. The weakness progresses to the muscles of mastication and the intrinsic/extrinsic laryngeal muscle.

> The progressive loss of muscle function in patients with bulbar involvement produces difficulty controlling oral contents, including secretions, food, and liquids, which may be observed as drooling, early spillage of the bolus into the pharynx, or pooling of residue in the gingivobuccal gutters.

Some patients are aware of these problems and respond to aspiration by clearing their throat or coughing when eating or drinking, suggesting a degree of preserved sensory functions. Others, however, may have minimal or absent sensory response, or the effectiveness of the reflexive cough may be weak and eventually ineffective, resulting in considerable penetration and aspiration of liquids and foods.

Dysphagia in the ALS patient leads to secondary complications such as nutritional deficiencies and dehydration, which can compound the deteriorating effects of the disease, and therefore requires careful monitoring such as that proposed by Yorkston et al[15] (Table 3–6). At least 73% of ALS patients have dysphagia before they require ventilatory support, and even a higher percentage experience swallowing difficulty subsequently. Patients have more problems with liquids and large pieces of food. For the ALS patient, pureed or soft foods are much easier to swallow. An investigation by Higo et al[16] reported

the progression of dysphagia in 50 patients with ALS using videofluoroscopy (VF), according to two different scales: the duration following bulbar symptom onset, and an ALS swallowing severity scale (ALSSS) related specifically to ALS. The authors found delayed bolus transport from the oral cavity to the pharynx and bolus stasis at the piriform sinus (PS) in about half of the patients with no bulbar complaints. In contrast, upper esophageal sphincter (UES) opening was relatively well maintained in the late stage of dysphagia. Other parameters, such as bolus holding in the oral cavity, constriction of the pharynx, and elevation of the larynx, became worse over time following bulbar symptom onset and as the disease advanced.

Table 3–6. Swallowing Severity Scale

Normal Eating Habits	10	*Normal Swallowing:* Patient denies any difficulty chewing or swallowing. Examination demonstrated no abnormality.
	9	*Nominal Abnormality:* Only patient notices slight indicators such as food lodging in the recesses of the mouth or sticking in the throat.
Early Eating Problems	8	*Minor Swallowing Problems:* Complains of some swallowing difficulties. Maintains an essentially regular diet. Isolated choking episodes.
	7	*Prolonged Time or Smaller Bite Size:* Mealtime has significantly lengthened and smaller bite sizes are necessary. Patient must concentrate on swallowing liquids.
Dietary Consistency Changes	6	*Soft Diet:* Diet is limited primarily to soft foods. Requires some special meal preparation.
	5	*Liquefied Diet:* Oral (PO) intake is adequate. Nutrition is limited primarily to a liquefied diet. Adequate thin liquid intake usually a problem. Patient may force self to eat.
Needs Tube Feeding	4	*Supplemental Tube Feeding:* PO intake alone is no longer adequate. Patient uses or needs a tube to supplement intake. Patient continues to take significant (greater than 50%) of nutrition PO.
	3	*Tube Feeding with Occasional PO Nutrition:* Primary nutrition and hydration are accomplished by tube. Patient receives less than 50% of nutrition PO.
NPO	2	*Secretions Managed with Aspirator/Medication:* Patient cannot safely manage any PO intake. Secretions are managed by an aspirator, medications, or both. Patient swallows reflexively.
	1	*Aspiration of Secretions:* Secretions cannot be managed noninvasively. Patient rarely swallows.

Source: Adapted from Yorkston KM, Strand E, Miller R, Hillel A, Smith K. Speech deterioration in amyotrophic lateral sclerosis: implications for the timing of intervention. *J Med Speech Language Pathol.* 1993;1(1):35–46.

> ALS patients in a group with normal eating habits showed disturbed bolus transport from the mouth to the pharynx, weak constriction of the pharynx, and bolus stasis at the piriform sinus.

Similar results were reported in Leder et al[17] using FEES. They suggested that serial FEES evaluations prior to implementing diet changes or therapeutic strategies provide safe treatment.

Drooling can be an early and disturbing symptom of bulbar ALS, often leading to social isolation. Many therapeutic approaches have been suggested over the years to reduce salivary production, including the tricyclic amitriptyline. Some ALS patients benefit from treatment with beta antagonists to help control and thicken secretions.

In patients with prominent bulbar weakness, a palatal lift (see the discussion about prosthodontics in Chapter 7) is sometimes useful to improve the velopharyngeal sphincter. Spasticity may complicate the bulbar contribution to dysarthria and dysphagia in the ALS patient. In occasional patients, baclofen can be effective in relieving some of the upper motor neuron (UMN) impairment. Diazepam can occasionally be useful, but sedation and increased weakness limit its use.

Cerebrovascular Accident

Stroke is the third most common cause of death in the US each year. Between 30% to 40% of stroke victims will demonstrate symptoms of significant dysphagia. Twenty percent of stroke victims die of aspiration pneumonia in the first year following a stroke. In addition, 10% to 15% of stroke victims who die in the years following the stroke will die of aspiration pneumonia. Cerebrovascular disease is the most common cause of neurogenic oral and pharyngeal dysphagia.

> Dysphagia, aspiration, and aspiration pneumonia are devastating sequelae of stroke, accounting for nearly 40,000 deaths from aspiration pneumonia each year in the United States.

Although the correlation of site and size of the stroke with subsequent dysphagia is variable, the trend is that the larger the area of infarction, the greater the impairment of swallowing. In general, brain stem strokes produce dysphagia more frequently and more severely than cortical strokes. Robbins et al[18] suggest that the severity of dysphagia in patients with left hemisphere strokes seem to correlate with the presence of apraxia and the reported deficits are more significant during the oral stage of swallowing. Right hemisphere patients have more pharyngeal dysfunction, including aspiration and pharyngeal pooling.

Infarct size and distribution define the clinical presentation of the CVA and are dependent on the degree and site of interrupted arterial blood supply. Arterial supply to the brain stem is based in the vertebrobasilar complex. The bilateral internal carotid arteries give rise to the majority of the anterior and middle cerebral blood supply. Each anterior cerebral artery supplies the ipsilateral orbital and medial frontal lobe and the medial parietal lobe. Each middle cerebral artery supplies the ipsilateral orbital and medial frontal lobe and the medial parietal lobe. Branches to the middle cerebral artery also penetrate the brain and supply the ipsilateral basal nuclei, internal capsule region, and most of the thalamus and adjacent structures. Each posterior cerebral artery supplies portions of the ipsilateral brain stem and cerebellum and the inferior temporal and medial occipital lobes. Spinal arteries supply branches to the medulla.

Patients with only small vessel infarcts had a significantly lower occurrence of aspiration compared to those with both large and small vessel infarcts.

Dysphagia after unilateral hemispheric stroke is related to the magnitude of pharyngeal motor representation in the affected hemisphere. Patients with right hemisphere stroke show longer pharyngeal transit and higher incidences of laryngeal penetration and aspiration of liquid, as compared to patients with left-sided strokes. Lesions in the left middle cerebral artery territory are known to produce aphasia, motor and verbal apraxia, hemiparesis, and dysphagia. More than half of patients with bilateral strokes aspirate. However, dysphagia, with its attendant risk of aspiration, decreases over time in most patients.

Dysarthria and dysphagia, when associated with emotional lability, is suggestive of pseudobulbar palsy, a condition characterized by weakness of muscles innervated by the medulla (tongue, palate, pharynx, and larynx) because of interruption of corticobulbar fibers, as may be seen with multiple bilateral strokes.

Patients with posterior circulation strokes are more likely to aspirate and show an abnormal cough, abnormal gag, and dysphonia. Lateral medullary syndrome (Wallenberg syndrome) is due to thrombosis of the posteroinferior cerebellar artery, which results in ischemia of the lateral medullary region of the brain stem. It differs from many other types of dysphagia in that the tongue driving force and oropharyngeal propulsion pump force are greatly increased, in part due to the failure of pharyngoesophageal sphincter opening during swallowing.

> Early screening and management of dysphagia in patients with acute stroke has been shown to reduce the risk of aspiration pneumonia, is cost-effective, and assures quality care with optimal outcome.

The Burke Dysphagia Screening Test (BDST) is highly sensitive in identifying stroke patients at risk for developing pneumonia and recurrent upper airway obstruction.[19] The BDST and other tests of screening for swallowing disorders are discussed in Chapter 5. Direct therapy programs for chronic neurogenic dysphagia resulting from brain stem stroke show that functional benefits are long lasting without related health complications.

Parkinson Disease

Parkinson disease is a progressive degenerative disorder characterized by loss of striatal dopamine. Oral and pharyngeal dysphagia in Parkinson disease is multifactorial. Prepharyngeal abnormalities, including cognitive impairment, drooling, jaw rigidity, head and neck posture during meals, upper extremity dysmotility, impulsive feeding behavior, and lingual transfer are common in patients with advanced disease.

Pharyngoesophageal motor abnormalities also play a role in dysphagia in Parkinson patients. Abnormalities include limited pharyngeal contraction, abnormal pharyngeal wall motion, impaired pharyngeal bolus transport, and manometric abnormalities with incomplete upper esophageal sphincter relaxation. Dysfunction of the lower esophageal sphincter (LES) includes an open LES or a delayed opening of the LES and gastroesophageal reflux. Other esophageal abnormalities include delayed transport, stasis, bolus redirection, and tertiary contractions.

Pneumonia is one of the most prevalent primary causes of death in patients with Parkinson disease. The disease is characterized by a release of subcortical inhibitory centers within the indirect (extrapyramidal) motor system, which modulate motor function. This is thought to occur due to the degeneration and depigmentation of dopamine-containing neurons found in the substantia nigra and its connections to the basal nuclei. The result is depletion of dopamine in the caudate nucleus and putamen, causing a motor disturbance that includes, among other signs, rigidity and resting tremor.

Disorders of the oral phase of swallowing, especially for solid foods, are common in Parkinson disease. Excessive lingual rocking or pumping, incomplete transfer of a bolus from oral to pharyngeal cavity, preswallow loss of bolus containment with spillage into the pharynx and/or larynx, and swallow hesitation are seen. Deficits during the pharyngeal phase include pooling of residue within the pharyngeal recesses and delayed onset of the pharyngeal response, predisposing the patient to aspiration before the swallow. Figure 3–3 shows the result of pooling after the swallow in a patient with Parkinson disease.

Reduced lingual range of motion and rigidity contribute to diminished hypolaryngeal excursion. This results in an inadequate or incomplete distension of the upper esophageal segment and incomplete airway protection, which is often followed by aspiration. Esophageal motor abnormalities are also commonly detected in Parkinson patients.

Cricopharyngeal myotomy improves swallowing in Parkinson patients with coexisting Zenker diverticulum, but is not recommended to treat other causes of dysphagia.

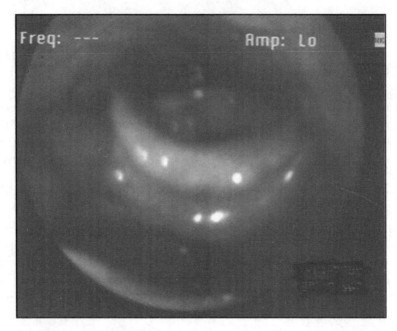

Figure 3–3. *Mucous pooling (white matter) after the swallow in patient with Parkinson disease.*

Data by Sapir et al[20] and by Plowman-Prine et al[21] suggest that Parkinson patients develop multiple neuromuscular deficiencies and that many of them may exhibit some improvement when given exercises to do, medications, and/or a medication adjustment.

The recent work by Miller et al[22] reviews the neurological functioning of Parkinson disease with implications for swallowing disorders. The challenges in treating the Parkinson patient with a progressive disease are such that the combined team must continually reassess the patient's status and his/her medications and adjust the treatment according to the patient's functional level.

Myasthenia Gravis

Adult-onset **myasthenia gravis** is an acquired autoimmune disorder of neuromuscular transmission in which acetylcholine receptor antibodies attack the postsynaptic membrane of the neuromuscular junction. This reaction reduces the available muscle-activating neurotransmitter, producing rapid fatigability of all muscles. Myasthenia gravis is the most common of the diseases of the neuromuscular junction. Others include **Eaton-Lambert syndrome**, **botulism**, and extensive use of aminoglycosides.

Swallowing problems occur in approximately one-third of patients with myasthenia gravis. Dysphagia is the usual presenting sign in neonates and in 6% to 15% of adult patients. Bulbar and facial muscles are frequently affected, causing dysphagia, dysarthria, nasal regurgitation, and weakness of mastication. Examination may show masseter weakness, bifacial weakness, poor gag reflex and palate elevation, dysarthria, or dysphonia. In addition, most patients have ptosis, diplopia, dysarthria, and dysphagia. Tongue weakness is very common when the bulbar musculature is involved and the oropharyngeal transit time (posterior tongue) is especially affected.

Liquids may be swallowed more easily than solids and patients may fatigue with chewing because of masseter weakness. Patients typically do well at the beginning of a meal but tire at the end. Some patients deteriorate to a point where there is total loss of the ability to chew and swallow, causing aspiration. Patients should take meals when muscle strength is best, possibly 1 hour after medication such as Mestinon®.

Compensatory training involves posture modification, alteration of food consistencies, frequent smaller meals, and other voluntary maneuvers designed to circumvent the health consequences of the oropharyngeal deficit.

Myopathies

Duchenne Dystrophy

Duchenne dystrophy is the most common childhood form of muscular dystrophy, with a usual age of onset at 2 to 6 years. The inheritance is X-linked and, thus, only males are affected.

Virtually all Duchenne dystrophy patients have severe dysphagia by 12 years of age. Episodes of aspiration pneumonia are common by age 18. For individuals with Duchenne dystrophy, deficits of oral preparatory and oral phases of swallowing, including increased mandibular angle and weakness of masticatory muscles, contribute to dysphagia.

Pharyngeal impairment in Duchenne dystrophy is associated with the appearance of macroglossia and weakness of the pterygoid and superior constrictor muscles. Weakness of lip and cheek muscles and tongue elevators may become more pronounced as the disease progresses. Pharyngeal swallowing reflexes are eventually delayed because of impaired elevation and retraction of the tongue. Aspiration of food and saliva, weight loss, and pulmonary complications ultimately occur as dysphagia progresses.

Facioscapulohumeral Muscular Dystrophy

Facioscapulohumeral muscular dystrophy is a slowly progressive, autosomal dominant neuromuscular disorder, with onset in adolescence or early adulthood. Less than 10% of individuals with facioscapulohumeral muscular dystrophy have dysphagia.

Inflammatory Myopathies

Inflammatory myopathies involve the inflammation and degeneration of skeletal muscle tissues. Inflammatory cells surround, invade, and destroy normal muscle fibers, eventually resulting in muscle weakness.

Dermatomyositis

Dermatomyositis usually presents with a rash characterized by patchy, bluish-purple discolorations on the face, neck, shoulders, upper chest, elbows, knees, knuckles, and back, accompanying, or more often preceding, muscle weakness. Dysphagia occurs in at least one-third of dermatomyositis patients, who typically present with oral dryness, delayed pharyngeal transit, and even aspiration.

High-dose prednisone is an effective treatment for many patients. In addition, other nonsteroidal immunosupressants such as azathioprine and methotrexate are often used, and even intravenous administration of immunoglobulins (Ig) has also proven effective.

Inclusion Body Myositis

Inclusion body myositis is an inflammatory muscle disease characterized by slow and relentlessly progressive muscle weakness and atrophy, similar to polymyositis. Indeed, inclusion body myositis is often the correct diagnosis in cases of polymyositis that are unresponsive to therapy.

Unfortunately, there is as yet no known treatment for inclusion body myositis. The disease is unresponsive to corticosteroids and other immunosuppressive drugs. Intravenous immunoglobulins have shown some preliminary evidence for a slight beneficial effect in a small number of cases.

Polymyositis

Polymyositis does not have the characteristic rash of dermatomyositis. As with dermatomyositis, dysphagia is common in polymyositis and its symptoms also include dryness of the mouth and prolonged pharyngeal transit. Treatment is also similar to that of dermatomyositis and other autoimmune diseases with medications such as prednisone, azathioprine, methotrexate, and Ig.

Limb-Girdle Muscular Dystrophy

Limb-girdle muscular dystrophy is a slowly progressive form of muscular dystrophy with both autosomal recessive and dominant forms. Males and females are equally affected, with onset usually in adolescence or early adulthood.

Swallowing abnormalities are demonstrated in up to one-third of patients, who show dysfunction of the pharyngeal muscles.

Myotonic dystrophy

Myotonic dystrophy is an autosomal dominant disorder that results in skeletal muscle weakness and wasting, myotonia, and numerous nonmuscular manifestations including frontal balding, cataracts, gonadal dysfunction, cardiac conduction abnormalities, respiratory insufficiency, and hypersomnolence.

Radiological features of dysphagia in myotonic dystrophy include a marked reduction in resting tone of both the upper and lower esophageal sphincters, and a reduction in contraction pressure in the pharynx and throughout the esophagus. Contrast radiography shows hypotonic pharynx with stasis and a hypomotility, and often esophageal dilation and gastroesophageal reflux disease.

Oculopharyngeal Dystrophy

Oculopharyngeal dystrophy is a progressive neurological disorder characterized by gradual onset of dysphagia, ptosis, and facial weakness. Oculopharyngeal dystrophy is an autosomal dominant disorder that affects both males and females, with onset of symptoms in the fourth or fifth decade. Dysphagia is slowly progressive and may be a presenting symptom before a diagnosis is made.

Both striated skeletal and smooth muscle are affected, leading to very low pharyngeal manometric pressures, cricopharyngeal bar, and lower esophageal sphincter pressure. Cricopharyngeal myotomy is an effective treatment of dysphagia secondary to cricopharyngeal achalasia. However, a cricopharyngeal myotomy does not modify the final prognosis and is contraindicated in cases with weak pharyngeal propulsion.

Spinal Muscular Atrophies

Spinal muscular atrophies constitute a group of neuromuscular disorders defined pathologically by degeneration of the anterior horn cells in the spinal cord.

Swallowing difficulties occur in over one-third of patients with spinal muscular atrophies. Bulbar and respiratory involvement is a prominent feature only in early-onset, more severely affected patients, with respiratory insufficiency, difficulty sucking and swallowing, accumulation of secretions, and a weak cry.

Progressive Supranuclear Palsy

Progressive supranuclear palsy (PSP) is a progressive, degenerative extrapyramidal disease that often masquerades as Parkinson disease. Almost all patients with progressive supranuclear palsy show multiple abnormalities in swallowing, including uncoordinated lingual movements, absent velar retraction or elevation, impaired posterior lingual displacement, and copious pharyngeal secretions. Tongue-assisted mastication, noncohesive lingual transfer, excessive spillage of the oral bolus into the pharynx prior to active transfer, vallecular bolus retention, abnormal epiglottic positioning, and hiatal hernias are also noted in about one-half of PSP patients. Unfortunately, PSP patients do not respond to dopaminergic pharmacological treatment as well as Parkinson disease patients do. Likewise, their dysphagia is more life-threatening and resistant to treatment. Early and aggressive swallowing evaluation and treatment are mandatory in PSP patients.

Traumatic Brain Injury

Following a traumatic brain injury, swallowing disorders generally consist of delayed or absent pharyngeal response, reduced lingual control, reduced pharyngeal clearance, and aspiration during and after the swallow. Due to its sudden onset, swallowing function may change rapidly after the initial traumatic event and may require repeated assessment with each change of neurological status. Cranial nerves can be affected due to skull base fractures and/or acceleration-deceleration injuries. Late effects of concussion fall into this latter category and are often the results of sports injuries not immediately detected.

Cognitive deficits in this population that may impact upon safe oral intake are disorders of attention, impulsivity, agitation, memory deficits, and reduced higher-level reasoning skills.

CONDITIONS FOUND IN CRITICAL CARE PATIENTS

Patients in critical care units often exhibit a variety of swallowing disorders. These patients, who are often elderly, are usually affected by multiple medical conditions and are frequently debilitated and deconditioned. Patients in surgical intensive care units are monitored continuously by the medical staff and a close communication between the medical staff and the swallowing rehabilitation staff must be maintained to ensure that a swallowing disorder does not adversely affect the recovery from surgery. Patients in both medical and surgical intensive care units often need nasogastric or endotracheal intubation and/or mechanical ventilation, which contribute to the swallowing difficulty and to aspiration or aspiration pneumonia.

> Nasogastric tubes reduce pharyngeal sensitivity, predispose the patient to gastroesophageal reflux, and may produce inflammation and pain, which interfere with laryngeal elevation and increase the risk for swallowing difficulties.

Simonian and Goldberg[23] listed an extensive number of signs of dysphagia in this group (see Table 2–3).

ESOPHAGEAL DISORDERS

The esophagus is a muscular, mucosal-lined tube that is generally thought to begin at the caudal end of the pharynx just inferior to the cricopharyngeus sphincter. It extends inferiorly through the thoracic cavity, the diaphragm muscle, and opens into the stomach. The wall of the esophagus consists of two types of muscle tissue, smooth muscle fibers in the alimentary canal and striated fibers at the junction of the pharynx and esophagus. Because of these two muscle types, a wide variety of diseases and injuries may affect the esophagus.

Esophageal Cancer

The most common manifestation of esophageal cancer is progressive dysphagia. Other symptoms include odynophagia, regurgitation, weight loss, and aspiration pneumonia. The barium swallow esophagogram is the preferred diagnostic tool and serves as a "road map" of the esophagus, providing diagnostic information on the site of luminal narrowing, the degree and length of obstruction, and the presence of concomitant tracheoesophageal fistula. The modified barium swallow (as discussed in Chapter 5) provides functional information for the clinician in managing dysphagia in the patient with a diagnosis of esophageal disease.

It is important for the clinicians treating the swallowing disorders of the esophagus to understand the conditions under which the esophageal cancer is identified and treated. The primary methods for palliating dysphagia involve endoscopic techniques. Endoscopic modalities include the ablation of the tumor using Nd:YAG laser or bipolar electrocautery, photodynamic therapy, pulsed dye laser (PDL), balloon dilatation, placement of expandable metal stents, and endoesophageal brachytherapy.

One of the simplest, but least effective, methods of endoscopic palliation is balloon dilatation. Dilatation is simple, relatively inexpensive, and easy to perform. However, it involves the risk of perforation, and the benefits are usually short-lived. Dilatation to the esophagus must be done carefully so as not to perforate the esophagus. Reports of esophageal perforation have suggested that the risk/benefit of this procedure must be assessed carefully as the treatment of esophageal perforation may require extensive treatment and slow down the treatment for the primary disease.[24]

In one large study, Nd:YAG was used as a palliative treatment for malignant dysphagia in 224 patients over a period of 8 years. The esophageal lumen was successfully reopened in 98.2% of patients, and 93.7% were able to ingest at least semisolids following the therapy.[25] Photodynamic therapy (PDT) is an alternative modality approved by the Food and Drug Administration for palliation of obstructive esophageal carcinoma.[26] External beam radiation therapy (EBRT) has been one of the most common approaches in the management of obstructing esophageal cancer. Brachytherapy involves inserting a radioactive source close to the tumor to maximize the delivery of radiation while minimizing its side effects.

Surgical bypass is an option for palliating dysphagia in a patient with good performance status, for whom conventional palliative methods have been ineffective. Minimally invasive esophagectomy utilizes laparoscopic and/or thoracoscopic techniques to perform the esophagectomy. Alternatively, a gastrostomy or jejunostomy tube can be surgically placed to provide enteral feedings.

Esophageal cancer is rapidly rising in western civilization and explanations for this have been offered by numerous sources, from nonmedical websites to advertisements for esophageal health foods to pathological studies of tissues from patients deceased from esophageal cancer. The answers leave the reader with more questions than in the past. Suffice to say that esophageal phase dysphagia may remain persistent despite medications, swallowing exercises, and/or further surgery.[27] The treatment of swallowing disorders associated with esophageal cancer are reviewed in Chapters 6 and 8.

Other Esophageal Disorders

Motility Disorders

Achalasia. Achalasia means "failure to relax." Achalasia is characterized by the degeneration of neural elements in the wall of the esophagus, particularly at the LES. The distal segment of the esophagus tapers, giving the appearance of a "bird's beak" (Figure 3–4).

Achalasia may be suspected in patients who complain of the sensation of food remaining in the throat that they cannot clear on repetitive swallowing. If the esophagus ultimately relaxes, the food is passed. The common treatments for this are balloon dilation or injection of botulinum toxin to the cricopharyngeus muscle. The diagnosis of achalasia, however, is confirmed manometrically with esophageal manometry studies, which are discussed in Chapter 5.

Curling. Curling is an alteration in esophageal motility frequently seen in elderly individuals. Curling represents tertiary contractions, which are nonpropulsive. This condition may occur as a result of scarring in the esophagus following surgery or bleeding.

Diffuse Esophageal Spasm. Diffuse esophageal spasm is characterized by intermittent dysphagia, chest pain, and repetitive contractions of the esopha-

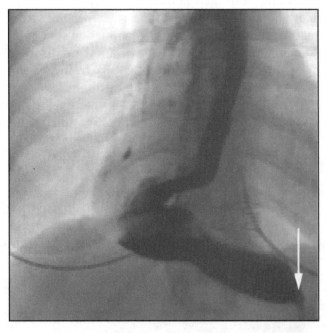

Figure 3–4. Barim esophagram of patient with achalasia showing the distal segment of the esophagus tapering into a "bird's beak."

gus. Dysphagia is present in 30% to 60% of patients with DES. Clinically, dysphagia is intermittent, with severity varying from mild to severe.

The distorted radiographic appearance of the esophagus is that of a "corkscrew" or of a "rosary bead" (Figure 3–5).

Nonperistaltic or simultaneous contractions following a majority of the swallows is the most reliable criteria in the identification of diffuse esophageal spasm.

Nonspecific Esophageal Motility Disorder. Nonspecific esophageal motility disorders may be found during esophageal manometry in patients with dysphagia who have no evidence of other systemic diseases. Patients with nonspecific esophageal motility disorders constitute approximately 25% to 50% of the abnormal motility studies performed during the evaluation of chest pain.

Systemic diseases such as diabetes mellitus, amyloidosis, and most notably progressive systemic sclerosis (PSS) can produce esophageal dysmotility and dysphagia. An estimated 50% to 90% of patients with PSS have esophageal involvement.

Diverticula. Esophageal **diverticula** are outpouchings of one or more layers of the esophageal wall. These diverticula occur: (1) immediately above the upper esophageal sphincter (Zenker diverticulum); (2) near the midpoint of the esophagus (traction diverticulum); or (3) immediately above the lower esophageal sphincter (epiphrenic diverticulum) or at the gastroesophageal junction. The outpouching seen in Figure 3–6 shows folds of tissue commonly known as a hiatal hernia found near the lower esophageal sphincter.

Webs/Rings. Patients with intermittent dysphagia for solids may have esophageal webs or rings. Esophageal webs are reported in 7% of the patients presenting with dysphagia. **Schatzki ring** is a lower esophageal mucosal ring that is located at the level of the squamocolumnar junction (Figure 3–7).

Esophageal Inflammatory Disorders

Gastroesophageal Reflux Disease. Gastroesophageal reflux disease (GERD) is defined as the retrograde movement of gastric contents from the

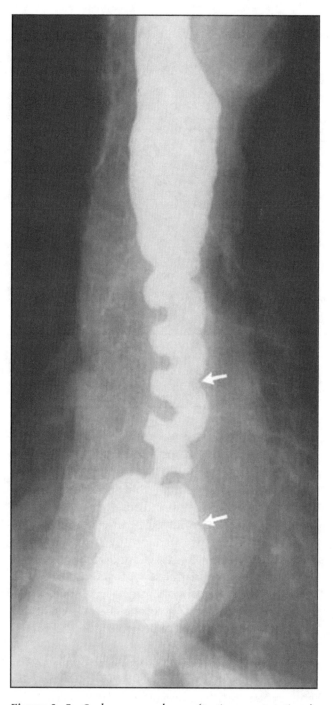

Figure 3–5. Corkscrew esophagus (tertiary contractions). Oblique view of the thoracic esophagus shows irregularly spaced contractions (arrows) causing indentations of the thoracic esophagus. At fluoroscopy, this was transient but recurred and the bolus was ineffectively propelled through the thoracic esophagus. Source: Adapted from Weissman JL. Chapter 11. In: Carrau RL, Murry T, eds. Comprehensive Management of Swallowing Disorders. *San Diego, CA: Singular Publishing Group; 1999:73, Figure 11–12.*

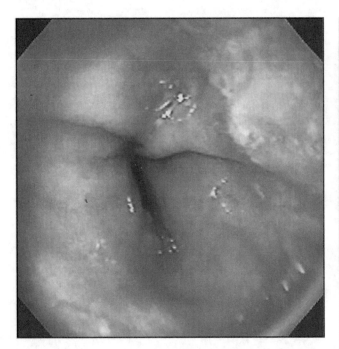

Figure 3–6. Hiatal hernia seen on esophagram. Patient with Zenker diverticulum was examined for hiatal hernia. The outpouching is near the upper esophageal sphincter.

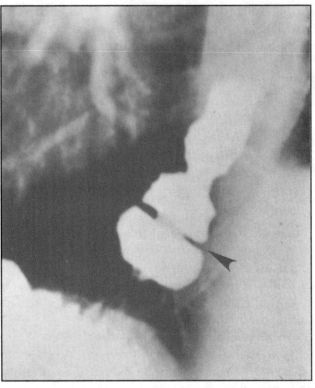

Figure 3–7. This barium esophagram shows a typical Schatzki's ring (arrow) in the distal esophagus. **Source:** *Adapted from Padda S, Young MA. The radiographic evaluation of dysphagia. In: Carrau R, Murry T, eds.* **Comprehensive Management of Swallowing Disorders.** *San Diego, CA: Plural Publishing; 1999:192, Figure 27–4.*

stomach through the lower esophageal sphincter and into the esophagus. The most common symptom is "heartburn." A study that surveyed presumably normal hospital staff and employees found that 7% of the people interviewed experience daily heartburn. The prevalence of monthly heartburn was estimated to be 36% to 44%. A randomized study of 2000 subjects demonstrated a prevalence of 58.1% of white patients with symptoms of heartburn and/or acid regurgitation. The prevalence of weekly or more frequent episodes of heartburn or acid regurgitation was 19.4%.[28]

Persons with GERD frequently complain of noncardiac chest pain, regurgitation of gastric contents, waterbrash (stimulated salivary secretion by esophageal acid), dysphagia, and sometimes **odynophagia** (pain upon swallowing).

> GERD has also been associated with numerous extraesophageal symptoms including pharyngitis, laryngitis, hoarseness, chronic cough, asthma, and pulmonary aspiration.

Acid reflux–induced symptoms referable to the oropharyngeal, laryngeal, and respiratory tracts are termed "extraesophageal reflux" or "atypical reflux" or, more commonly, laryngopharyngeal reflux disease (LPRD; see Chapter 11) and are discussed below.

Some investigators and clinicians feel that GERD may be the underlying etiology of **globus** (sensation of a lump in the throat). Gastroesophageal reflux disease was reported in 64% of patients reporting globus that were studied by ambulatory pH monitoring. GERD has also been implicated in the etiology of oropharyngeal dysphagia, the difficulty in passing a food bolus from the oropharynx into the upper esophagus. Cervical dysphagia is often linked to inflammation of the esophagus.

GERD occurs through one of three mechanisms: (1) inappropriate or transient lower esophageal sphincter relaxation; (2) increased abdominal pressure or stress-induced reflux; or (3) incompetent or reduced lower esophageal sphincter pressures or spontaneous free reflux. Lower esophageal sphincter competence is the most important barrier to esophageal reflux. Transient relaxation of the lower esophageal sphincter is probably the most important cause of GERD, both in healthy individuals and in patients with **esophagitis**.[27] Table 3–7 lists the protective and injurious determinants of esophageal function as it relates to inflammation and control of inflammation.

Acid, **pepsin**, and **bile** acids are the active components of the refluxate contributing to GERD, as they are potentially damaging to the esophageal mucosa and submucosa. Table 3–8 lists the substances that influence the pressures in the lower esophagus and affect lower esophageal pressure. The degree of mucosal damage by hydrogen seems to be potentiated by adding pepsin to the reflux material. The amount of time that the refluxed material is in contact with the esophageal mucosa might be a determining factor in the formation of esophagitis.

Upper esophageal dysfunction may contribute to GERD. The cricopharyngeus muscle has been implicated in the development of **Zenker diverticulum**, which is formed by the protrusion of the posterior hypopharyngeal mucosa between fibers of the

Table 3–7. Determinants of Reflux Injury

Protective
Competency of antireflux barrier:
LES
UES?
Esophageal acid clearance
Esophageal motility
Saliva
Epithelial tissue resistance
Injurious
Reflux constituents
Acid
Pepsin
Bile

Source: Adapted from Levy N, Young MA. Pathophysiology of swallowing and gastroesophageal reflux. In: Carrau RL, Murry T, eds. *Comprehensive Management of Swallowing Disorders.* San Diego, CA: Singular Publishing Group; 1999:175–185.

inferior constrictor and cricopharyngeus muscles. Figures 3–8A and 3–8B show an x-ray of the upper esophageal sphincter prior to surgery for Zenker diverticulum and following the surgery. The surgery to close the Zenker pouch may be done endoscopically or through an open surgical procedure. When the barium esophagram shows no evidence of Zenker diverticulum, the tight cricopharyngeus may be relaxed temporarily with injection of **botulinum toxin**.[29]

Laryngopharyngeal Reflux Disease. Laryngopharyngeal reflux disease (LPRD) is actually an inflammatory disease of the larynx, but it originates in the stomach like other reflux disorders. Acid from the stomach rises up to the level of the larynx and targets the laryngeal tissues to cause a number of disorders such as hoarseness, vocal process granulomas, and coughing. Reflux of acid into the hypopharynx is a very common and potentially debilitating disease. A healthy person complaining of hoarseness, throat clearing, and excess phlegm in the throat is typically describing the common symptoms of laryngopharyngeal reflux disease. In more severe cases, the symptoms might also include excessive coughing, occasional choking of liquids or foods, and globus. It differs from GERD in that it is an upright disease, occurring in the daytime and presenting with the common symptoms noted above and usually without the specific complaint of heartburn. GERD, on the other hand, usually results in complaints of heartburn, abdominal pain, and regurgitation.

The most common symptoms of LPRD have been quantified systematically by Belafsky et al.[30] From a list of common symptoms, they developed the Reflux Symptom Index (RSI; see Appendix III), a patient self-assessment questionnaire of the severity of common symptoms of reflux. Heartburn and regurgitation, the classic symptoms of GERD, are unusual symptoms in patients with LPRD, occurring in as few as 10% of patients with LPRD symptoms, according to Belafsky et al.[30] Although the reasons for this are not completely understood, most investigators suspect that it relates to the lack of acid-clearing mechanisms in the laryngopharynx.

The physical exam findings of LPRD have also been quantified by Belafsky et al,[30] and are referred

Table 3–8. Substances Influencing Lower Esophageal Sphincter Pressure

	Increase LES Pressure	Decrease LES Pressure
Hormones	Gastrin	Secretin
	Norepinephrine	Cholecystokinin
	Acetylcholine	Glucagon
	Motilin	Nitric Oxide
		Pancreatic Polypeptide
		Intestinal Polypeptide
		Substance P
		Progesterone
Pharmacological Agents	Metoclopramide	Cholinergic Agonists
	Cisapride	Cholinergic Antagonists
	Domperidone	Alpha Adrenergic Agonists
	Prostaglandin F2	Alpha Adrenergic Antagonists
		Beta Adrenergic Antagonists
		Beta Adrenergic Agonists
		Antacids
		Barbiturates
		Diazepam
		Calcium Channel Blockers
		Theophylline
		Morphine
		Dopamine
		Prostaglandin E2, I2
Diet	Protein	Fat
		Chocolate
		Caffeine
		Peppermint
		Spearmint
		Ethanol

Source: Adapted from Levy N, Young MA. Pathophysiology of swallowing and gastroesophageal reflux. In: Carrau RL, Murry T, eds. *Comprehensive Management of Swallowing Disorders.* San Diego, CA: Singular Publishing;1999:180.

to as the Reflux Finding Score (RFS; see Appendix II).[31] The RFS is determined by a clinician after the transnasal flexible laryngoscopic (TFL) examination. A score of 9 or greater is significant and strongly suggests LPRD. Rarely are the signs of LPRD seen in isolation, meaning it would be very unusual for a patient to have only a pseudosulcus vocalis as the sole manifestation of their LPRD. Typically, the patient with LPRD has multiple laryngeal indicators. Edema of the larynx, not erythema, is the clinical hallmark of LPRD, as seen in Figure 3–9.

Traditionally, the diagnosis of LPR is made by a combination of patient history, physical examination of the larynx, and diagnostic instrumental testing.

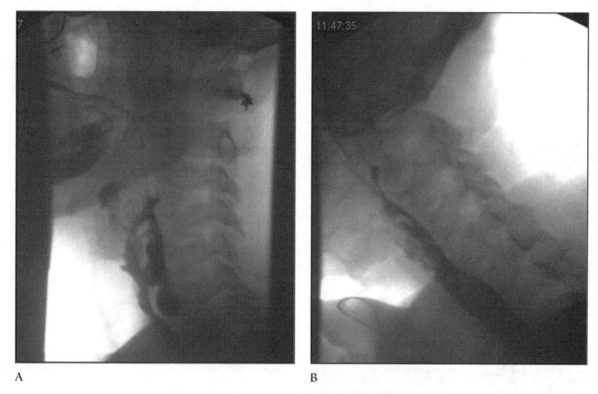

A

B

Figure 3–8. This barium esophagram allows easy delineation of the dilated esophagus. A. Shows the Zenker diverticulum prior to surgery. B. Shows the same esophageal segment following successful surgery.

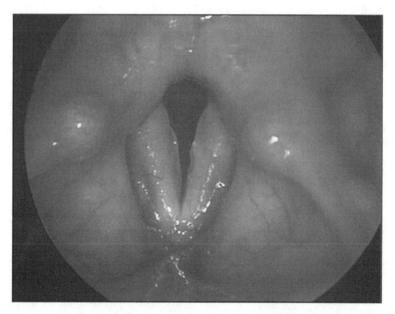

Figure 3–9. Patient with significant edema at the level of the larynx and vocal folds.

The test may consist of a 24-hour pH test or an in-office sensory test that takes minutes to perform and may be much more appealing to a patient.[32]

Table 3–9 summarizes the salient differences between GERD and LPRD, as reported by Levy and Young.[33]

Barrett Esophagus. **Barrett esophagus** (sometimes referred to as Barrett metaplasia), is a compensatory change in the esophageal mucosa from squamous to specialized intestinal epithelium, and it occurs in up to 15% of patients with atypical presentations of GERD. This disease often presents as a swallowing problem with nonspecific complaints of heartburn and dyspepsia. Moreover, there is evidence that the condition predisposes one to esophageal adenocarcinoma, cancer of the lower esophagus, which is rapidly increasing in the western world.[26]

INFECTIOUS DISEASES

Oral Cavity/Oropharynx

Bacterial infections of the oropharynx that result in dysphagia include tonsillitis, pharyngitis, and abscesses that may be associated with primary mucosal or lymphoid inflammation that causes pain and odynophagia. **Candidiasis** may also involve the oral cavity and the oropharynx in both immunocompetent and immunocompromised individuals. It is more common, however, in the latter group of patients and in those who require prolonged treatment with broad spectrum antibiotics.

Esophagitis

Primary esophageal infections are unusual in the general population. When they arise, these are typically due to **candidiasis** or **herpes simplex virus (HSV)**. Esophagitis, however, is a major cause of morbidity in individuals with impaired immunity caused by **human immunodeficiency virus (HIV)** infection, chemotherapy, or solid organ or bone marrow transplantation.

Chagas Disease

Chagas disease is a parasitic infectious disease that leads to achalasia. Chagas disease, endemic in the Amazon basin, is caused by *Trypanosoma cruzi*, a parasite. It can lead to achalasia that, in severe cases, results in megaesophagus as a result of destruction of the parasympathetic innervation.

Deep Neck Infections

Deep neck infections are typically the result of polymicrobial infections. In addition to symptoms of the primary infection site, patients may present with dysphagia, odynophagia, drooling, fever, chills, neck stiffness, and swelling. Treatment includes empiric therapy with broad spectrum agents, airway protection, and, often, surgical intervention.

Laryngeal Infections

Adult **epiglottitis** may cause life-threatening supraglottic edema that can progress to a delay in diagnosis and treatment. Common symptoms of supraglottic infection include a sore throat that is out of proportion to the findings of a pharyngeal examination, dysphagia, odynophagia, and dysarthria. Epiglottitis is diagnosed via endoscopic examination.

Table 3–9. *Symptoms of Gastroesophageal Reflux (GERD) and Laryngopharyngopharyngeal Reflux Disease (LPRD)*

Esophageal (GERD)	Laryngopharyngeal (LPRD)
Heartburn	Pharyngitis
Acid regurgitation	Laryngitis
Waterbrash	Hoarseness
Dysphagia	Globus
Odynophagia	Chronic cough
	Shortness of Breath
	Air hunger
	Pulmonary aspiration

MEDICATIONS

The effects of medications are influenced by sex, age, body size, metabolic status, individual biological response, and concurrent use of other medications. A variety of medications, including those obtained over the counter and those medically prescribed, affect swallowing, impairing consciousness, coordination, motor and sensitivity functions, and the lubrication of the upper aerodigestive tract (Table 3–10).

Analgesics

Salicylates (aspirin) and nonsteroidal antiinflammatory agents cause ulceration of the mouth, throat burning, mucosal hemorrhage, glossitis, and dry mouth.

Antibiotics

Side effects such as **glossitis**, **stomatitis**, and **esophagitis** have been described for penicillin, erythromycin, chloramphenicol, and the tetracyclines. Sulfa can cause a Stevens-Johnson syndrome-type reaction resulting in extensive mucosal ulceration and glossitis. Aminoglycosides can increase parkinsonian symptoms of weakness.

Antituberculous medications such as isoniazid, rifampin, ethambutol, and cycloserine can cause confusion, disorientation, and dysarthria. Antiviral agents such as acyclovir, amantadine, gancyclovir, and vidarabine can indirectly cause dysphagia with confusion, asthenia, and lingual facial dyskinesia. Amantadine can cause severe xerostomia and xerophonia in some patients. Zidovudine (AZT7), an antiviral drug, causes dysphagia in approximately 5% to 10% of patients and tongue edema in 5% of

Table 3–10. Common Medications Affecting Swallowing

Product Category	Examples	Common Indications	Possible Effects
Neuroleptics			
antidepressants	Elavil (tricyclic)	Relief of endogenous depression	Drying of mucosa, drowsiness, cough
antipsychotics	Haldol Thorazine	Management of patients with chronic psychosis	Tardive dyskinesia
Sedatives			
barbiturates	Phenobarbital Nembutal	Treatment of insomnia	CNS depressant (drowsiness causing decompensation of patients with cognitive deficits)
Antihistamines	Cold and cough preparations	Relief of nasal congestion and cough	Drying mucosa, sedative effects
Diuretics	Lasix	Treatment of edema (eg, associated with congestive heart failure)	Signs of chronic dehydration (dryness of mouth, thirst, weakness, drowsiness)
Mucosal anesthetics	Hurricaine (contains benzocaine)	Topical anesthetic used to aid passage of fiberoptic nasopharyngoscopes, control of dental pain	Suppresses gag and cough reflex
Anticholinergics	Cogentin	Adjunct in Parkinson disease therapy	Dry mouth and reduced appetite

Source: Adapted from Perlman AL, Schulze-Delrieu K. *Deglutition and Its Disorders.* San Diego, CA: Singular Publishing; 1997:139.

patients. Chloroquine (Plaquenil), mostly used for treating malaria, can cause stomatitis.

Antihistamines

Antihistamines (H_1-receptor antagonists) are commonly used to treat allergies. However, because of their anticholinergic side effects, this class of medications commonly exerts a drying effect on the aerodigestive tract mucosa, causing difficulty in gastrointestinal motility during the swallowing process.

Other side effects include sedation, disturbed coordination, and gastric distress. Central nervous system effects include ataxia, incoordination, convulsions, dystonia, and bruxism, which can lead to poor oral intake.

Antimuscarinics, Anticholinergics, and Antispasmodics

Antimuscarinics and antispasmodics, used for a variety of reasons such as bradycardia, excessive oral secretions, motion sickness, and diarrhea, diminish the production of saliva and mucus. Salivary secretion is particularly sensitive to inhibition by antimuscarinic agents, which can completely abolish the copious water secretions induced by the parasympathetic system. The mouth becomes dry, and swallowing and talking become difficult.

Prokinetic agents improve motility and speed gastric emptying. The two major drugs in this category are metoclopramide (Reglan®) and cisapride (Propulsid®); however, the latter is no longer available in the United States. The former is associated with greater antihistamine-like side effects and must be taken carefully to avoid confounding the swallowing disorder.

Mucolytic Agents

Mucolytics can be used to counter the effects of drying agents such as antihistamines. However, no medications, including mucolytic agents, are a substitute for adequate hydration and, indeed, these medications are dependent on adequate water intake.

Antihypertensives

Almost all of the antihypertensive agents have some degree of parasympathomimetic effects and thus dry the mucous membranes. Hydration is the first step to improve swallowing when taking these medications.

Antineoplastic Agents

These agents affect swallowing mainly through the mechanism of inflammation, sloughing, and occasionally causing superinfection of the aerodigestive tract mucosa. This effect results in mucositis, stomatitis, pharyngitis, esophagitis, and esophageal ulceration. Common antineoplastic agents are cisplatin and tamoxofen, both used in chemotherapy protocols to treat cancer in various organs.

Vitamins

Overdosage of vitamin A causes hypervitaminosis, a condition that includes dermatological, gastric, skeletal, and cerebral and optic nerve edema. Fissures of the lips, dry mouth, and abdominal discomfort can result. A similar stomatitis can result with vitamin E overdosage.

Neurological Medications

Anticonvulsants

Phenobarbital is a sedative and anticonvulsant with side effects similar to the tricyclic antidepressants: dry mouth, sweating, hypotension, and tremor. Phenytoin's (Dilantin®) adverse effects include central nervous system signs such as ataxia, slurred speech, incoordination, and dystonia.

Carbamazepine (Tegretol®) is an anticonvulsant used primarily for seizures. Digestive symptoms can also be serious, such as glossitis, stomatitis, and dryness of the mouth.

Anti-Parkinson Disease Agents

Levodopa may improve all symptoms of Parkinson disease, including swallowing, but it can cause gastrointestinal discomfort, dyskinesia, and oral dryness.

Antipsychotics

Antipsychotic medications primarily work by dopamine antagonism. Commonly used drugs in this class include haloperidol (Haldol), chlorpromazine (Thorazine), thioridazine (Mellaril), and prochlorperazine (Compazine). These medications can have anticholinergic effects, such as dry mouth, nasal congestion, and hypotension.

> Approximately 14% of patients receiving long-term antipsychotic medications will develop tardive dyskinesia, with symptoms ranging from tongue restlessness, disfiguring choreiform, and/or athetoid movements, leading to significant swallowing and feeding problems.

Life-threatening dysphagia can occur after prolonged neuroleptic therapy. Neuroleptic drugs can induce extrapyramidal symptoms such as **dystonia**, **akathisia**, and **tardive dyskinesia**. Contrast radiography has revealed poor contractions in the upper esophagus, a hypertonic esophageal sphincter, and hypokinesia of the pharyngeal muscles.

Anxiolytics

Significant dysphagia can result from chronic use of benzodiazepines. Reported effects include hypopharyngeal retention, cricopharyngeal incoordination, aspiration, and drooling. Benzodiazepines can inhibit discharges from interneurons in the nucleus of the tractus solitarius or nucleus ambiguus, both of which are critical to the pharyngeal phase of swallowing.

NEOPLASMS

Neoplasia causes distortion, obstruction, reduced mobility, or neuromuscular and sensory dysfunction of the upper aerodigestive tract. **Exophytic** **tumors** interfere with swallowing principally by distorting or obstructing the aerodigestive tract. Tumors with an infiltrating growth pattern may cause reduced mobility or fixation of the tongue, soft palate, pharynx, or larynx (Table 3–11). Tumors also affect swallowing by interfering with the afferent fibers (sensory input) from the mucosa of the upper aerodigestive tract by invasion and destruction of mucosal nerve endings, or sensory nerves such as the trigeminal (V), glossopharyngeal (IX), and vagus (X) cranial nerves and their branches.

Neoplasms of the floor of the mouth, tongue, or buccal mucosa may by mass effect or by restricting mobility of the tongue and floor of the mouth impair a patient's ability to interpose food between the teeth. Tumor invasion of the dorsum of the tongue or involvement of the lingual nerve (CN V) may affect sensory input causing premature spillage of the bolus into the pharynx and, consequently, aspiration.

Tumors of the pharynx may cause an adynamic segment that interferes with peristalsis or laryngeal elevation or may cause mechanical obstruction. Tumor invading or destroying the larynx may cause either an incompetent laryngeal sphincter or sensory denervation of the larynx.

Table 3–11. *Pathophysiology of Swallowing in Accordance with Tumor Origin and Growth Pattern*

Tumor	Swallowing Pathophysiology
Intrinsic tumor	
Exophytic growth	Obstruction
	Distortion
	Anesthesia/hypesthesia
Infiltrating growth	Fixation
	Pain
	Trismus
	Cranial nerve deficits
Extrinsic tumor	Compression
	X Obstruction
	X Distortion
	Cranial nerve deficits
	Fixation

Source: Adapted from Falestiny MN, Yu VL. Chapter 55. In: Carrau RL, Murry T, eds. *Comprehensive Management of Swallowing Disorders.* San Diego, CA: Singular Publishing; 1999:38.

SWALLOWING DISORDERS FOLLOWING RADIATION THERAPY

The head and neck areas include numerous structures, each with an inherent response to radiation that is largely governed by the presence or absence of mucosa, salivary glands, or specialized organs within that site. Irradiated mucocutaneous tissues demonstrate increased vascular permeability that leads to fibrin deposition, subsequent collagen formation, and eventual fibrosis.

Dysphagia is a common side effect of radiation therapy for cancers of the upper aerodigestive tract and the head and neck regions. It is further complicated by the effect of surgical procedures that may be done prior to radiation. The etiology of dysphagia following radiation therapy is multifactorial and can be divided into acute and late effects. Acute effects present during and immediately following a course of irradiation, and late effects manifest themselves from several months to as many as 5 to 10 years after completion of radiation therapy.

Irradiation produces mitotic death of the basal cells of the mucosa, as this is a rapidly renewing system. With a standard course of radiation therapy (180–200 cGy/fraction; 5 daily fractions per week for approximately 6 weeks), there is a 2-week delay from the start of therapy before the onset of mucositis.

The acute phase of dysphagia is primarily due to radiation effects on mucosa (erythema, pseudomembranous mucositis, ulceration), taste buds (decreased, altered, or loss of taste acuity), and salivary glands (thickened saliva secondary to decreased serous secretions). These conditions tend to last for several months after the completion of radiation, especially if the dosage exceeds 60 Gy.

Late effects of radiation to the head and neck have been examined by Lazarus et al[34] and by Jensen et al.[35] The long-term effects of external beam radiation therapy include loss of tongue strength and thus disrupt the timing of the swallow. Late effects also include injury to salivary glands resulting in **xerostomia** and damage to connective tissue (fibrosis) resulting in **trismus** and poor pharyngeal motility.

Late complications involving the mucosa of the upper aerodigestive tract are primarily related to atrophy, manifested by pallor and thinning, submucosal fibrosis, manifested as induration and diminished pliability, and occasionally chronic ulceration and necrosis with resultant exposure of the underlying bone/soft tissue.

In humans, the parotid glands are purely serous, the submandibular glands are made of serous and mucous acini, and the minor salivary glands are predominantly mucous secreting. The normal human salivary glands produce approximately 1000–1500 cc of saliva per day. The parotid gland accounts for about 60% to 65% of the salivary flow; the submandibular gland contributes 20% to 30% and sublingual glands 2% to 5%. Irradiation of the normal salivary glands results primarily in injury to the serous acini, with no significant effect on the mucous acini.

A decrease in the salivary flow can be detected 24 to 48 hours after initiation of standard fractionated irradiation and it continues to decline through the course of therapy. In addition to the decrease in flow there is increase in viscosity and decreased pH and IgA in saliva. Because the serous acini are primarily affected, the saliva becomes thick, sticky, and ropy, resulting in dry mouth and difficulty with mastication and swallowing. Most patients are unable to clear these thick secretions. These changes allow for an increased yeast flora of the oral cavity.

Irradiated salivary tissue degenerates after relatively small doses, leading to markedly diminished salivary output. This, in turn, affects the teeth by promoting dental decay, which in turn affects the integrity of the mandible. Details of these changes, including their pathophysiology, clinical syndromes, and potential treatment, are presented by Cooper et al.[36] The dose at which 50% of patients develop xerostomia at 5 years after irradiation was 7000 cGy. Figure 3–10 shows the larynx following external beam radiation therapy (XRT) for laryngeal cancer. Note the heavy white secretions.

Xerostomia results from permanent injury to the salivary glands. The most effective treatment for xerostomia is prevention. Once xerostomia develops, its treatment primarily consists of saliva substitute (water and glycerin mixture) and salivary gland stimulants such as pilocarpine hydrochloride, bromohexine, and anethole-trithione.

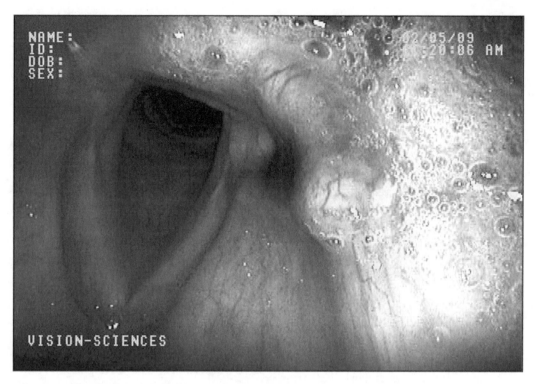

Figure 3–10. The larynx following radiation therapy (XRT) for laryngeal cancer.

Pilocarpine is a cholinergic agonist that simulates the smooth muscle and exocrine glands; it affects the postganglionic cells. This results in increased excretion of saliva and sweat.

INTUBATION

> The minimum requirements for a patient to actively participate in the dysphagia evaluation process include the ability to maintain alertness, follow basic commands, and ideally be 24 hours postextubation or 48 hours posttracheotomy.

Swallowing evaluation in orally or nasally intubated patients is usually deferred, although possible in selected cases (eg, young patients with normal upper aerodigestive tract). If swallowing evaluation is done using transnasal flexible endoscopy, ie, FEES or FEESST, it may be easier to pass the endoscope on the side of the nasogastric tube.

AUTOIMMUNE DISEASES

The diagnosis and treatment of swallowing disorders in patients with autoimmune disorders and diseases is complex and commonly limited by their primary condition or by the other treatments that they may be receiving.

Autoimmune diseases are characterized by the production of antibodies that react with host tissue or immune effector T cells that react to self-peptides. Autoimmune diseases may affect swallowing by causing intrinsic obstruction, external compression, abnormal motility, or inadequate lubrication.

Crohn Disease

Crohn disease produces lesions throughout the digestive tract that vary in appearance, often resembling apthous ulcers or cheilitis. Dysphagia is the most common presenting symptom of esophageal Crohn disease.

Epidermolysis Bullosa

Epidermolysis bullosa is a rare disorder characterized by blistering of the mucosal lining, often elicited by minimal trauma. It has a variable onset and no racial or gender predilection. The oral cavity, pharynx, larynx, and esophagus may be severely affected, resulting in severe dysphagia. Pharyngeal and esophageal webs and/or scarring may be severe, necessitating a gastrostomy or jejunostomy. The disease is often refractory to standard therapy using corticosteroids.

Giant Cell Arteritis

Giant cell arteritis, also known as temporal arteritis, is an inflammatory disorder affecting large- and medium-size vessels. The arteries that originate from the arch of the aorta are the most affected. Pharyngeal, tongue, or jaw claudication may occur when the ascending pharyngeal, lingual, deep temporal, or massenteric arteries are affected. Systemic corticosteroids often resolve these all within 1 to 2 weeks.

Mixed Connective-Tissue Disease

Mixed connective-tissue disease (MCTD) is characterized by clinical findings that may be found in progressive systemic sclerosis, systemic lupus erythematous, and polymyositis/dermatomyositis. Similarly, the swallowing disorders described under each of these disorders can be part of MCTD.

Esophageal motility is severely affected and the majority of the patients have little or no peristalsis, or they have low amplitude peristalsis contributing to gastroesophageal reflux disease. Heartburn and dysphagia are present in up to 50% of the patients with MCTD. The treatment of GERD in these patients may reduce the dysphagia.

Myositis

Polymyositis and **dermatomyositis** are characterized by inflammation of the skeletal muscle. Thus, muscles of the pharynx are often affected while the esophageal smooth muscle is spared. Endoscopic evaluation of swallowing with transnasal flexible laryngoscopy (TFL) may reveal prominence of the cricopharyngeus muscle, decreased epiglottic tilt, and moderate to severe residue in the pharynx, which fails to pass into the esophageal inlet even with multiple swallows. Two-thirds of these patients have demonstrable delayed esophageal transit. Polymyositis and dermatomyositis are treated with corticosteroids.

Pemphigus Vulgaris

Pemphigus vulgaris is a rare, chronic intraepidermal bullous disease. Blisters most commonly develop on the soft palate but can occur anywhere on the oral cavity. Painful ulcerations that can become infected follow the ruptured blisters. Ulcerations heal by secondary intention, often leading to scarring. Distal involvement of the pharynx, larynx, and esophagus is possible and may account for the dysphagia noted by some patients.

Ocular Cicatricial Pemphigoid

Ocular cicatricial pemphigoid is a chronic blistering disease that affects the oral mucosa in almost all cases. Typical lesions are characterized by erosion of the gingiva and buccal mucosa that usually are not as painful as those associated with pemphigus vulgaris. As the targeted proteins are found in the basement-membrane zone, the lesions heal with submucosal scarring. Treatment of ocular cicatricial pemphigoid is primarily with corticosteroids.

Rheumatoid Arthritis

Rheumatoid arthritis (RA) is a chronic, relapsing inflammatory arthritis, usually affecting multiple diarthrodial joints with a varying degree of systemic involvement. The female to male ratio is 3:1.

Rheumatoid arthritis is associated with xerostomia, temporomandibular joint (TMJ) syndrome, a decrease in the amplitude of the peristaltic pressure complex in the proximal, striated part of the esophagus, as well as from cervical spine arthritic disease, all of which cause or contribute to swallowing problems. Rheumatic laryngeal involvement can result in cricoarytenoid joint fixation. Objective functional testing is necessary to determine the contributions of the oral phase and pharyngeal phase to the swallowing disorder. Patients may benefit from a modified barium swallow to identify the oral phase components amenable to therapeutic exercises.

Treatment of the dysphagia is focused on hydration and artificial saliva and/or pilocarpine for the xerostomia. TMJ dysfunction (ie, trismus, mastication problems) is treated with nonsteroidal antiinflammatory agents and exercises with mechanical devices. Laryngeal closure exercises may also be useful. These are further described in Chapter 6.

Sarcoidosis

Sarcoidosis is a chronic systemic disorder presumed to have an autoimmune pathogenesis. Sarcoidosis may cause laryngeal lesions, extrinsic compression of the esophagus by mediastinal adenopathy, and esophageal dysmotility due to myopathy, infiltration of Auerbach plexus, or granulomatous infiltration of the esophageal wall, which may produce long esophageal strictures.

Scleroderma

Systemic sclerosis (**scleroderma**) is a disorder characterized by progressive fibrosis and vascular changes. The most common and the earliest symptom in people with progressive systemic sclerosis is Raynaud disease, characterized by pallor and sweating of the fingers or hands that progresses to cyanosis and pain. Dysphagia, which is the second most common symptom of this disorder, is usually first noticed while swallowing solids.

Dysphagia is most often due to poor motility through the inferior two-thirds of the esophagus. The process starts affecting the Auerbach plexus, which coordinates the smooth muscle. This is followed by a myopathy, which is then followed by fibrosis and strictures secondary to the effects of gastroesophageal reflux.

The dysphagia can be minimized by adequate chewing and by reducing the bolus size. Esophageal motility can be improved by prokinetic agents, which, other than Reglan®, were taken off the market several years ago.

Sjögren Disease

Sjögren disease includes dry eyes and mouth. Xerostomia, oral pain, glossodynia, and **dysgusia** are prominent features of the disease.

> **Xerostomia** also increases the incidence of GERD, because it decreases the ability of the esophagus to clear gastric refluxate and the bicarbonate antacid effect of saliva is diminished.

Treatment of xerostomia is often palliative and includes saliva preparations, pilocarpine, antacids, and H_2 blockers. Diet modification to a mixed thickened and slippery combination of foods also is helpful.

Systemic Lupus Erythmatosus

Systemic lupus erythematous is an inflammatory disorder that is associated with a variety of auto antibodies against many different tissue components. The vast majority of patients with systemic lupus erythematous do not experience dysphagia and have normal esophageal transit studies. Dysphagia and/or chest pain is most often attributed to esophageal dysmotility associated with lower esophageal sphincter insufficiency and thus gastroesophageal reflux disease (GERD).

Wegener Granulomatosis

Wegener granulomatosis is characterized by a granulomatous arteritis involving the upper and lower respiratory tracts, a progressive glomerulonephritis, and extrarespiratory symptoms attributable to systemic small-vessel arteritis. Wegener granulomatosis often affects the hard and soft palate and may lead to extensive ulceration, oronasal fistulas, and velopharyngeal insufficiency.

SUMMARY

A brief summary of the phases of swallowing along with the critical cranial nerve involvement at these phases is summarized here.

Oral Phase

Retention and Mastication—retention of the bolus in the mouth (CN VII)

Sensation—feel, taste, temperature (CN VII, CN IX)

Salivation—needed to form the bolus (CN VII, CN IX)

Oral and Lingual Transit—Cranial nerves operating motorically (CN X, CNXII)

Pharyngeal Phase

Sensation—perception of bolus at posterior pharyngeal wall (CN IX)

Transit—oral cavity to pharynx (CN IX, CN X, CN XII)

Transit—pharynx to esophagus (CN X, CN XII)

Esophageal Phase

Sensation—perception of bolus at or below the cricopharyngeus muscle (CN X)

Transit—to lower esophagus (CN X)

Reverse Transit (regurgitation)—UES and LES pressure irregularities

The conditions and diseases encountered by the members of the swallowing rehabilitation team extend from occasional coughing or choking while eating to obvious debilitating diseases such as esophageal cancer or Parkinson disease. The clinician should not be fooled, however, into thinking that a patient complaining of occasional choking does not have a significant swallowing disorder or a disease or disorder that is being reflected in its early stages. In this chapter, conditions and diseases that give rise to swallowing disorders or that foretell future dysphagia are reviewed. It should be pointed out that causal relationships are not the hallmark of many swallowing disorders. Rather, the swallowing disorder may develop shortly after the disease or disorder or may develop long after a condition, such as a swallowing disorder years after radiation therapy to the larynx or pharynx. The astute clinician, regardless of his or her medical or paramedical specialty, should work as a team member with other clinicians who are also treating the patient. In some cases, this may be the general practitioner, whereas in other cases, the team may include an entire surgical or neurological group.

STUDY QUESTIONS

1. Aspiration occurs when:
   A. Food or liquid remains at the entrance to the laryngeal inlet
   B. Food or liquid is regurgitated up from the esophagus into the oral cavity
   C. Food or liquid enters the airway below the vocal folds
   D. The patient coughs following drinking or eating

2. Aspiration pneumonia:
   A. Is a swallowing disorder resulting from food or liquid residing in the trachea or lungs
   B. Is a condition of the elderly who recently had a CVA and continued to be fed orally without assessment of their swallowing status
   C. Is a condition in which a chemical inflammation or bacterial infection results in entry of foreign materials into the bronchi of the lungs
   D. Is diagnosed with a modified barium swallow or fiberoptic endoscopic evaluation of swallowing test (FEEST)

3. The swallowing problems associated with cerebrovascular accidents (CVAs):
   A. Usually end shortly after the acute period has passed

B. May occur during the first 24 hours after a CVA or may develop weeks or even months after the occurrence

C. Are generally not life threatening if the CVA is on the right side of the brain

D. Are primarily dangerous if the patient is also elderly

4. Autoimmune disorders of swallowing are generally due to:

A. Obstruction along the passageway of food or liquid

B. Inflammation within the esophagus causing regurgitation or choking

C. Inadequate lubrication for the normal passage of food or liquid from the oropharynx to the hyopharynx

D. All of the above

5. Gastroesophageal reflux disease and laryngopharyngeal reflux disease are:

A. Inflammatory disorders of the lower esophagus

B. Inflammatory disorders of the esophagus that affect structures within and above the esophagus

C. Not true swallowing disorders because they rarely cause aspiration or aspiration pneumonia.

D. Usually exist in patients with dysphagia but rarely require specialized treatment

DISCUSSION QUESTIONS

1. Discuss the possible complications of treating a patient with a swallowing disorder who has: (a) advanced Parkinson disease or (b) advanced ALS. What are some of the differences in these patients that affect treatment?

2. The current literature on reflux disease (GERD and LPRD) suggests that both may contribute to swallowing disorders. Why is it important for the speech-language pathologist (SLP) to understand the importance of GERD and LPRD as they relate to the treatment of swallowing disorders? See, for example: Fletcher KC,

Goutte M, Slaughter JC, Garrett CG, Vaezi MF. Significance and degree of reflux in patients with primary extraesophageal symptoms. *Laryngoscope*. 2011 Dec;121(12):2561–2565; and Altman KW, Prufer N, Vaezi MF. The challenge of protocols for reflux disease: a review and development of a critical pathway. *Otolaryngol Head Neck Surg*. 2011 Jul;145(1):7–14.

REFERENCES

1. Aviv JE, Murry T. *FEESST Flexible Endoscopic Evaluation of Swallowing with Sensory Testing*. San Diego, CA: Plural Publishing; 2005.

2. Coelho CA. Preliminary findings on the nature of dysphagia in patients with chronic obstructive pulmonary disease. *Dysphagia*. 1987;2:28–31.

3. Kendall KA, Leonard RJ, McKenzie S. Airway protection: evaluation with videofluoroscopy. *Dysphagia*. 2004;19:65–70.

4. Vu KN, Day TA, Gillespie MB, et al. Proximal esophageal stenosis in head and neck cancer patients after total laryngectomy and radiation. *ORL*. 2008;70:229–235.

5. Nguyen NP, Frank C, Moltz CC, et al. Long term aspiration following treatment for head and neck cancer. *Oncology*. 2008;74:25–30.

6. Mendelsohn N. New concepts in dysphagia management. *J Otolaryngol*. 1993;22(suppl 1):9–10.

7. Falestiny MN, Yu VL. Aspiration pneumonia. In: Carrau RL, Murry T, eds. *Comprehensive Management of Swallowing Disorders*. San Diego, CA: Singular Publishing Group; 1999:383–388.

8. Pou AM, Carrau RL. In: Carrau RL, Murry T, eds. *Comprehensive Management of Swallowing Disorders*. San Diego, CA: Singular Publishing; 1999:155–158.

9. White AC, O'Connor HH, Kirby K. Prolonged mechanical ventilation: review of care settings and an update on professional reimbursement. *Chest*. 2008;133:539–545.

10. Ludlow C. Recent advances in laryngeal sensorimotor control for voice, speech and swallowing. *Curr Opin Otolaryngol Head Neck Surg*. 2004;12:160–165.

11. Kunibi I. Nonaka S, Katada A. The neuronal circuit of augmenting effects on intrinsic laryngeal muscle activities induced by nasal air jet stimulation in deceregrate cats. *Brain Res*. 2003;978:83–90.

12. Perlman A, Shultze-Delrieu K. *Deglutition and Its Disorders*. San Diego, CA: Singular Publishing; 1997:352–359.

13. Coyle JL, Rosenbek JC, Chignell KA. Pathophysiology of neurogenic oropharyngeal dysphagia. In: Carrau RL, Murry T, eds. *Comprehensive Management of Swallowing Disorders*. San Diego, CA; Singular Publishing Group; 1999:93–108.

14. Siddique T, Donkervoort S. Amyotrophic lateral sclerosis overview. In: Pagon RA, Bird TC, Dolan CR, Stephens K. *Gener Reviews* (Internet). Seattle: University of Washington. Updated 7/28/2007.

15. Yorkston KM, Strand E, Miller R, Hillel A, Smith K. Speech deterioration in amyotrophic lateral sclerosis: implications for the timing of intervention. *J Med Speech-Lang Pathol.* 1993;1:35–46.

16. Higo R, Tayama N, Nito T. Longitudinal analysis of progression of dysphagia in amyotrophic lateral sclerosis. *Auris Nasus Larynx.* 2004 Sep;31(3):247–254.

17. Leder SB, Novella S, Patwa H. Use of fiberoptic endoscopic evaluation of swallowing in patients with amyolateral sclerosis. *Dysphagia.* 2004;19:177–181.

18. Robbins J, Levine RL, Maser A, Rosenbek JC, Kempster JB. Swallowing after unilateral stroke of the cerebral cortex. *Arch Phys Med Rehabil.* 1993;74:1295–1300.

19. DePippo KL, Holas MA, Reding MJ. The Burke Dysphagia Screening Test: validation of its use in patients with stroke. *Arch Phys Med Rehabil.* 1994;75:1284–1286.

20. Sapir S, Ramig L, Fox C. Speech and swallowing disorders in Parkinson disease. *Curr Opin Otolaryngol Head Neck Surg.* 2008 Jun;16(3):205–210.

21. Plowman-Prine EK, Sapienza CM, Okun MS, et al. The relationship between quality of life and swallowing in Parkinson's disease. *Mov Disord.* 2009 Jul 15;24(9):1352–1358.

22. Miller N, Noble E, Jones D, Burn D. Hard to swallow: dysphagia in Parkinson's disease. *Age Aging.* 2006;35:6614–6618.

23. Simonian MA, Goldbert AN. Swallowing disorders in the critical care patient. In: Carrau RL, Murry T, eds. *Comprehensive Management of Swallowing Disorders.* San Diego, CA: Singular Publishing; 1999:363–369.

24. Ferri L, Lee JK, Law S, Wong KH, Kwok KF, Wong J. Management of spontaneous perforation of esophageal cancer with covered self expanding metallic stents. *Dis Esophagus.* 2005;18(1):67–69.

25. Houghton A, Mason R, Allen A, McColl I. NdYAG laser treatment in the palliation of advanced oesophageal malignancy. *Br J Surg.* 1989 Sep;76(9):912–913.

26. Mognissi K, Dixon K. Photodynamic therapy (PDT) in esophageal cancer: a surgical view of its indications based on 14 years experience. *Technol Cancer Res Treat.* 2003 Aug;2(4):319–326.

27. Belafsky P, Rees CJ. Esophageal phase dysphagia. In: Leonard R, Kendall K, eds. *Dysphagia Assessment and Treatment Planning: A Team Approach.* 2nd ed. San Diego, CA: Plural Publishing; 1997:63–65.

28. Aviv JE, Liu H, Parides M, Kaplan ST, Close LG. Laryngopharyngeal sensory deficits in patients with laryngopharyngeal reflux and dysphagia. *Ann Otol Rhinol Laryngol.* 2000;109:1000–1006.

29. Murry T, Wasserman T, Carrau RL, Castillo B. Injection of botulinum toxin A for the treatment of dysfunction of the upper esophageal sphincter. *Am J Otolaryngol.* 2005;26:157–162.

30. Belafsky P, Postma GN, Amin MR, Koufman JA. Symptoms and findings of laryngopharyngeal reflux. *Ear Nose Throat J.* 2002; 81(9 suppl 2):10–13.

31. Belafsky PC, Postma GN, Koufman JA. The validity and reliability of the reflux finding score (RFS). *Laryngoscope.* 2001;111:1313–1317.

32. Botoman VA, Hanft KL, Breno SM, et al. Prospective controlled evaluation of pH testing, laryngoscopy and laryngopharyngeal sensory testing (LPST) shows a specific post inter-arytenoid neuropathy in proximal GERD (P-GERD). LPST improves laryngoscopy diagnostic yield in P-GERD. *Am J Gastroenterol.* 2002;97(9 suppl):S11–12.

33. Levy B, Young MA. Pathophysiology of swallowing and gastroesophageal reflux. In: Carrau RL, Murry T, eds. *Comprehensive Management of Swallowing Disorders.* San Diego, CA: Singular Publishing; 1999:175–186.

34. Lazarus C, Logemann JA, Pauloski BR, et al. Effects of radiotherapy with or without chemotherapy on tongue strength and swallowing in patients with oral cancer. *Head Neck.* 2007;29:632–637.

35. Jensen K, Lambertsen K, Grau C. Late swallowing dysfunction and dysphagia after radiotherapy for pharynx cancer; frequency, intensity and correlation with dose and volume parameters. *Radiother Oncol;* 2007;85(1):74–82.

36. Cooper JS, Fu K, Marks J, Silverman S. Late effects of radiation therapy in the head and neck. *Int J Radiat Oncol Biol Phys.* 1995;31(5):1141–1164.

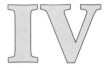

Swallowing Disorders Arising From Surgical Treatments

CHAPTER OUTLINE

    I. INTRODUCTION
   II. ANTERIOR CERVICAL SPINAL SURGERY (ACSS)
  III. HEAD AND NECK SURGERY
  IV. FLOOR OF THE MOUTH SURGERY
   V. PARTIAL GLOSSECTOMY
  VI. PALATE SURGERY
 VII. LIP SURGERY
VIII. MANDIBULAR SURGERY
  IX. OROPHARYNGEAL SURGERY
   X. HYPOPHARYNGEAL SURGERY
  XI. SKULL BASE SURGERY
 XII. TRACHEOTOMY
       A. Airway Pressure Changes
       B. Expiratory Speaking Valves
       C. Laryngeal Elevation
       D. Glottic Closure
       E. Pharyngeal Transit
XIII. ZENKER DIVERTICULUM
XIV. SUMMARY
 XV. STUDY QUESTIONS
XVI. DISCUSSION QUESTIONS
XVII. REFERENCES

INTRODUCTION

Virtually all patients surgically treated for head, neck, or other disorders of the upper respiratory tract experience some difficulty in swallowing postoperatively. Dysphagia may be short term, requiring neither special tests nor the implementation of diet modifications, or long term due to severe nerve damage or tissue destruction, requiring the involvement of the entire dysphagia rehabilitation team.

ANTERIOR CERVICAL SPINAL SURGERY (ACSS)

Anterior cervical spinal surgery (ACSS) is a common surgical approach. Surgeons approach the spinal cord anteriorly, using a cervical incision to mobilize the laryngotracheal complex away from the great vessels of the neck to reach the prevertebral space to allow inspection and repair of the cervical spine.

Postoperative dysphagia is found in almost all patients who undergo ACSS. Although the dysphagia is of short duration in most patients, in 5% to 10% it can persist longer than 12 months. A report by Hart et al[1] found that dysphagia was the most frequent complication of surgical spine surgery, accounting for 46% of the complications. Most of the complications reported were minor; however, percutaneous endoscopic gastrostomy (PEG) feeding was required in 15% of the patients and long-term vocal fold paralysis requiring surgical correction was found in 7% of the patients.

There are several possible etiologies for dysphagia following ACSS in addition to vocal fold paralysis. The patient may have dysphagia preoperatively, which may worsen after the surgery. Thus, there is a need for assessment of the swallow function prior to ACSS. The patient may become more aware of symptoms postoperatively, leading to fear of swallowing. Neurological damage may result from direct trauma or retraction trauma to the recurrent laryngeal nerve, superior laryngeal nerve, or glossopharyngeal nerve.

> Another major complication is airway edema, reducing sensation and the ability to manage the bolus in the oral or oropharyngeal stage of swallowing.[2]

A list of common complications identified by Drennen et al[3] are summarized in Table 4–1. A host of surgical complications, side effects, and sequelae that may affect deglutition include edema, hematoma formation, infection, and denervation. The following are the most common:

1. Prevertebral soft tissue swelling and associated reduced epiglottis inversion may result in dysphagia following ACSS. Swelling of the posterior pharyngeal wall or a prevertebral **hematoma** may cause displacement of the pharyngeal wall toward the epiglottis, preventing it from inverting. This causes a transient obstruction that traps the bolus, resulting in residue at the valleculae and piriform sinuses.
2. Hypertonicity of the upper esophageal sphincter (UES), as diagnosed by manometry, results in dysphagia following ACSS. Hypertonicity of the UES may prevent passage of the bolus into the esophagus, resulting in pharyngeal residue. It may be caused by direct inflammation to the muscle caused by retraction or dissection or by parasympathetic (vagal) denervation. Hypertonicity of the UES may be secondary to gastro-

Table 4–1. *Complications of Anterior Cervical Approach*

Early dysphagia (≤1 month): 100%
Prolonged dysphagia (≥12 months): 5%–11%
Hematoma: 1%–3%
RLN injury: 1%–16%
SLN injury: 1%
Esophageal perforation: 0.2%–0.9%

RLN = recurrent laryngeal nerve; SLN = superior laryngeal nerve
Source: Adapted from Drennen K, Welch W, Carrau RL. Chapter 25. In: Carrau RL, Murry T, eds. *Comprehensive Management of Swallowing Disorders.* San Diego, CA: Singular Publishing; 1999:166, Table 25–1.

esophageal reflux disease (GERD); therefore, this should also be ruled out.

3. Esophageal perforation is a rare but serious cause of dysphagia following ACSS (approximately 1 in 500). A perforation often is not recognized until the patient develops an abscess or tracheoesophageal fistula in the immediate postoperative period.

4. Size and positioning of the bone graft and/or plate during ACSS must be optimal so there is not impingement on or compression of the posterior pharyngeal wall. Use of bone grafts or plates that produce a bulge of the posterior pharyngeal wall may lead to dysphagia.

5. Screw or plate displacement or extrusion following ACSS also may result in dysphagia. This may not be readily noticed if the screw loosens slowly. When dysphagia occurs some time after surgery, a loose or loosening screw must be considered. This is corrected by repeating the surgical procedure and removing or replacing the screw.

In some cases, dysphagia after ACSS can be addressed immediately and no long-term treatment is necessary. The assessment process ultimately may lead to long-term treatments, which are discussed in Chapter 6. Table 4–2 summarizes the initial assessment process from which treatment may be initiated.

A detailed analysis of complications and mortality associated with cervical spine surgery in the United States was reported by Wang et al in 2008.[4]

> Wang et al found that complications increased according to age of the patient, posterior fusion, surgery related to cervical spondylosis and other spine degenerative diseases, and combined anterior/posterior procedures.

Short-term effects were seen in almost all of the 932,000 patients whose hospital discharge records were reviewed. The highest morbidity and mortality were found following posterior procedures. Dysphagia was the most common short-term and long-term complication, regardless of the patient's age, type of surgery, or preoperative diagnosis.

Table 4–2. Etiological Factors for Postoperative Dysphagia After Anterior Cervical Spine Surgery

Pain	Muscles of Tongue, Pharynx/ Larynx (post-ET)
Edema	Tongue, pharynx, larynx, neck
Hematoma	Retropharyngeal space
Infection/abscess	Retropharyngeal space
Interruption of motor innervations	Ansa cervicalus
	RLN
	Pharyngeal plexus
Interruption of neuromuscular function	Anterior tongue
	Base of tongue
Injury to sensory innervations	SLN
	Pharyngeal plexus
Mechanical factors	Perforation
	Bulky reconstruction plate
	Adhesions—posterior pharyngeal wall
Velopharyngeal incompetence	Palatal shortening
	Wound breakdown

ET = endotracheal tube; RLN = recurrent laryngeal nerve; SLN = superior laryngeal nerve

Source: Adapted from Drennen K, Welch W, Carrau RL. Chapter 25. In: Carrau RL, Murry T, eds. *Comprehensive Management of Swallowing Disorders.* San Diego, CA: Singular Publishing; 1999:169, Table 25–2.

HEAD AND NECK SURGERY

Head and neck surgery for neoplasms of the upper aerodigestive tract alters the anatomy, causes scarring, and may injure motor and sensory nerves. All these factors contribute to the presence of dysphagia in the postoperative period. In addition, many of these patients require reconstruction with insensate tissue flaps that can contribute to the incoordination of the swallowing mechanism or even cause mechanical obstruction or diversion of the bolus into the airway. Head and neck surgery may result in dysphagia at any stage. In Chapters 6, 7, and 8 the various swallowing problems and treatment options will be outlined.

With regard to cancers in the oral cavity, Table 4–3 lists the causes of abnormal oral phase swallowing related specifically to surgical resection of the lip, floor of the mouth, palate, or mandible. It should be kept in mind that there is not a direct correlation between surgery in one area and a specific dysphagia problem as evidenced from the information seen in Table 4–3. However, identification of dysphagia after surgery must begin with the assessment of the site affected by surgery. It should be noted that two-thirds of patients with head and neck cancer have dysphagia at the time of their diagnosis. Table 4–4 summarizes the common dysphagias after oropharyngeal resection.

In 2009, a systematic review of the speech and swallowing problems following oral and oropharyngeal cancer was reported by Kreeft et al.[5]

They found that speech production in patients 1 year after treatment (surgery and/or radiation therapy) was reported to be moderately impaired to good.

Aspiration rated from liquids varied from 12% to 50%, and was higher after oropharyngeal resection. Postoperative radiotherapy was found to increase swallow function in the groups reviewed.

The hypopharynx is generally considered the inferior portion of the pharynx, between the epiglottis and the larynx. It corresponds to the height of the epiglottis. This area is critical to maintaining control of liquids during swallowing. Hypopharyngeal cancer usually requires extensive surgery plus radiation therapy. The resected tumor may require additional surgery to form a swallow tube. The radial forearm free flap (RFFF) is one of the optimal choices for hypopharyngeal reconstruction.[6] Table 4–5 presents the common problems after surgery in the hypopharynx. Reports indicate that if the flap survives, oral swallow may follow.

Table 4–3. Causes of Abnormal Oral Phase Swallowing After Head and Neck Surgery

Loss of oral sphincter
a. Resection of lip
b. Poor reapproximation of orbicularis oris
c. Marginal mandibular and lingual nerve section
Dental extractions
Floor of mouth resection
a. Loss of glossoalveolar sulcus
b. Tethering of anterior tongue
Tongue resection
a. Improper bolus preparation
Hard palate resection
a. Loss of oronasal separation
b. Nasal regurgitation
Mandibulectomy
a. Loss of dentition
b. Altered oral sphincter

Table 4–4. Dysphagia After Oropharyngeal Resection

Soft palate
a. Loss of glossoalveolar sulcus
b. Loss of oropharyngeal suction pump
c. Velopharyngeal insufficiency
Tonsil
a. Altered mobility of lateral pharyngeal wall
Tongue base
a. Loss of laryngeal protection
b. Loss of sensation
c. Loss of laryngeal elevation

Table 4–5. Dysphagia After Surgery of the Hypopharynx

Piriform Sinus
a. Scarring of lateral pharyngeal wall
b. Injury to superior laryngeal nerve and loss of sensation
Posterior Pharyngeal Wall
a. A dynamic insensate flap reconstruction
b. Scarring and aspiration

FLOOR OF THE MOUTH SURGERY

The floor of the mouth acts as a sulcus for saliva and food particles that aids in the preparation and direction of the bolus. When obliterated by surgery, the lack of this sulcus and the loss of mobility of the anterior tongue become a major impairment during the preparation of the food bolus. To preserve sensation in the tongue, all efforts should be made to protect the lingual nerve.

PARTIAL GLOSSECTOMY

Following partial glossectomy surgery, near-normal swallowing and normal speech can be predicted if the patient can protrude the tongue past the sublabial crease. Small defects of the mobile tongue are repaired primarily. Large defects, however, lead to the loss of tongue driving force and inability to propel the bolus posteriorly. The bolus is often improperly prepared and, due to the lack of proper control, may be presented to the oropharynx prematurely, or the patient may not be able to drive the bolus back effectively, requiring an extension of the head to move the bolus by gravity. Food and saliva will spill out of the oral cavity because of poor tongue mobility, a problem worsened if the oral sphincter (lips) has been altered or if the patient's lower lip has no feeling (anesthetic).

PALATE SURGERY

Tumors of the hard palate that require partial or total maxillectomy affect both speech and swallowing. Resection results in loss of oronasal separation, which will cause leakage of food into the nose (nasal regurgitation) and hypernasal speech. Unilateral maxillectomy is usually best reconstructed with a dental prosthesis. Free microvascular flaps can be used to reconstruct large palatal defects in edentulous patients in whom a prosthesis would not be retained. The reconstruction options, however, are limited and offer no sphincteric action. Defects in the soft palate are best managed by dental prostheses with extensions to close the nasopharyngeal isthmus.

LIP SURGERY

The orbicularisoris muscle is crucial to the sphincteric function of the lips. This muscle is divided during lip splitting procedures and must be carefully reapproximated during closure to restore function. The loss of lower lip sensation secondary to mental nerve injury makes sphincteric control difficult if not impossible. Lip resection may hinder swallowing by creating difficulty in getting food into the mouth (microstomia). Motor denervation of the lower lip secondary to sacrifice of the marginal mandibular nerve often manifests itself as loss of sphincteric control, resulting in drooling.

MANDIBULAR SURGERY

Mandibular defects of the midline arch cause problems with proper chewing, oral sphincter control, laryngeal suspension and elevation, and the driving force of the tongue.

OROPHARYNGEAL SURGERY

Resection of the lateral pharyngeal wall leads to decreased pharyngeal wall mobility, which alters oropharyngeal propulsion. The muscles of the base of the tongue assist in elevation of the larynx and are essential for the oropharyngeal propulsion pump and for adequate oral cavity–pharyngeal separation. Although resection is usually well tolerated, large defects often cause dysphagia. Reconstruction of up to one-third of the base of the tongue is best accomplished with a sensate flap. Resection of even limited portions of the soft palate produces **velopharyngeal insufficiency**, alters the propulsion of the bolus, and can lead to poor oral cavity–pharyngeal separation, with early spillage of the bolus and aspiration before the pharyngeal swallow is initiated.

HYPOPHARYNGEAL SURGERY

Resection of hypopharyngeal tumors arising on the posterior pharyngeal wall poses several problems for swallowing rehabilitation. Small defects (less than 2 cm) can be closed primarily or the edges can be stitched to the prevertebral fascia. Reconstruction with a split-thickness skin graft or radial forearm free flap provides a satisfactory closure of larger defects. However, neither technique restores the gliding action of the posterior wall on the vertebral fascia, because of scarring of the posterior hypopharyngeal wall to the prevertebral fascia. Impairment of pharyngeal contraction leads to significant retention at the hypopharynx, leading to postprandial aspiration.

> Reconstructive grafts and flaps are also almost always devoid of sensation, which further weakens laryngeal protection.

Reconstruction using a radial forearm free flap or a split-thickness skin graft frequently results in scarring that forms horizontal shelves along the posterior pharyngeal wall. These shelves divert the food bolus anteriorly, into the larynx, and may retain secretions and ingested food. When enough food or saliva accumulates, the material is dumped anteriorly into the introitus of the larynx. That may result in significant aspiration, especially if the patient lacks sensation due to injury or sacrifice of the sensory nerves during surgery. Commercial products may be used to thicken liquids and other thin foods so that the transit time is increased, possibly increasing the opportunity for laryngeal protection.

SKULL BASE SURGERY

Patients undergoing skull base surgery are at risk for injury to the lower cranial nerves, brain stem, brain parenchyma, and soft tissues of the upper aerodigestive tract, depending on the location and nature of the tumor. Injury to these vital structures can lead to dysfunction of speech, swallowing, and airway protection. In addition to these deficits, patients undergoing skull base surgery frequently need reconstruction with insensate soft tissue flaps, which may compound the motor and sensory deficits by the mechanical obstruction caused by their bulk. After skull base surgery, patients frequently need enteral tubes, prolonged intubation and ventilation, and tracheotomies that further compound the swallowing deficits. Lower cranial neuropathies are common sequelae and/or complications of skull base surgery or of the tumor itself.

> A high vagal injury leads to ipsilateral laryngeal anesthesia and vocal fold paralysis. In addition, it also produces paralysis of the ipsilateral soft palate, loss of vagus-mediated relaxation of the cricopharyngeus muscle, discoordination of the pharyngeal musculature, esophageal dysmotility, and gastroparesis.[7]

Therefore, a high vagal lesion, in addition to other cranial nerve or neurological deficits, produces marked postoperative deglutition and airway morbidity. This can be compounded by injury to other lower cranial nerves such as IX or XII. Table 4–6 summarizes the clinical manifestations of cranial nerve deficits following head and neck and/or skull base surgery.[7] Changes in the anatomical structures and the neurological complications will affect the treatment of dysphagia. These patients will benefit from surgical procedures that optimize the compensatory mechanisms of the remaining function (see Chapter 8).

TRACHEOTOMY

Between 43% to 83% of patients with tracheotomy tubes will manifest signs of aspiration or aspiration pneumonia. Dysphagia is produced by the physiological changes associated with opening the trachea to atmospheric pressure, not merely the presence of the tube in the neck. Table 4–7 summarizes the most common physiological changes following tracheostomy.

Table 4–6. Clinical Manifestations of Cranial Nerve Deficits

Dysfunctional Cranial Nerve	Clinical Manifestations
V	Impaired oral preparation and transport
VII	Drooling
	Impaired oral preparation
	Retention in gingivobuccal sulcus
IX & X	Delayed initiation of pharyngeal phase
	Nasal reflux
	Pharyngeal stasis and pooling
	Voice weakness or loss
	Aspiration
XII	Lack of awareness of food in mouth
	Impaired oral preparation
	Impaired oral transport

Source: Adapted from Fagan J. Chapter 30. In: Carrau RL, Murry T, eds. *Comprehensive Management of Swallowing Disorders.* San Diego, CA: Singular Publishing; 1999:212, Table 30–2.

Table 4–7. Physiological Changes Following Tracheotomy

Loss or change in airway resistance.
Inability to generate subglottic air pressure during the swallow.
Reduced ability to produce an effective cough.
Loss of sense of smell.
Loss of phonation.
Reduced mucosal sensitivity.
Reduced true vocal fold closure and coordination.
Disruption of the respiration/swallowing cycle.
Foreign body effect.
Reduced laryngeal elevation during deglutition.

Airway Pressure Changes

A major factor contributing to aspiration is that a tracheotomy results in a reduction of airway resistance. Expiratory resistance during respiration is provided by the vocal folds, with a constant resistance of about 8 to 10 cm H_2O/liter/min. This "valving" helps maintain lung inflation through physiological prolongation of the expiratory phase. Pressure measurements during swallowing in patients with an occluded tracheotomy are similar to those of normal individuals and are significantly diminished with an open tracheotomy. This pressure is present in the trachea following glottic closure during swallowing, and peaks at about 8 to 10 cm H_2O. Subglottic air pressure seems to be critical to swallow function. Its restoration reverses, at least in part, the disordered swallowing function that accompanies tracheotomy.

Expiratory Speaking Valves

Decannulation or tube occlusion will enhance swallowing function in a patient with a tracheotomy. However, this is not feasible in all patients. An alternative strategy is to place an expiratory speaking valve on the open tracheotomy tube, which restores subglottic air pressure during swallowing (Figure 4–1). The beneficial effect of a valve strengthens the fact that subglottic air pressure is a critical factor in swallowing efficiency, probably through restoring proprioceptive cues.

Laryngeal Elevation

The vertical motion of the larynx is dependent on the function of the suprahyoid musculature, and results in shortening of the pharynx and simultaneous active opening of the cricopharyngeal sphincter. Laryngeal elevation is reduced following tracheotomy, and probably plays a significant role in the dysphagia associated with the procedure.

Glottic Closure

Lung protection is provided by cessation of respiration and the maintenance of glottic closure. In the typical individual, swallowing is timed to occur during expiration. This relationship is lost in patients with severe respiratory disease and is probably also lost in the presence of a tracheotomy. Glottic closure

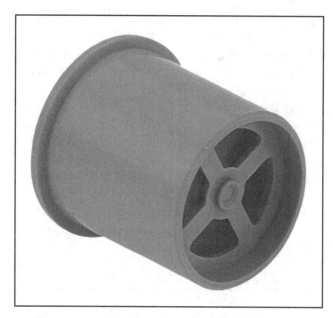

Figure 4–1. An expiratory speaking valve designed to fit over the open tracheostomy tube to restore subglottic air pressure during swallowing.

during swallowing is an extremely basic reflex mediated by the superior laryngeal nerve (uncrossed) and requiring from approximately 18 to 40 ms.[8] This rapid response demonstrates that the reflex arc is located in the lower brain stem and does not require input from higher centers. The laryngeal surface of the epiglottis and the other supraglottic structures are richly endowed with receptors, including water receptors.

> Interruption of this sensory input by superior laryngeal nerve or high vagal nerve interruption will limit reflex glottic closure and contribute to aspiration.[3]

Disruption of the integrity of the subglottic airway by the presence of a tracheotomy will also blunt or eliminate this reflex.

Pharyngeal Transit

Bolus transit from the tongue base to the esophagus typically requires less than a second in normal swal-lowing. Prolongation of bolus transit time, as well as disruption of the glottic closure, will result in food or liquid being in the pharynx while the glottis is open, thus placing the individual at risk for aspiration. It has been demonstrated that this transit time can be prolonged in the presence of a tracheotomy and that this effect is reversible. Restricted range of motion of pharyngeal structures due to the tethering of the larynx by the presence of a tracheotomy tube also affects transit time.

ZENKER DIVERTICULUM

Zenker diverticulum is a pulsion diverticulum that forms above the cricopharyngeal sphincter muscle through areas of lesser muscle strength, such as Killian triangle. The diverticulum (pouch) is created by failure of the upper esophageal sphincter to open before the propulsive wave, and by failure of active opening of the cricopharyngeal muscle due to weakness of the laryngeal elevators. As surgery is the only effective therapeutic option for Zenker diverticulum, the decision to operate is driven by the degree of the patient's symptoms. Typical symptoms are summarized in Table 4–8.[9] These include: regurgitation of partially digested food, which may lead to a foul smell and halitosis, dysphagia, coughing, and choking on swallowing; malnutrition and weight loss; obstruction; and recurrent aspiration pneumonia. Symptomatic patients who desire excision and can tolerate anesthesia are candidates for excision. The indications and contraindications are shown in Table 4–9. Surgical treatment options are many and include a range of options, from cricopharyngeal myotomy to myotomy and excision of the pouch (diverticulectomy). Small diverticula can be observed if symptoms are tolerated by the patient. Absolute contraindications to surgery include inability to tolerate anesthesia (a significant consideration in the elderly population in which Zenker diverticula are found) and carcinoma of the esophagus (which has rarely been reported within the actual diverticular pouch). The presence of untreated severe gastroesophageal reflux disease (GERD) is a relative contraindication.

Table 4–8. Symptoms of Zenker Diverticulum

Symptom	Patients (%)
Dysphagia	48 (100)
Aspiration	20 (42)
Postdeglutitive cough	17 (35)
Regurgitation	14 (29)
Noisy swallowing	13 (27)
Weight loss (> 10 lbs)	13 (27)
Recumbent cough	10 (21)
Sore throat	8 (17)
Unable to swallow	8 (17)
Halitosis	2 (4)

Source: Adapted from Schmidt PJ, Zuckerbraun L. Treatment of Zenker's diverticula by cricopharyngeal myotomy under local anesthesia. *Am Surg.* 1992;58:710–716.

Table 4–9. Zenker Diverticulum: Surgical Indications and Contraindications

Indications	Contraindications
Coughing and choking during swallowing	Inability to withstand general anesthesia
Recurrent aspiration pneumonia	Carcinoma of the esophagus
Regurgitation/halitosis	Untreated severe GERD (relative)
Inanition/weight loss	
Dysphagia	
Esophageal obstruction	

External approaches to Zenker diverticulum have been used with considerable success since the beginning of the 20th century. Cricopharyngeal **myotomy** is performed sometimes prior to the removal, pexy, or imbrication of the diverticulum.[9] Endoscopic approaches for the management of a Zenker diverticulum have been performed successfully for the last 40 years. During the endoscopic approach, the mucosa and muscle that make up the party wall between the diverticular pouch and the esophagus are divided with an electrocautery laser or an automatic stapler.[10] Prolonged follow-up of the patient is recommended, though no specific guidelines for reevaluation have been recommended. Yearly follow-up appears to be a logical interval.

SUMMARY

Surgery of the head and neck, skull base, and upper aerodigestive tract can have detrimental effects on the swallowing function. Removal or disruption of the soft tissues, including muscles and nerves, may lead to weakness, scarring, or incoordination of the swallowing apparatus. These problems are often predictable and their treatment should be included in the preoperative plan, as most patients will benefit from an early intervention.

STUDY QUESTIONS

1. Dysphagia after cervical spine surgery is:
   A. Common in the early postoperative period
   B. Often self-limited
   C. Often due to injury to the recurrent laryngeal nerve
   D. All of the above
   E. A and B

2. Dysphagia after cervical spine surgery is due to:
   A. Scarring of the retropharyngeal space
   B. Edema
   C. Disruption of the pharyngeal plexus
   D. Pain
   E. All of the above

3. After skull base surgery, patients may suffer aspiration due to:
   A. Injury to the vagus nerve
   B. Injury to the trigeminal nerve
   C. Deconditioning
   D. All of the above
   E. A and C

4. Patients with a Zenker diverticulum often present:
   A. Prandial aspiration
   B. Emotional lability
   C. Regurgitation
   D. Early onset of dysphagia to liquids
   E. All of the above

5. Dysphagia in patients with cancer of the upper aerodigestive tract is:
   A. Often present at the time of diagnosis
   B. Often intractable
   C. Corrected with the successful treatment of the cancer
   D. A and C
   E. All of the above

DISCUSSION QUESTIONS

1. Anterior cervical spine surgery may result in dysphagia in up to 15% of patients undergoing the surgery. Given the complications and the etiological factors that are shown in Tables 4–1 and 4–2, discuss the possible assessment and treatment modifications that must be considered when seeing these patients shortly after surgery.

2. Interactions between the speech-language pathologist and the head and neck surgeon have multiple benefits for the patient. At what times should the speech-language pathologist and the surgeon interact when a patient is scheduled for surgery in the oral cavity or pharynx? Why are these points in time important?

REFERENCES

1. Hart RA, Tatsumi RL, Hiratzka JR, Yoo JU. Perioperative complications of combined anterior and posterior cervical decompression and fusion crossing the cervicothoracic junction. *Spine.* 2008;33(26):2887–2891.
2. Emery S, Smith MD, Bohlman HE. Upper airway obstruction after multilevel cervical corpectomy for myelopathy. *Spine.* 1991;16:544–550.
3. Drennen K, Welch W, Carrau RL. Chapter 25. In: Carrau RL, Murry T, eds. *Comprehensive Management of Swallowing Disorders.* San Diego, CA: Singular Publishing; 1998: 165–174.
4. Wang MC, Chan L, Maiman DJ, Kreuter W, Deyo RA. Complications and mortality associated with cervical spine surgery for degenerative disease in the United States. *Spine.* 2007;32(3):342–347.
5. Kreeft AM, Van der Molen L, Hilgers FJ, Balm AJ. Speech and swallowing after surgical treatment of advanced oral and oropharyngeal carcinoma: a systematic review of the literature. *Eur Arch Otorhinolaryngol.* 2009;266:1687–1698.
6. Song M, Chen SW, Zhang Q, et al. External monitoring of buried radial forearm free flaps in hypopharyngeal reconstruction. *Acta Otolaryngol.* 2010 Oct 29. Epub ahead of print.
7. Fagan J. Neoplasia of the upper aerodigestive tract: primary tumors and secondary involvement. In: Carrau RL, Murry T, eds. *Comprehensive Management of Swallowing Disorders.* San Diego, CA: Singular Publishing; 1999: 211–215.
8. Sasaki CT, Hundal JS, Kim YH. Protective glottic closure: biomechanical effects of selective laryngeal denervation. *Ann Otol Rhinol Laryngol.* 2005;114(4):271–275.
9. Schmidt PPJ, Zuckerbraun L. Treatment of Zenker's diverticulum by cricopharyngeal myotomy under local anesthesia. *Ann Surg.* 1992;58:710–716.
10. Goldberg AN, Eibling DE. Pathophysiology of Zenker's diverticulum. In: Carrau. RL, Murry. T, eds. *Comprehensive Management of Swallowing Disorders.* San Diego, CA: Singular Publishing; 1999:195–198.

Evaluation of Dysphagia

CHAPTER OUTLINE

I. INTRODUCTION
II. DYSPHAGIA SCREENING
   A. Self-Assessments
   B. Screening Tests
III. CASE HISTORY AND BEDSIDE SWALLOW
   EVALUATION (BSE)
   A. Case History
   B. Bedside Swallow Evaluation
   C. The Oral, Pharyngeal, and Laryngeal Examination
   D. The Physical Examination
   E. Optimal Protocols
IV. INSTRUMENTAL TESTS OF SWALLOW FUNCTION
   A. Transnasal Flexible Laryngoscopy (TFL)
   B. Fiberoptic Endoscopic Evaluation of Swallowing
     (FEES)
   C. Flexible Endoscopic Evaluation of Swallowing with
     Sensory Testing (FEESST)
   D. Modified Barium Swallow (MBS)
   E. Instrumental Assessment and Predicting Aspiration
   F. Manometry and Videomanometry
   G. Ultrasound
   H. Magnetic Resonance Imaging (MRI)
   I. Positron Emission Tomography
   J. Other Instrumental Tests Associated With
     Swallowing Disorders
V. SUMMARY
VI. STUDY QUESTIONS
VII. DISCUSSION QUESTIONS
VIII. REFERENCES

INTRODUCTION

The evaluation of swallowing encompasses the case history, the clinical or bedside swallow examination, and the instrumental examination. Each aspect of the swallow evaluation is designed to address the issues of: (1) swallow safety, (2) nutritional status, (3) continuation or possible modification of present diet, (4) need for specialized treatments, and (5) referrals for additional tests based on the results of the specific swallow evaluation or the patient's general behavior.

New tools have been developed over the past 20 years to obtain information on swallowing from the patient's perspective. Data from the patient's perspective provide the clinician with a guide as to what the specific problems the patient is facing are and how severe they are. Moreover, when valid and reliable self-assessment tools are used prior to intervention and following intervention, an additional avenue of outcome data is available.

Patient self-assessment tools have also been proposed to quantify quality of life and specific aspects related to swallowing symptoms. In many assessment protocols, the case history and bedside swallow evaluation (BSE) are combined. In this chapter, the self-assessment tools are reviewed as part of dysphagia screening.

DYSPHAGIA SCREENING

Self-Assessments

The SWAL-QOL and SWAL-CARE

The SWAL-QOL and SWAL-CARE are two tools for assessing the swallowing quality of life and quality of care that are completed by the patient.[1,2,3] They can be used as outcome measures following treatment. The original assessment tool was exceptionally long (93 items), but it is now reduced to 44 items in the SWAL-QOL and 15 items in the SWAL-CARE. This is a pencil and paper tool that patients can respond to prior to treatment (SWAL-QOL) and after treatment (SWAL-CARE). The SWAL-QOL consists of 44 items

divided into 10 scales that assess quality of life concepts, and the SWAL-CARE consists of 15 items that assess quality of care and patient satisfaction. The scales differentiate individuals without swallowing problems from those with oropharyngeal swallowing disorders. In addition, the scales are sensitive to the severity of dysphagia in those with a swallowing disorder. Extensive work has been done to obtain validity and reliability for each of the scales. As with any self-assessment tool, its use is limited to those patients who are cognitively able to respond to the test items.

The SWAL-QOL and SWAL-CARE have been translated into French and validated with a group of 73 patients with post stroke or post surgery oropharyngeal dysphagia.[4] In addition, Bogaardt and colleagues[5] have recently produced a reliable and validated version of the SWAL-QOL in Dutch using 152 subjects from 7 different etiologies of swallowing disorders.

> Studies using the SWAL-QOL and SWAL-CARE have shown its value as an outcome measure following treatment.

McHorney et al[6] examined the results of videofluoroscopic studies of 386 subjects with oropharyngeal dysphagia. They used the SWAL-QOL and SWAL-CARE questionnaires as outcome measures and related them to the fluoroscopic findings. They found that the SWAL-QOL and SWAL-CARE scales were most related to measures of oral transit duration and total swallow duration. The scales were least related to pharyngeal transit duration. Their results were stronger for semisolid than for liquid trials. In general, the greater the bolus flow severity, the worse the quality of life according to the self-assessment. They concluded that observed modest correlations suggest that patient-centered quality of life measures such as the SWAL-QOL and clinician-driven bolus flow measures obtained from the videofluoroscopic examinations provide distinct yet complementary information and should both be a part of assessment of dysphagia assessment and outcomes.

Other researchers have shown the value and reliability of the SWAL-QOL in assessing outcomes in tongue cancer[7] and in a pre-/posttreatment study of lingual exercises in patients with dysphagia following stroke.[8] The SWAL-QOL and SWAL-CARE require approximately 20 minutes to complete. The scoring of the SWAL-QOL and SWAL-CARE take additional clinical time. Thus, in a busy clinical setting, these tools may be underutilized.

The MD Anderson Dysphagia Inventory

The MD Anderson Dysphagia Inventory (MDADI) is a self-assessment tool developed specifically to evaluate the impact of dysphagia on the quality of life of patients with head and neck cancer.[9] The MDADI is a multiple-scale assessment of patients' responses to questions involving their swallowing quality of life following treatment for head and neck cancer.

> The MDADI consists of four subscales that have an impact on quality of life: (a) a global measure of the individual's overall daily routine; and (b) emotional, (c) functional, and (d) physical statements related to swallowing and head and neck cancer.

Gillespie et al[10] demonstrated its usefulness in comparing a surgical treatment group with a chemoradiation treatment group of patients with head and neck cancer. Patients who received chemoradiation for various oropharyngeal cancers demonstrated better emotional and functional subscale scores than patients who received surgery/radiation. The MDADI has also been translated and validated in Italian.[11]

The EAT-10

The EAT-10 is a 10-item outcome measure of symptom severity, quality of life, and treatment efficacy.[12] The EAT-10 was validated on 7 groups of patients in various diagnostic categories. The instrument has excellent internal consistency, test-retest reproducibility, and criterion-based validity. The assessment tool uses a 5-point interval scale. The authors suggest that the EAT-10 is not limited to one type of dsyphagia or to one diagnostic group. The EAT-10 is shown in Appendix I.

The Reflux Symptom Index (RSI) and Reflux Finding Score (RFS)

The **Reflux Symptom Index (RSI)** is a 10-statement patient self-assessment measure that quantifies a patient's perception of his/her reflux symptoms.[13] The RSI has been validated using 24-hour pH metry and has been found to be a valid index of reflux severity. Gastroesophageal reflux disease (GERD) or laryngopharyngeal reflux disease (LPRD) is often associated with dysphagia and, when treated maximally, the improvement of GERD and/or LPRD is usually related to an improvement in swallow function.

The RSI has been studied in relation to the reflux finding score (RFS), a clinician-based assessment tool used to score the severity of reflux symptoms as seen on laryngeal endoscopy. The RSI and RFS are shown in Appendices II and III.

Other Self-Assessments of Dysphagia

Other self-assessment tests have been reported.[14,15] Future studies are needed to identify the strength of these tests and their relationship to physical findings. Also, the use of all of the above tests is restricted to patients who have the cognitive abilities to respond reliably to the statements in the assessments. Thus, the clinician must be aware of when to use these assessments and how to interpret the results in lieu of the patient's condition. Although self-assessment tools may provide a way of assessing current status or severity from the patient's perspective as well as for outcomes following intervention, the clinician must be aware of their limitations in neurologically disadvantaged patients, as well as in patients who demonstrate the need to want to swallow despite obvious safety concerns.

Screening Tests

Burke Dysphagia Screening Test (BDST)

Prior to a formal bedside swallowing evaluation (BSE), and in some settings in place of the complete BSE, the use of a dysphagia screening test may be appropriate. This is usually done by a speech-language pathologist (SLP), but may also be done be a nurse trained in the procedure. The **Burke Dysphagia Screening Test (BDST)** reported by DePippo et al[16] is a quick screening test that consists of 7 items shown in Table 5–1. If the patient has a positive response to one or more of the items in the test, he/she is considered to have failed and referral for a complete BSE is made.

The Dye Test

The **dye test,** also known as the **Evans Blue Dye Test,** may be used to determine the presence of aspiration in a tracheotomized patient. A few drops of methylene blue or vegetable coloring are placed in the mouth, the tracheotomy cuff is deflated, and the tracheotomy tube is deep suctioned for secretions that may have been resting on or above the level of the cuff. The patient's tracheotomy tube is then deep suctioned again, this time looking for evidence of dyed material in the airway.

> In two studies using the dye test with tracheotomized and nontracheotimized patients, the results suggest that the blue dye test is highly sensitive in detecting aspiration in tracheotomized patients.

It is less sensitive in patients without a tracheotomy.[17,18] The dye test, however, may not detect trace amounts of aspirated materials. Alternatively, a Dextrostix test may be used to detect the presence of glucose (ie, food) in the tracheal secretions.[19]

Chest Auscultation

Auscultation of the chest and cervical airway is done by placing a stethoscope over various parts of the airway. Placing the stethoscope gently on the lateral aspect of the larynx and listening to the airflow during normal breathing, swallowing, and speech provides the listener with indirect evidence of penetration and/or aspiration. Other tests such as the Toronto Bedside Swallowing Screening Test (TOR-BSST) have been shown to have high validity for specific groups of patients.[20]

Limitations of Screening Tests for Dysphagia

Observations of patients swallowing water or coughing after swallowing various amounts of water may grossly identify dysphagia. However, accurate detection of the presence or absence of penetration and/or aspiration is difficult with patients who are

Table 5–1. The Burke Dysphagia Screening Test

Patient Name:	
ID Number:	
Date of Evaluation:	
1. Bilateral stroke	_____
2. Brainstem stroke	_____
3. History of pneumonia following acute stroke phase	_____
4. Coughing associated with feeding or during a 3 oz. water swallow test	_____
5. Failure to consume one-half of meals	_____
6. Prolonged time required for feeding	_____
7. Non-oral feeding program in progress	_____
Presence of one or more of these features is scored as failing the Burke Dysphagia Screening Test.	
Results: **Pass** **Fail** Signature _____	

Source: Reprinted from DePippo KL, Holas MA, Reding MJ. The Burke dysphagia screening test: Validation of its use in patients with stroke. *Arch Phys Med Rehab.* 1994;75:1284–1286.

severely ill, who have had a stroke and cannot follow exact directions, or who have lost sensitivity in part of the swallowing organs and aspirate without any observable evidence.

CASE HISTORY AND BEDSIDE SWALLOW EVALUATION (BSE)

Case History

Table 5–2 summarizes the critical components of the case history. Prior to any assessment of the patient, the clinician should identify the **chief complaint** or define the **current status** of the patient. The detailed history should account for the current physical status, any recent surgeries, or conditions from previous surgeries that may contribute to the dysphagia. The onset of the dysphagia should be documented and related to events such as surgery, neurological changes, medicines, or trauma (physical or emotional). Based on the patient's input, family input, and medical records, the severity of the problem should be assessed prior to swallowing liquids or foods. Time since oral food intake, anatomical changes to the swallowing mechanism, neurological status, and degree of alertness help to make those determinations.

Clinical findings noted in the medical records should be considered. Common clinical findings that are associated with dysphagia and/or aspiration are shown in Table 5–3. It should be pointed out that even when the majority of these symptoms are absent, swallow safety may still be an important issue.[21] Table 5–3 emphasizes that **observing** the patient, **reviewing** the case history, and **acquiring** information from caregivers are important aspects of the BSE.

Table 5–2. *Critical Components of the Clinical Case History*

- Identify the chief complaint or define the current status
- Type of dysphagia — liquids, foods, pills
- Onset, progression
- Recent pneumonia and probable cause(s)
- Recent hospitalizations — reasons
- Associated symptoms — voice changes, weakness
- Present and past — illnesses, surgery, trauma
- Medications
- Trauma
- Social history/habits
- Family history
- Review of systems — pulmonary, cardiac, digestive, etc

Source: Adapted and revised from Carrau RL. Chapter 4. Carrau RL, Murry T, eds. *Comprehensive Management of Swallowing Disorders.* San Diego, CA: Singular Publishing; 1999:34, Table 4–2.

Table 5–3. *Common Clinical Findings in Dysphagic Patients*

- Coughing/Choking — swallowing food, liquid, or own saliva
- Frequent throat clearing — with or without a productive cough
- Multiple swallow pattern
- Wet vocal quality
- Edentulous
- Drooling
- Increased oral or pharyngeal secretions
- Cyanosis
- Shortness of breath
- Weight loss
- Bronchorrhea
- Increased time to consume meal
- Spiking
- Pulmonary infiltrate
- Resistance to eating or drinking
- Food sticking in mouth
- Changes in taste
- Difficulty in managing foods of specific textures or sensation
- Aberrant behavioral patterns when food is presented

Source: Adapted from Simonian MA, Goldberg AN. Chapter 52. Carrau RL, Murry T, eds. *Comprehensive Management of Swallowing Disorders.* San Diego, CA: Singular Publishing; 1999:368, Table 52–2.

The clinician should be prepared to answer the following questions as a result of conducting a thorough case history and bedside swallow evaluation:

1. Is the patient currently eating by mouth or is he/she relying on nonoral feeding?
2. Is there a history of aspiration pneumonia?
3. Is there a risk of aspiration given the present nutritional status and diet?
4. What is the anatomical and functional status of the oral mechanism?
5. Is the patient thriving or maintaining his general health and nutrition status based on the current diet and method of eating?
6. Should the patient be referred for further evaluation of his/her swallowing based on the information gleaned at the BSE?
7. Is the patient cognitively capable of participating in instrumental testing and rehabilitation?
8. What changes in the treatment plan should be anticipated or planned given the outcome of the BSE?

Bedside Swallow Evaluation

The clinical **bedside swallow evaluation (BSE)** provides a roadmap for the diagnosis and treatment of swallowing disorders. Nonetheless, the clinician must understand that the BSE has significant limitations, because it does not include an examination of the pharynx and larynx nor does it accurately determine if the patient is aspirating silently. Moreover, depending on the status of the patient (eg, severe impairment from stroke or extensive trauma), a complete BSE is sometimes not possible.

Detecting the presence of penetration and aspiration is an important part of the BSE because the potential consequences of health status and recovery are dependent on nutrition and safe swallowing. Several investigators have examined the sensitivity and specificity of the BSE for predicting aspiration. McCullough, Wertz, and Rosenbek[21] examined 60 stroke patients and found that the BSE was not highly predictive of patients who subsequently aspirated during the modified barium swallow instrumental examination. Ramsey and colleagues[22] found that the BSE had highly variable specificity

and sensitivity and also concluded that the BSE was poor at detecting silent aspiration. Peruzzi and colleagues[23] compared the use of a colored bedside dye test to the videofluoroscopic studies of swallowing and found that in 20 consecutive patients with tracheotomy, the videofluoroscopic exam was significantly better at detecting aspiration than the colored bedside dye test.

Although the majority of BSE reports focus on stroke patients, there are reports that relate findings from the clinical bedside assessment of swallowing to other patient groups. In general, these findings suggest that for surgical patients, the larger the surgical excision, the more likely the patient will exhibit a longer course of dysphagia. Patients in these categories will require more extensive evaluation and treatments.

Bedside Swallow Examination with Pulse Oximetry

A relatively new approach to monitoring swallowing and possibly increasing the sensitivity of the bedside swallow evaluation for detecting aspiration is **pulse oximetry**. Pulse oximetry is suggested by some as a well-tolerated and inexpensive option to endoscopy and videofluoroscopy.[24,25] Pulse oximetry to identify aspiration is based on the principle that reduced and oxygenated hemoglobin exhibit different absorption characteristics to red and infrared light emitted from a finger or ear probe. Pulse oximetry is noninvasive, simple, and may be repeated often. It easily measures oxygen desaturation of arterial blood, a condition that is thought to occur as a result of aspiration. Thus, although this test does not provide diagnostic information to formulate treatment plans, its use as a part of the BSE may offer diagnostic information regarding the presence and possibly the severity of aspiration. It is suggested for use with patients who cannot easily be transferred, in patients whose cognition is suspect and cannot tolerate instrumental testing, or those who are in nursing homes where radiological or endoscopic instrumental examinations are not available. Pulse oximetry added to the BSE offers an alternative to a group of patients who might otherwise only receive a bedside swallow assessment and no further diagnostic test.

Lim et al[26] found that by combining the BSE with the measurement of oxygen desaturation before and after drinking 50 ml of water, a test they called the bedside aspiration test, sensitivity rose to 100% and specificity was almost 71%. They concluded that the bedside aspiration test was a suitable screening test to identify acute stroke patients at risk for aspiration and in need of further evaluation and management. These results were similar to those of Smith et al,[25] who studied 53 acute stroke patients at bedside using pulse oximetry. They found that by comparing bedside screening using desaturation assessments with modified barium swallow assessments, they detected 86% of aspirators or penetrators who required follow-up testing and management.

Despite the limitations of the BSE, for patients who are unable to be tested more thoroughly or when instrumental facilities are not available, a limited BSE may be the only basis for the decision to begin or suspend oral feeding or to recommend a nasogastric (NG) or **percutaneous endoscopic gastrostomy (PEG)** feeding tube. Adding pulse oximetry to the bedside protocol appears to increase an examiner's ability to detect penetration and or aspiration. This procedure requires the examiner's knowledge of how to administer and report the results of pulse oximetry and the cooperation of the patient. Thus, the BSE, with its case history component and the addition of pulse oximetry, should be considered an important first step in the diagnostic process despite its caveats.

Trial Swallows

The final portion of the BSE consists of trial swallows of water. This can be combined with measurement of oxygen saturation, as reviewed above. The clinician should be consistent in the amount of water to be swallowed. The majority of reports suggest that beginning with a 5-ml bolus is appropriate.[27] Depending on the results, one can advance to 10- and 20-ml boluses. Laryngeal elevation, identified by palpation of the thyroid prominence, should be monitored for each swallow. After each swallow, the patient is asked to sustain the /a/ vowel for a few seconds or count from 1 to 5 to determine if there is wet hoarseness or other drainage in voice quality. Daniels and her associates[28] suggest that wet hoarse-

ness and a weak cough are two signs of increased risk for aspiration.

Mann Assessment of Swallowing Ability

A noninvasive assessment protocol for quantifying the severity of swallowing impairment was developed by Mann.[29] This protocol, called the Mann Assessment of Swallowing Ability (MASA), is a comprehensive clinical examination of oropharyngeal dysphagia consisting of 24 items. The MASA is one clinical measure of dysphagia that has demonstrated strong reliability and has been validated against videofluoroscopic and videoendoscopic swallowing examinations in several populations. It provides a numerical score reflecting the severity of dysphagia symptoms, and is sensitive to change in patient performance over time.

> The MASA exam has been extensively evaluated for use as a bedside swallowing assessment for stroke patients. The MASA demonstrates strong psychometric properties compared to radiographic swallowing studies and it provides good interobserver reliability for assessing dysphagia and aspiration.

The 24 items in the MASA combine to provide a total score and cutoff criteria for dysphagia and aspiration severity. It is considered simple to use and score.

The MASA has been followed with the Modified Mann Assessment of Swallowing Ability (MMASA), a 12-item assessment tool for use by physicians, nurses, and SLPs.[30] The MMASA is a quick but reliable screening tool for use in acute patients to accurately identify patients with stroke who need intervention for safety reasons.

Silent Aspiration and the Bedside Swallow Evaluation

The clinician must always be aware of the possibility of silent aspiration.

> Silent aspiration is the penetration of food, liquid, or saliva to the subglottic area without the elicitation of a cough.

It has been estimated that silent aspiration may be as high as 40% in patients with dysphagia, and it is not generally identifiable during the BSE. However, a history of pneumonia, a weak or absent cough, changes in body temperature after eating, and a voice that has a "wet hoarse" quality suggest the possibility of silent aspiration. Additionally, the use of sensory testing (described below) provides an objective test of sensory awareness that may be the best indicator that the patient is a silent aspirator.[31,32]

The Oral, Pharyngeal, and Laryngeal Examination

A thorough examination of the oral, laryngeal, and pharyngeal structures should include an assessment of lip closure, tongue strength and mobility, facial symmetry, and voice and volitional cough strength. Table 5–4, modified from Daniels, McAdam, Brailey and Foundas,[28] provides a comprehensive orderly approach to the oropharyngeal examination. Clinicians, even those with extensive experience in oral examination, may profit from this structure, as it provides an orderly approach to assessing muscular function related to the cranial nerves most important for swallowing.

Prior to the oropharyngeal examination, the clinician should have a general knowledge of the patient's characteristics that may interfere with parts of the examination. These include:

A. Airway
B. Cognition/alertness/endurance
C. Ability to follow instructions
D. Body tone/size/posture/positioning
E. Self-feeding potential

Oral Examination

The oral examination should include assessment of the range of motion, strength, and sensory function of all oral structures. Prominent atrophy and **fasciculation** of the tongue should raise the possibility of **amyotrophic lateral sclerosis (ALS)**.

1. *Reflexes and responses*
   - The **gag reflex** includes a head and jaw extension, rhythmical tongue protrusions, and pharyngeal contractions in response to stimulation at the posterior part of the oral cavity. Recent literature suggests that the gag reflex may not be important for normal swallowing to occur.
   - The **bite reflex** is clamping of the teeth or up and down movement of the jaw in response to stimulation of the gum, molar, or other dental surfaces.
   - The **transverse tongue response** is a lateral movement in response to tactile stimulation at the lateral border.
2. *Sensation.* Assess by light touch of lips and tongue.
3. *Structural anatomy.* Look for abnormalities of lips and oral cavity.
4. *Movement*
   - Jaw—ability to open and close the jaw.
   - Lips—labial closure and compression at rest and during swallowing.
   - Tongue—anterior lingual movement may be assessed by having the patient extend, lateralize, elevate, and depress the tip and by having the patient sweep the tongue from front to back along the roof of the mouth.
   - Velum—movement of the velum, or soft palate, may be assessed by having the patient open the mouth, and then observing palatal movement during production of a sustained /a/ sound.
5. *Secretions.* Note location and amount.
6. *Articulation.* Screen with sentences or words containing tongue tip and posterior tongue consonants (p,t,b,d,th,k,g).
7. *Resonance.* Note presence of hypernasal quality.

Pharyngeal and Laryngeal Examinations

1. Vocal quality/changes—listen to patient talking before and after swallowing. Note the difference, if any.
2. Pitch control/range—is the pitch of the voice appropriate and does the patient have variation in his pitch range? A voice without pitch changes may be indicative of a sensory paralysis.
3. Breathing—is the patient experiencing labored breathing or is there an audible noise associated with inhalation or exhalation?
4. Volitional cough/throat clear—can the patient produce a normal cough and clearing of the

Table 5–4. *The Oropharyngeal Examination for the Bedside Swallow Examination*

Name _____ Date _____

Diagnosis _____

Mandible (CN V)

Symmetry on Extension _____ Strength _____

Lips (CN VII)

Symmetry: Rest _____ Retraction _____ Protrusion _____

Strength _____

Nonspeech Coordination: Repetitive Movement _____ Alternating Movement _____

Speech Coordination: Repetitive (/p,w/) _____ Alternating (/p-w/) _____

Tongue (CN XII)

Symmetry: Rest _____ Protrusion _____ Lateralization _____

Elevation **Yes/No** Lateralization **Yes/No** Fasciculations **Yes/No**

Strength _____

Nonspeech Coordination: Repetitive Movement _____ Alternating Movement _____

Speech Coordination: Repetitive (/t,k/) _____ Alternating (/t-k/) _____

Alternating Movement (/p^t^k^/) _____

Multisyllabic Word Repetition (tip top, baseball player, several, caterpillar, emphasize) _____

Conversation: (speech, voice, coordination characteristics) _____

Laryngeal Function: Isolated Movement (/i-i-i/ on one breath) _____

Alternating Movement (/u-i/) _____

Buccofacial Apraxia: "Blow out the candle" _____ "Lick an ice cream cone" _____

"Lick milk off your top lip" _____ "Sip through a straw" _____ "Kiss a baby" _____

Velum (CN IX, X, XI)

Symmetry: Rest _____ Elevation _____

Coordination: Repetitive Movement (/a/) _____

Appearance of Hard Palate _____

Dentition _____

Reflexes (CN IX, X, XI)

Gag (Abnormal: **Yes/No**) _____

Swallow (Cough: **Yes/No**) _____

Voice Change (**Yes/No**) _____

Additional information

c/o Facial Numbness or Tingling: **Yes/No** Light Touch _____

Dysphonia: **Yes/No** (mild, moderate, severe) _____

Dysarthria: **Yes/No** (mild, moderate, severe) _____

Breath Support _____

Resonance _____

Volitional Cough (Abnormal: **Yes/No**) _____

Clinician _____ Date _____

Source: Adapted with permission from: Daniels SK, McAdam CP, Brailey K, Foundas AL. Clinical assessment of swallowing and prediction of dysphagia severity. *Am J Speech Lang Path.* 1997;6(4):17–24.

throat? Lack of this ability may suggest poor vocal fold closure.

5. Saliva swallow: laryngeal management—does the patient continue to feel saliva or mucous in the throat, sometimes a sign of reflux or a more serious problem called Zenker diverticulum?

6. Laryngeal elevation—by placing your finger on the thyroid cartilage, feel the larynx elevate when the patient is asked to swallow. Lack of laryngeal elevation usually suggests a nerve injury at the laryngeal level.

The Physical Examination

The physical examination should include a basic head and neck and neurological examination, with assessment of gait, balance, sensory and motor function of the extremities, deep tendon reflexes, and full assessment of the cranial nerves, as outlined in Table 5–5. This may be done by an SLP, neurologist, or otolaryngologist, or these professionals may do it as a team. For those patients with a weak or breathy voice, a consultation with an otolaryngologist is recommended. The otolaryngologist may perform an examination of the larynx and vocal folds using a **flexible endoscope**.

Optimal Protocols

Other options for measuring swallowing function in place of the BSE have been proposed by DePippo et al.[33] They found that cough or voice change during or directly after drinking 3 oz of water was a sensitive and valid screening tool for aspiration following a stroke. It should be remembered that the clinical swallow assessment with water should be tried only after the findings from the patient history and oropharyngeal examination are taken into account. Patients unable to tolerate their secretions, patients who have a limited attention span such as those shortly after a severe stroke, or patients who resist for some other reason may not be candidates for the clinical water swallow test.

Once the clinical evaluation is completed, the clinician will be able to establish a reasonable differential diagnosis and determine which other tests are needed (Table 5–6).

Table 5–5. Bedside Clinical Evaluation: Physical Examination

Oral
Oral continence
Lip pursing
"Trumpeter" maneuvers
Drooling
Tongue range of motion
Extends beyond lower lip
Approximates to gingivobuccal area
Can push against tongue blade
Tongue sensation
Oropharynx
Motion of soft palate
Sensation
Tongue blade/swab
Cold laryngeal mirror
Gag reflex
Swallow reflex
Flexible Laryngoscopy
Anatomy of base of tongue, vallecula, hypopharynx, endolarynx
Pooling of secretions
Penetration/aspiration of secretions
Motion (symmetry, range) of base of tongue, arytenoid, epiglottis, false vocal folds, true vocal folds (fixation vs paralysis)
Velopharyngeal closure
Lateral walls
Passavant ridge
Velum
Neck
Laryngeal elevation
Adenopathy
Thyroid
Other masses
Neurological
Cranial nerves
Gait/balance
Motor function/fine skills
Deep tendon reflexes

Source: Adapted from Carrau RL. Chapter 4. Carrau RL, Murry T, eds. *Comprehensive Management of Swallowing Disorders.* San Diego, CA: Singular Publishing; 1999:35, Table 4–3.

Table 5–6. *Differential Diagnosis*

Type	Possible Etiology
Congenital	Dysphagia lusoria
	Tracheoesophageal fistula
	Laryngeal clefts
	Other foregut abnormalities
Inflammatory	GERD
Infections	Lyme disease
	Neuropathies/encephalitis
	Chagas disease
Trauma	CNS—Multiple
	Upper aerodigestive tract
	Surgical injury
Endocrine	Goiter
	Hypothyroid
	Diabetic neuropathy
Neoplasia	Upper aerodigestive tract
	Thyroid
	Central nervous system
Systemic	Autoimmune: Dermatomyositis
	Scleroderma
	Sjogren
	Amyloidosis
	Sarcoidosis
Iatrogenic	Surgery
	Chemotherapy
	Other medications
	Radiation

Source: Adapted from Carrau RL. Chapter 4. Carrau RL, Murry T, eds. *Comprehensive Management of Swallowing Disorders.* San Diego, CA: Singular Publishing Group; 1999:33, Table 4–1.

INSTRUMENTAL TESTS OF SWALLOW FUNCTION

Screening assessments of dysphagia, case histories, and clinical bedside assessments of swallowing are important steps in learning about the patient, his/her concerns regarding swallowing, his/her ability to follow instructions, and his/her ability to cooperate in more detailed examinations of the swallowing mechanisms. However, none of the procedures in these preliminary screening or bedside assessment measures offer direct information about the safety of swallowing—namely, if the patient aspirated on the bolus. For that reason, it is often necessary to do an instrumental test of swallowing to verify the impressions of the bedside assessment and to offer direct guidance regarding the safety of oral nutrition. Table 5–7 summarizes the more commonly used tests used to study dysphagia along with their application and utility.

Transnasal Flexible Laryngoscopy (TFL)

The standard method for examining the larynx and vocal folds is with a transnasal flexible laryngoscope. During the flexible laryngoscopy, the anatomy of the pharynx and larynx should be observed during quiet and forced respiration, coughing, speaking, and swallowing. Attention is also given to the motion of the base of the tongue, pharyngeal walls, arytenoids, and other endolaryngeal structures. Symmetry, coordination, and range of movement between the two sides of the upper aerodigestive tract are also noted. Pooling of secretions or food residue in the vallecula or piriform sinuses is noted. The laryngeal closure reflex can be tested by gentle touch of the epiglottis or aryepiglottic folds with the tip of the endoscope. This maneuver requires some experience and should be as gentle as possible to avoid eliciting a **gag reflex** or **laryngospasm**. With the advent of air pulse sensory testing (described below), touching the epiglottis or the aryepiglottic folds is no longer recommended. A more detailed assessment of sensation is presented later in this chapter. The neck is examined for swelling or masses. Observation of the thyroid movement and prominence upon swallowing reflects laryngeal evaluation.

Fiberoptic Endoscopic Evaluation of Swallowing (FEES)

The **fiberoptic endoscopic evaluation of swallowing (FEES)** assessment was first described by Langmore and colleagues.[34] FEES is an assessment that uses a transnasal flexible laryngoscope to evaluate the swallow before and after the pharyngeal swallow (Figure 5–1). The assessment of swallowing using this tech-

Table 5–7. *Functional Evaluation of Swallowing: Tests Most Commonly Used and Their Usefulness for Identifying Various Aspects of Swallowing Disorders*

	Defines Anatomy	Detects Aspiration	Quantifies Aspiration	Detects Etiology	Availability	Cost[a]
BSE	—	+/–	—	+/–	++	1
FEES	++	+	—	+	++	2
FEESST[b]	++	++	—	++	+/–	3
MBS	+	++	+	+	+	4
Ultrasound	+/–	—	—	—	+/–	5
Manometry	—	+/–	—	+	+	6
Scintigraphy[c]	—	++	++	—	+/–	7

+ = Useful for evaluating; ++ = Highly desirable to make diagnosis

[a]Order from least to most expensive

[b]Can detect actual aspiration in patients with tracheotomies

[c]Quantifies reflux

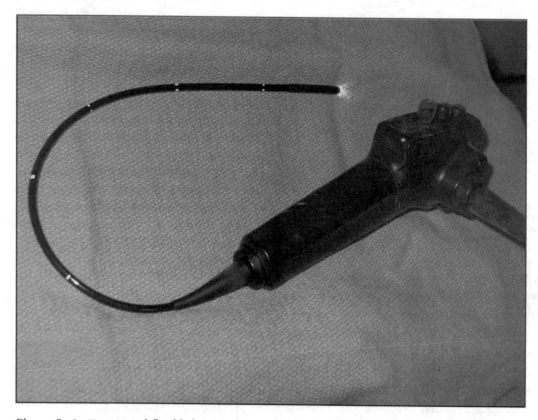

Figure 5–1. *Transnasal flexible laryngoscope used for FEES and FEESST examinations.*

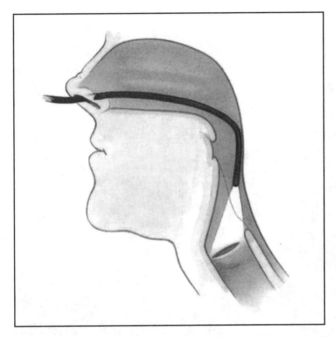

Figure 5–2. Drawing from lateral view showing proper placement of scope prior to feeding the patient. Note the scope is above the epiglottis.

nique requires the passage of a flexible laryngoscope into the nares, over the velum, and to a position above the epiglottis (Figure 5–2). Specific amounts of liquids and food consistencies treated with food dye are viewed as they pass the pharynx and larynx. The speed of the pharyngeal swallow, premature flow of food or liquid into the pharyngeal and laryngeal areas, and residual amounts of the bolus can all be seen during this examination. The endoscope may remain in place for long periods to monitor the residual bolus and examine anatomical structures. Swallowing, using compensatory strategies and changes in neck position, is easily accomplished while the endoscope is in place. With the addition of newer video chip endoscopes, the term "fiberoptic" is rarely used and this test is now referred to as a flexible endoscopic test of swallowing in current literature.

Flexible Endoscopic Evaluation of Swallowing with Sensory Testing (FEESST)

As noted above, the use of flexible endoscopy for swallowing assessment was first described in 1988 by Langmore and colleagues.[34] The FEES examination, however, lacked the ability to assess sensation in an objective manner. **Flexible endoscopic evaluation of swallowing with sensory testing (FEESST)**, a sensory and motor test of swallowing developed by Aviv[35] to quantify the sensory and motor deficiencies in dysphagia.

> **FEESST** is the only test of a swallow that examines airway protection and bolus transport.

Airway protection is determined by administering a pressure- and duration-controlled calibrated pulse of air to the hypopharyngeal tissues innervated by the internal branch of the superior laryngeal nerve (SLN) in order to elicit the **laryngeal adductor reflex (LAR)**, a fundamental brain stem–mediated airway protective reflex.[35] Figure 5–3 shows the examination procedure with a trained SLP conducting the examination.

Because swallowing is a complex process that involves interplay between two distinct but related phenomena, airway protection and bolus transport, a test that assesses both sensory and motor components of swallowing is highly advantageous, as opposed to a test that measures the motor component only. Almost all tests of swallowing—**videofluoroscopy** or modified barium swallow (MBS), barium swallow or **esophogram**, fiberoptic endoscopic examination of swallowing (FEES)—specifically look at bolus transport and ignore or infer airway protective capacity. Early research on transnasal flexible endoscopy for swallowing suggested the importance of sensitivity testing of the larynx during an endoscopic swallowing evaluation. What these early studies described was touching or tapping the laryngopharyngeal tissues with the tip of the endoscope and assessing the patient's reaction to such stimulation.[36] Touching or tapping tissues with an endoscope tip is an extremely subjective way to assess sensory capacity. Movement of the endoscope itself may cause a reaction prior to tapping the tissues. Furthermore, it is difficult to translate the reaction to a tissue tap from patient to patient or from the same patient one day to the next.

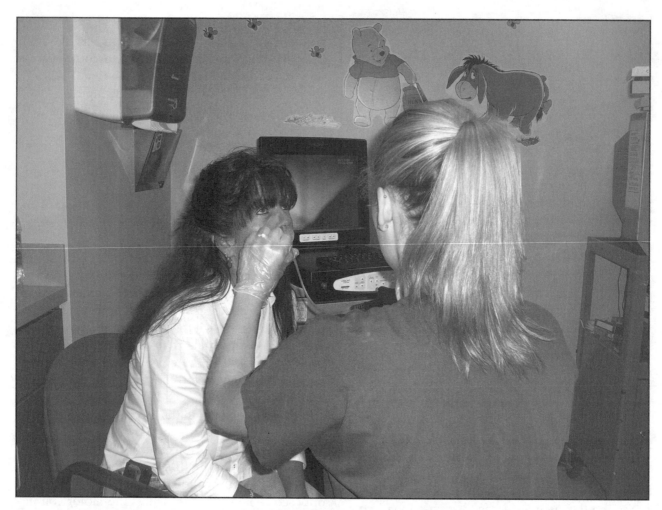

Figure 5–3. Student conducting FEESST exam on patient.

It has been shown that the afferent signal arising from the internal branch of the SLN is necessary for normal deglutition, especially for providing feedback to central neural circuits, which facilitate laryngeal adduction during swallowing.[37] With information obtained from the FEESST regarding both the patient's sensory and motor functions, the patient with aspiration is managed quite differently depending on what his sensory test results show. The sensory test, along with the food administration portion of the FEESST, provides comprehensive information regarding both sensory and motor functions of the swallowing mechanism. Neither FEES nor MBS alone allows the clinician to safely make decisions to feed the patient or to withhold feeding.[38]

To perform the test, an air pulse generator is used to send a pulse of air from a specially designed machine through a port in a specially designed flexible nasopharyngoscope. Air pulses can be delivered to the supraglottic larynx and pharynx areas. Using a calibrated puff of air from a specially designed machine, sensory thresholds can then be determined using one of the psychophysical testing methods. The twitch response of the mucosa suggests the sensory awareness of the stimulus. The FEESST provides an accurate indication of the sensory function or dysfunction of the aryepiglottic space, which in turn reflects the degree of awareness of bolus in the oropharynx and the need to protect the airway.

During the time of airway closure, the swallow cannot be visualized, as the pharyngeal walls contract over the bolus, collapsing the lumen over the endoscope (**whiteout phase**). Monitoring of the bolus is only possible after the pharyngeal swallow. However, the bolus can be monitored as it enters into view from the oral cavity to the pharynx. A video camera and recorder coupled to the endoscope provide a permanent record of the examination for later review by the clinician and patient and serve as a baseline to monitor the patient's progress. This test is often performed by an otolaryngologist and SLP. In selected cases, FEESST can provide a patient with visual feedback that may aid the rehabilitation process. Moreover, this test can be performed at bedside, in the clinic, or in an intensive care unit. A complete protocol for conducting the FEESST is currently available,[39] and it has been shown to be safe when performed following training.[40,41] Figure 5–4 shows the bolus penetrating below the epiglottis after the patient attempted to swallow.

Modified Barium Swallow (MBS)

The modified barium swallow (MBS) is also called a videofluorographic swallowing study. The term

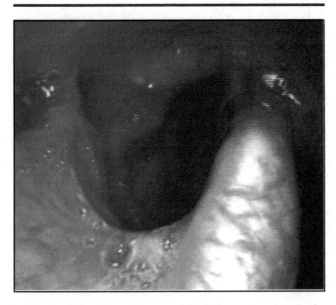

Figure 5–4. A large portion of the bolus remaining in the hypopharynx after patient attempted to swallow. View of larynx following swallow of liquid by a 58-year-old male with bilateral vocal fold paresis and atrophy.

"cookie swallow" has been used in the past to describe the MBS, but it is misleading and does not adequately describe the procedure. The test is more comprehensive than swallowing a cookie and involves the use of technical instrumentation and expertise to assess the results. The MBS is a multidisciplinary evaluation of the swallowing mechanism involving collaboration between a radiologist and an SLP, and was first described by Logemann.[27]

> The MBS offers a dynamic assessment of the oral, pharyngeal, and esophageal phases of swallowing by means of videofluoroscopy.

The MBS provides a comprehensive instrumental assessment of swallowing and follows the BSE when dysphagia risk factors are identified in the BSE. The decision to recommend an MBS test is often based on the findings of the clinical bedside evaluation. The test requires a fluoroscopic unit, video recorder, a chair suitable for stabilizing the patient, and various food and liquids that will be coated or mixed with barium.

Under **fluoroscopic observation,** controlled by the radiologist, the patient ingests barium-coated boluses or liquid barium of varying consistencies, offered at the discretion of the SLP. The MBS usually starts with a liquid barium preparation unless there is evidence of choking on liquids. Thickened barium liquid, pudding, and solids (usually pieces of cookie or a marshmallow coated with barium) are also commonly used in this test. These consistencies are chosen to approximate the consistencies of food that a patient is likely to encounter in his daily diet. Some clinicians use other preparations, such as deviled chicken and beef stew, to test the patient's ability to handle different consistencies of food.

Frontal and lateral dynamic x-rays are obtained with the fluoroscope in a fixed position during the MBS with the patient standing or sitting. The MBS is purely dynamic; the complete study is recorded on videotape or computer. The MBS can be used with various consistencies, different patient postures in swallowing, or different techniques to manage the bolus. With this recorded information, goals can be set and treatment can be defined.

MBS Test Observations

The MBS concentrates on the **oral**, **oropharyngeal**, and **hypopharyngeal** phases of deglutition, although it is useful to perform a brief evaluation of the esophagus. This dynamic study evaluates formation of the bolus in the mouth, tongue motion, coordination, timing and completeness of swallowing, movement of the epiglottis, elevation of the larynx, and cricopharyngeal contraction. Because of the potential danger of excessive exposure to radiation, the clinician must select consistencies wisely in order to limit radiation exposure. Often, the patient with a severe problem or a patient undergoing treatment for dysphagia will be given more than one MBS.

The MBS is an excellent test for evaluating the oral and pharyngeal phases of swallowing. Pathology that may explain the presence of dysphagia, such as abnormal movements of the tongue in forming the bolus and initiating deglutition, residual barium that pools in the valleculae or piriform sinuses, and aspiration of barium into the airway can be identified. Because the entire fluoroscopic study is recorded on videotape, the study can provide a highly detailed analysis of the coordination and timing of swallowing. The MBS may also include testing with compensatory and swallowing maneuvers, such as the chin-tuck, supraglottic swallow, or Mendelsohn maneuver, to name a few. These postures and maneuvers are discussed in Chapter 6.

Entry of barium into the airway may be the most important observation that the team performing the MBS can make. The clearest and most clinically useful solution to the problem of terminology to describe barium in the airway is to state the location of the barium that extends lowest into the airway. This may be as subtle as a coating of the laryngeal surface of the epiglottis (ie, penetration), or as obvious as gross aspiration of barium into the lower tracheobronchial tree, as shown in Figure 5–5. The location and extent of aspiration should be stated clearly.

Rosenbek and his colleagues[42] proposed an 8-step scale to evaluate the degree of penetration and aspiration seen in the MBS. That scale may be quite useful to monitor changes in a patient's ability to control aspiration and advance to another eating level.

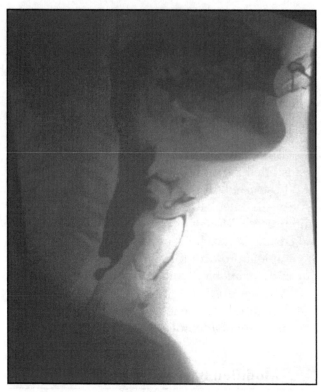

Figure 5–5. *A lateral radiograph during the modified barium swallow showing significant aspiration.*

The 8 steps of the Penetration-Aspiration Scale (PAS) are:

1. Material does not enter airway.
2. Remains above folds/ejected from airway.
3. Remains above folds/not ejected from airway.
4. Contacts folds/ejected from airway
5. Contacts folds/not ejected from airway.
6. Passes below folds/ejected into larynx or out of airway
7. Passes below folds/not ejected despite effort.
8. Passes below folds/no spontaneous effort to eject.

Although these steps may not be exact intervals, they do describe decreasing swallow safety, from no penetration to aspiration. As with the "traditional" barium swallow, nasopharyngeal reflux of barium should also be documented during the MBS.

Recent studies have shown the value of the Penetration-Aspiration Scale in the study of normal subjects to document the variability seen in the normal swallow.[43] In addition, the PAS has been used to track swallowing changes in Parkinson disease patients.[44]

Instrumental Assessment and Predicting Aspiration

The MBS can often provide information as to the cause of aspiration, but it does not necessarily predict aspiration. Silent aspiration may remain undetected on clinical (bedside) swallow examination and even after the modified barium swallow.

Martin-Harris et al[45] reviewed the findings of the MBS and found that with the number of studies reported in the past 30 years, the degree of validity, reliability, and interpretation of these measures in various patient populations was highly variable. From this review, she and her colleagues developed the MBS Measurement Tool for Swallowing Impairment (MBSImp). The MBSImp is a qualitative measurement tool based on previously validated instruments (such as the PAS, nutritional health status, etc.). The MBSImp scores are based on physiological observations and bolus flow measures. The MBSImp scores were found to correlate significantly with intake recommendations made by SLPs, the Penetration-Aspiration Scale, and measures of quality of life. The authors suggest that the MBSImp demonstrates the importance of obtaining a validated measure of swallowing using a standardized set of terms, a standardized protocol for interpreting the MBS, and a standardized reporting system that can be transferred from institution to institution.

The advent of sensory testing has further provided increased predictive value of instrumental testing. Abnormal motion of the epiglottis, diminished contractions of the pharyngeal constrictor muscles, and abnormal laryngeal "rise" can all be identified on the modified barium swallow, FEES, or FEESST.

> Silent aspiration is aspiration into the tracheobronchial tree that fails to elicit a normal cough response to clear the barium and can only be measured objectively using FEESST.

Silent aspiration offers evidence of an underlying neurological dysfunction related to the loss or diminution of sensation. Leder and Espinosa[46] examined a cohort of subjects using the FEES technique following clinical examination. They found that the clinical examination underestimated aspiration risk in patients who were at risk for aspiration but overestimated aspiration risk in patients who did not exhibit aspiration risk. A retrospective review of the results from the FEESST and videofluoroscopic examinations of 54 subjects by Tabaee et al[47] revealed complete agreement in 52% of the examinations done within a 5-day period. In the other 48%, the disagreements were related to the amount of pooling, penetration, and aspiration. The FEESST tended to lead observers to identify higher percentages of pooling, penetration and minor aspiration than the videofluorographic exam. In this study, no reports of treatment recommendations or outcomes of treatment based on the observers' findings were given.

Manometry and Videomanometry

Esophageal manometry with video recording consists of simultaneously recording video radiographic images and solid-state manometry to determine the relationships between intraluminal pressures and movement of the anatomical structures while the bolus passes through the swallowing structures. It provides a qualitative as well as a quantitative assessment of esophageal motility, pressures, and coordination. Manometry is used in the evaluation of **esophageal motility disorders**, including achalasia and diffuse esophageal spasm. It is also important in the identification of motor abnormalities associated with other systemic diseases such as scleroderma, diabetes mellitus, and chronic intestinal pseudo-obstruction.

Pharyngeal manometry can be performed in conjunction with esophageal motility studies. Normally, the response of the oropharynx to swallowing has two components. First, compression of the catheter against the pharyngeal wall by the tongue results in a high, sharp-peaked amplitude pressure wave followed by a low-amplitude, long-duration wave that reflects the initiation of pharyngeal peristalsis. Second, there is contraction of the middle and inferior pharyngeal constrictor muscles to provide the midpharyngeal response to swallowing, resulting in a rapid, high-amplitude pressure upstroke ending in a single, sharp peak, followed by a rapid return to baseline.

The pharynx is not symmetrical and, therefore, the measurements obtained during standard manometry vary with the catheter placement. Nonetheless, measurements of intrabolus pressures during the pharyngeal phase of swallowing may predict which patients will respond to a surgical **myotomy**.

Manometry is performed with a polyvinyl catheter, a thin tube about 35 cm long made of a flexible polyvinyl material and constructed with multiple pressure sensors, which is passed transnasally, and the patient is instructed to perform a series of wet and dry swallows. LES pressure is measured at baseline and in response to a swallow. Figure 5–6 shows

the manometry catheter in place. LES pressure is measured as a step up in pressure from the gastric baseline referenced as atmospheric. Complete LES relaxation with a swallow is demonstrated by a decrease in pressure to gastric baseline for approximately 6 seconds. Basal UES sphincter pressures can be identified as a rise in pressure above the esophageal baseline. Due to the asymmetry of the UES, this is normally 50–100 mm Hg depending on the direction of the pressure sensor, ie, whether lateral or anterior/posterior. Evaluation of UES relaxation and correlation of sphincter relaxation with pharyngeal contraction is obtained by instructing the patient to perform a series of wet swallows.

Videomanometry has been used to document the effects of swallow maneuvers such as the supraglottic swallow, the effortful swallow, and the chin-tuck swallow posture to determine if they are beneficial to patients with oropharyngeal dysphagia.[48] Bulow and colleagues[48] found that none of the three techniques reduced the number of misdirected swallows, but the effortful swallow and the chin-tuck posture did reduce the depth of penetration. Kawahara et al[49] showed that anatomical variations in the esophagus such as the corkscrew esophagus

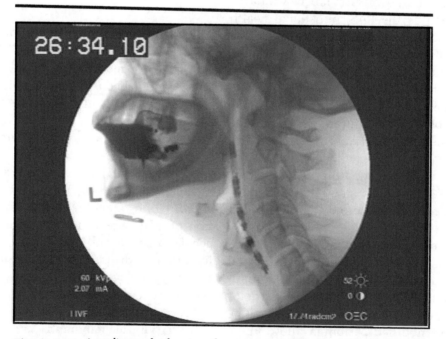

Figure 5–6. *A radiograph showing the manometry sensing tube in place for study of esophageal motility.*

or esophageal atresia are related to abnormal pressure changes that occur in children with esophageal motility disorders. It is apparent that the use of videomanometry has value both for the study of esophageal motility disorders as they are related to dysphagia symptoms and for identifying treatment options once an accurate diagnosis is made.

Ultrasound

Ultrasound uses high frequency sounds (>2 MHz) from a transducer held or fixed in contact with skin to obtain a dynamic image of soft tissues. As ultrasound does not penetrate bone, its use is limited to the soft tissues of the oral cavity and parts of the oropharynx.

> Ultrasound is completely noninvasive and does not use ionizing radiation; therefore, repeated studies can be done without risk.

It is highly efficient in studying the oral aspects of bolus preparation and bolus transfer. These characteristics render ultrasound as highly useful for children or when multiple studies are required to make a diagnosis. However, if dysphagia due to pharyngeal or laryngeal dysfunction is suspected, ultrasound offers little diagnostic or treatment information.

In ultrasound studies of swallowing, a handheld transducer is placed sub mentally and is rotated 90°. The swallowing functions of the upper surface of the tongue, the intrinsic tongue muscles, and the soft tissue anatomy of the mouth are within the view of the transducer. Ultrasonography does not require the use of any special bolus or contrast (real food can be used).

Endoscopic Ultrasound

Endoscopic ultrasound is especially important in the evaluation of submucosal lesions, which cannot be adequately assessed with standard endoscopic techniques. Throughout the GI tract, the wall layer echo structure is examined endosonographically (Figure 5–7).

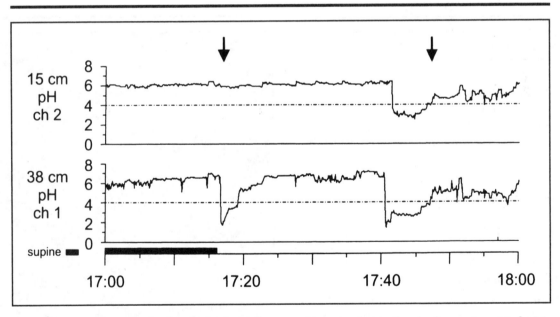

Figure 5–7. *A photograph of an endoscopic ultrasound image taken in the esophagus. Layer 1 depicts the superficial mucosa, layer 2 is the deep mucosa, layer 3 corresponds to the submucosa, layer 4 corresponds to the muscularis propria, and layer 5 corresponds to surrounding fat in the esophagus, as there is no serosa in the esophagus.* Source: *Adapted from Padda S, Young MA. Chapter 13. Carrau RL, T Murry, eds.* Comprehensive Management of Swallowing Disorders. *San Diego, CA: Singular Publishing; 1999:82, Figure 13–1.*

Intraluminal probes are invasive and thus are not tolerated by all patients. The use of ultrasound intraluminal probes requires a high degree of experience and sometimes the probe cannot be passed through a tight stricture. Endoluminal ultrasonography has been used for the study of esophageal and cricopharyngeal diseases, including esophagitis, strictures, and motility disorders.

Magnetic Resonance Imaging (MRI)

High-speed **magnetic resonance imaging (MRI)**, such as **fast low angle shot (FAST)** or **echoplanar imaging**, has permitted a dynamic analysis of the pharyngeal phase of swallowing that was impossible using conventional MRI. The pharyngeal oral cavity, laryngeal lumen, and musculature can be evaluated during motion, allowing the assessment of the swallowing mechanism.

During a FAST MRI, images are obtained as a bolus containing a contrast substance is swallowed. This technique is particularly useful for assessing rapid activity of the oral cavity.

> MRI has the advantage of not involving exposure to radiation.

However, temporal and spatial resolution of MRI is inferior to videofluoroscopy, producing images with poor resolution. MRI is costly, and swallowing in the supine position may not reflect the true physiological mechanism of swallowing.

Functional Magnetic Resonance Imaging

Functional magnetic resonance imaging (fMRI) attempts to track motion during magnetic resonance imaging. Using this technique, it is now possible to investigate the neural mechanisms of motion-induced tasks such as speaking and swallowing. Although early studies were confounded by motion artifacts, it is now possible to examine the neural bases of various motion events such as swallowing using fMRI.[50] In doing so, functional neural mapping of the events such as swallowing provide information about the neural control under normal conditions and how control may be reestablished after injury to the primary cortical control center.[51] Figure 5–8 shows the activation areas during vocal fold movement in an fMRI.[52]

Positron Emission Tomography

Positron emission tomography (PET), like fMRI, provides a method of examining neural activity associated with specific motions. Although it is noninvasive, it has the disadvantage of exposure to radiation. Using PET, Smithard[53] demonstrated that swallowing has numerous representations in the brain for both normal healthy volunteers and patients suffering from stroke. Moreover, he demonstrated that recovery of swallowing following stroke may be spontaneous or may be enhanced by medications. Smithard suggests that recovery of cortical function does not necessarily follow the same path despite nearly the same location of CVA.

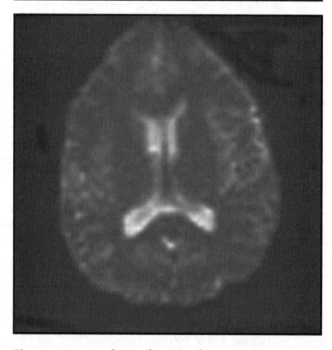

Figure 5–8. *An fMRI showing the activation areas in white during vocal fold movement.*

Other Instrumental Tests Associated With Swallowing Disorders

Esophogram (Barium Swallow)/Upper Gastrointestinal Series (UGIS)

Table 5–8 summarizes other tests associated with dysphagia and gastroesophageal reflux disease. The traditional barium swallow evaluates the upper aerodigestive tract between the oral cavity or oropharynx and the gastric fundus or cardia. It is not intended to identify swallow dysfunction, nor dictate treatment, as in the modified barium swallow (MBS). The single contrast esophogram series fills and distends the lumen with thin liquid barium. Intrinsic minor irregularities and masses and extrinsic impressions are visible. An air contrast study provides the same information, but also allows a more detailed view of the mucosa. For an air contrast barium study, the patient ingests effervescent crystals followed by thick barium. A barium swallow has both dynamic and static components. The dynamic portion, fluoroscopy, can be recorded on tape (videofluoroscopy, cineradiography) for later review. The static portion is recorded on a series of rapid still frames.

The barium swallow can identify intrinsic and extrinsic pathology. Intrinsic abnormalities include tumors, cricopharyngeal dysfunction, and aspiration of barium into the airway or reflux into the nasopharynx, diverticula, webs, and esophageal dysmotility. Extrinsic masses such as cervical osteophytes, as seen in Figure 5–9, and an enlarged thyroid gland may be visualized directly or suspected by their effect on the barium column.

The subjective location of dysphagia does not always correspond to the anatomic location of

Table 5–8. Diagnostic Tests of Dysphagia and Gastroesophageal Reflux Disease

Test	Indication
Barium Esophagram	Structural lesions
Videoradiography	Pharyngeal function
Scintigraphy	Aspiration
Endoscopic Ultrasound	Submucosal lesions
Endoscopy	Structural and mucosal lesions
Esophageal Manometry	Motility disorders
24-hour pH-metry	Gastroesophageal reflux disease
Sensory Testing	Laryngopharyngeal reflux disease
	Cough, throat clearing, excess mucus

Source: Adapted and expanded from Padda S, Young MS. Chapter 7. Carrau RL, Murry T, eds. *Comprehensive Management of Swallowing Disorders.* San Diego, CA: Singular Publishing; 1999:48, Table 7–1.

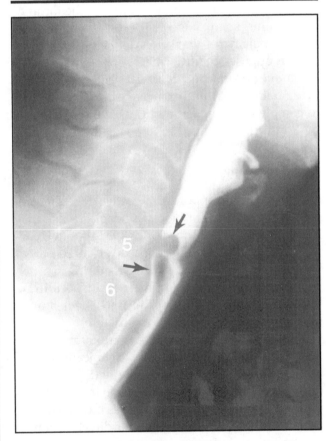

Figure 5–9. Lateral view of a barium swallow shows the impression of a prominent cricopharyngeus muscle (arrow) on the barium column. An osteophyte at C5-6 causes a smaller impression. Source: *Adapted from Weissman JL. Chapter 11. Carrau RL, Murry T, eds.* **Comprehensive Management of Swallowing Disorders.** *Singular Publishing; 1999:67, Figure 11–2.*

pathology. Therefore, the barium study when used to evaluate dysphagia should extend as low as the gastric fundus or cardia. The UGIS evaluates the stomach and small bowel. Obstruction or dysfunction of these areas may cause or contribute to esophageal dysfunction (eg, GERD).

Computed Tomography (CT)

Computed tomography (CT) and MRI are used to delineate the anatomy of a particular region of the head, neck, or other components of the upper aerodigestive tract. The most common use is to identify the site of a lesion, as in the case of a cerebrovascular accident within the central nervous system, or to delineate the extent of a lesion in the intra- or extraluminal space. In general, CT offers direct axial and coronal images that better define the bony anatomy, as opposed to MRI, which better delineates the soft tissue (ie, brain, other neural structures, muscle) in sagittal, coronal, and axial planes, but takes longer to complete the images and thus is more prone to motion artifact.

Esophagoscopy

Endoscopy of the upper aerodigestive tract is recommended to rule out or biopsy a neoplasm that may be suspected as the cause of dysphagia or odynophagia. Occasionally, the endoscopy may be part of the treatment, as in those patients requiring injection of a paralyzed vocal fold, injection of **botulinum toxin**, or dilation of the esophagus for the treatment of cricopharyngeal achalasia or strictures.

Dysphagia and odynophagia are common indications for upper GI endoscopy, technically known as an **esophagogastroduodenoscopy (EGD)**, which may be performed as the initial test in the evaluation of these disorders. The esophagus is intubated with a handheld scope of 60 mm under direct visualization of the posterior hypopharynx. The endoscope is usually advanced through the upper esophageal sphincter (UES), which appears as a slitlike opening in the cricopharyngeus muscle at about 20 cm from the incisor teeth. The entire length of the esophagus is in direct view of the endoscope until its termination at the gastroesophageal junction, which lies at the diaphragmatic hiatus. The esophagus is usually closed at the gastroesophageal junction, but this is easily distended with air insufflation or swallowing. This allows the endoscope to easily advance through the LES into the stomach.

The EGD is the most specific test for identifying esophageal complications of gastroesophageal reflux disease (GERD), esophageal ulcers, infectious disorders, and benign and malignant neoplasms. It is, however, more useful in defining the cause of disease in those patients with solid food dysphagia (transit dysphagia). Contraindications for endoscopy include suspected perforation of the GI tract, lack of adequately trained personnel, and lack of informed consent. Figure 5–10 shows a summary of pictures from a typical EGD exam.

Recently, a modification of the traditional EGD has been proposed. Transnasal esophagoscopy (TNE)[54] examines the esophagus by passing a small flexible scope through the nose, similar to laryngeal endoscopy. However, the scope is long enough to examine the entire length of the esophagus and the stomach. This test is done with the patient awake; thus, no general anesthesia is needed. Postma and colleagues[55] have shown the value of this test when nonspecific symptoms of difficulty swallowing, hoarseness, intermittent heartburn, and cough are present.

Scintigraphy

Scintigraphy is a procedure used to track movement of the bolus and quantify the residual bolus in the oropharynx, pharynx, larynx, and trachea. The patient swallows a small amount of a **radionuclide material** such as Technetium 99m combined with liquid or food. A special camera (**gamma camera**) records images of the organs of interest over time to obtain a quantitative image of the transit and metabolic aspects.

Scintigraphy can be used to identify trace aspiration and quantify the aspiration over short or long periods of time. Scintigraphy can also be used to calculate the transit time and residual "pooling" of a bolus, before and after treatment, in patients suffering degenerative neuromuscular diseases.

Scintigraphy is typically performed in the **nuclear medicine test suite** by trained personnel. Acquisition of data from the oral cavity to the tho-

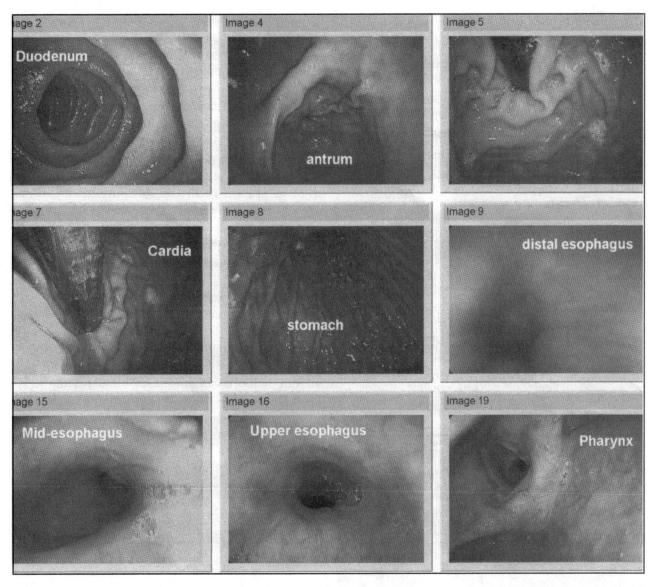

Figure 5–10. *During the EGD, numerous pictures are taken at various locations along the esophagus and into the stomach. Images can be seen from the hypopharynx (where there is excessive mucous down through the esophagus and into the stomach).*

racic and even upper abdominal cavities may be dynamic during the swallow and then followed by static images over longer time periods ranging from several minutes to several hours.

The precise amount of aspiration or residual bolus may be identified through computer analysis of the scans made at various time intervals. With the use of scintigraphy, the amount of aspiration in each region may be quantified. Scintigraphy may be more sensitive than barium swallow or MBS studies for long-term assessment of bolus location, and it has the added advantage of permitting the use of common food as the bolus.

Scintigraphy requires cooperation from the patient. Patients with known movement disorders, severe cognitive disorders, and the inability to remain standing or sitting in front of the gamma camera may not be candidates for this test.

Esophageal pH Monitoring

Prolonged (24-hour) esophageal pH monitoring is a test for diagnosing gastroesophageal reflux disease (GERD). In addition, ambulatory monitoring devices permit evaluation of the temporal relationship between reflux episodes and atypical symptoms. pH monitoring is especially important in the diagnostic evaluation of patients with atypical presentations of GERD. Figure 5–11 shows a reading from part of a dual probe 24-hour pH metry study. The test is relatively expensive, not available at all institutions, and may not be tolerated by some patients.

The identification of lesions that may be caused by GERD requires direct examination (ie, laryngoscopy, esophagoscopy), whereas pH monitoring identifies and quantifies the gastroesophageal reflux.

Dual probe 24-hour pH monitoring (the use of 2 catheters) is now an accepted protocol for identifying esophageal and gastroesophageal reflux. 24-hour pH monitoring is usually done following an overnight fast. The pH catheter is inserted transnasally into the esophagus. Standard placement of the distal probe is at a position that is approximately 5 cm above the proximal border of the LES. The proximal probe is located in the upper esophagus just below the esophageal inlet. The probes are attached to a recording device. Patients are asked to note in a diary, or in the recording device, the times that they eat, sleep, or perform any other activities. More importantly, patients will be asked to record any type of discomfort that they have, including heartburn, chest pain, wheezing, and coughing, and to record the time that these symptoms occurred. This information will be used to correlate the pH at the time a symptom or activity took place and a symptom index can be calculated. The most valuable discrimination between physiological and pathological reflux is the percentage of total time that the pH is less than 4. Normal values for the proximal probe have not yet been established. Dual probe 24-hour pH monitoring is considered to be the most sensitive and specific method of making a diagnosis of LPRD.[56] The difficulty with pH monitoring is the need to maintain a "routine daily schedule" for 24 hours while wearing a nasal probe. Many patients do not tolerate the probe or alter their daily schedule, which renders the data suspect. Alternatives to the 24-hour pH probe test have been developed. These alternatives involve inserting a small pilllike camera into the esophagus that then travels through the digestive system and out after 48 hours while sending information back to a small, battery-operated device that is worn on a belt. These devices are more easily tolerated than wearing the nasal probe.

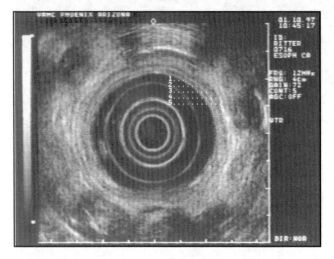

Figure 5–11. *One hour of a 24-hour ambulatory pH recording from the distal and proximal esophagus, which shows 2 episodes of reflux. Each reflux episode is labeled with an arrow. In the second reflux episode, acid reflux in the distal esophagus reaches the proximal esophagus or higher.* Source: *Adapted from Padda S, Young MA. Chapter 13. Carrau RL, Murry T, eds.* Comprehensive Management of Swallowing Disorders. *San Diego, CA: Singular Publishing; 1999:85, Figure 13–3.*

Laryngopharyngeal Sensory Testing, LPRD, and Dysphagia

Sensory testing (ST) has been shown to be a valid and reliable substitute for 24-hour pH monitoring. A report by Aviv[57] indicated that edema is the clinical hallmark of LPRD and that this edema can be quantified with laryngopharyngeal sensory testing. Furthermore, patients with dysphagia who reflux during a FEESST have measurable sensory deficits in the posterior larynx. Also, the effect of proton pump inhibitor PPI therapy on the posterior laryngeal edema can be quantified.

A second controlled study was carried out to examine the relationship between dual probe

24-hour pH testing, laryngopharyngeal sensory testing, and TFL findings.[58] Seventy-six patients were enrolled in a tightly controlled study. All patients underwent dual pump 24-hour pH testing 7 days after PPI treatment, laryngopharyngeal sensory testing, and TFL by otolaryngologists who were blinded to pH status and laryngopharyngeal sensory testing results. There were 3 patient groups: Group A—patients with GERD who had LPRD symptoms (study group); Group B—patients with GERD but no LPRD symptoms (GERD control group); and Group C—patients with no GERD or LPR symptoms (normal group).

Patients with GERD and LPRD symptoms (Group A) had significantly higher posterior laryngopharyngeal sensory thresholds than both patients with GERD but no LPRD symptoms and patients with no GERD or LPRD symptoms. Sensitivity of blinded TFL findings versus dual probe 24-hour pH testing was 50%, and specificity was 83%. However, adding laryngopharyngeal sensory thresholds greater than 5 mm Hg air pulse pressure to the TFL findings increased the sensitivity of TFL versus dual probe 24-hour pH testing from 50% to 88%, and specificity from 83% to 88%. This study showed that LPRD is associated with a posterior laryngeal sensory neuropathy with impairment of the laryngeal adductor response LAR. The investigators reasoned that because greater air pulse strength was required to elicit the LAR in the patients with documented acid reflux compared to the patients without acid reflux, it effectively represented an alteration in laryngeal sensory nerve function—hence their use of the term "neuropathy." Furthermore, adding sensory testing, specifically a sensory deficit greater than 5 mm Hg air pulse pressure, to the TFL findings was essentially as sensitive and specific as dual probe 24-hour pH testing to diagnose reflux disease.[58]

Electromyography

Electromyography (EMG) is the measurement of electrical activity within a muscle. EMG is recommended to ascertain the presence of specific nerve or neuromuscular unit deficits, such as that accompanying vocal fold paralysis or to elucidate or corroborate the presence of a systemic myopathy or degenerative neuromuscular disease. When used

for the diagnosis of vocal fold paralysis, laryngeal electromyography (LEMG) may also provide information regarding the prognosis for spontaneous recovery.

The goals of direct LEMG are to detect normal from abnormal activity and localize and assess the severity of a focal lesion by determining whether there is neuropraxia (physiological nerve block or focal injury, with intact nerve fibers) or **axonotmesis** (damage to nerve fibers leading to complete peripheral degeneration).

> Needle LEMG can also evaluate prognosis, providing valuable information to either proceed to definitive surgical correction for a permanent or long-term deficit, or implement temporary measures if spontaneous recovery is likely.

The thyroarytenoid muscle is approached by insertion of a monopolar or concentric electrode through the cricothryoid ligament midline 0.5–1.0 cm, then angled superiorly 45° and laterally 20° for a total depth of 2 cm. The cricothyroid muscle is reached by inserting the electrode 0.5 cm off the midline, then angling superiorly and laterally 20° toward the inferior border of the thyroid cartilage. Figure 5–12 shows a normal recruitment pattern.

Reduced motor unit recruitment is observed with focal demyelinating (neuropraxic) lesions such as found after intubation injuries (Figure 5–13). Patients with axon loss lesions, such as partial nerve transection after surgical procedures, will also exhibit decreased motor unit recruitment with normal configuration within the first 6 weeks after injury. However, axonal injuries will exhibit positive waves and fibrillation potentials at rest, which begin three to four weeks postinjury. Laryngeal nerve regeneration following axon loss lesions can be observed between 6 weeks to 12 months postinjury and is characterized by polyphasic motor unit potentials with wide duration.

LEMG is useful in differentiating neurological vocal fold paralysis from laryngeal joint injury. LEMG may also confirm the diagnosis of joint dislocation when a normal recruitment pattern is seen with vocal fold immobility.

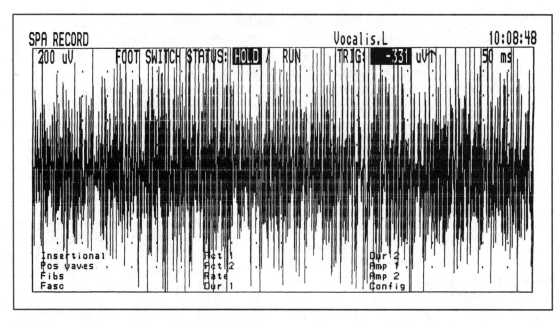

Figure 5–12. *Normal voluntary motor unit recruitment of the vocalis muscle using the Valsava maneuver. Note the full interference pattern that obliterates individual motor unit analysis when the sweep speed is set at 50 ms per division.* Source: *Adapted from Munin MC, Rainer M. Chapter 14. Carrau RL, Murry T, eds.* Comprehensive Management of Swallowing Disorders. *San Diego, CA: Singular Publishing Group;1999:88, Figure 14–1.*

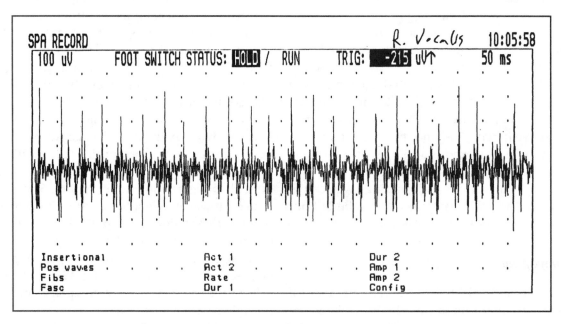

Figure 5–13. *Decreased motor unit recruitment with the primary unit firing at 24 Hz. Note that there is a decreased interference pattern with the Valsava maneuver. The sweep speed is 50 ms/division.* Source: *Adapted from Munin MC, Rainer M. Carrau RL, Murry T, eds.* Comprehensive Management of Swallowing Disorders. *San Diego, CA: Singular Publishing; 1999:89, Figure 14–2.*

The three areas of interest for electrodiagnostic evaluation of swallowing are the laryngeal sphincter, the sensory ability of the supraglottic larynx and pharynx (indirectly evaluated through cricothyroid muscle function), and the cricopharyngeal sphincter.

EMG, however, has several pitfalls: the precise site of the lesion cannot be determined, only whether it involves the vagus nerve or brain stem, the superior laryngeal nerve, or the recurrent laryngeal nerve. The posterior cricoarytenoid, which is the main abductor muscle, can be technically difficult to localize. Systemic neuromuscular diseases cannot be differentiated from focal lesions without full neurological evaluation in conjunction with EMG studies of other muscles and nerves.

SUMMARY

Normal swallowing consists of a series of well-coordinated neuromuscular movements beginning with placement of a bolus in the mouth. From that point, bolus transport and bolus awareness become an integrated neural process. Although originally thought to be a serial processing pattern, we now know that the 4 phases of swallowing (described in detail in Chapter 1) overlap considerably in a parallel processing paradigm. This chapter pointed out the importance of the case history to guide further evaluation of the swallowing complaints. Depending on the types of complaints the patient has and using self-assessment techniques and case history information, tests may be selected by one or more specialists involved in the patient's care. It should be noted that the diagnosis of swallowing disorders extends into many disciplines and that there is no single gold-standard test for all swallow complaints. Different disciplines may opt for specific tests based on their initial evaluation. New tests have been developed in the past 25 years to guide the treatment of swallowing disorders. Some tests remain experimental or may be extremely costly to use on a regular basis. Nonetheless, clinicians should be aware of all of the possible tests for identifying the basis of the swallowing disorder and how the test may aid in treating the problem.

STUDY QUESTIONS

1. Patient self-assessment in the management of swallowing disorders has limitations related to:
   A. The number of tests now available
   B. The lack of construct validation of scales or charts now being used
   C. The condition of the patient when asked to complete the assessment
   D. The length of assessment scales

2. In conducting various assessments of swallowing function, a false positive test is:
   A. Better because it will suggest conservative treatment procedures
   B. Indicates the patient is having problems that he really does not have
   C. Suggests that feeding or oral eating be stopped due to aspiration
   D. Requires another test to verify the results

3. Laryngeal electromyography is useful in assessing swallowing as it:
   A. Provides a prediction of penetration and aspiration
   B. Indicates the status of vocal fold closure during swallowing
   C. Provides a measure of activity in the vocal folds
   D. May be used to replace the clinical bedside assessment in patients who are not cooperative

4. The primary difference between FEES and FEESST is:
   A. One cannot assess sensation
   B. One cannot assess oral function
   C. One provides a calibrated measure of sensory function
   D. One can be done by an SLP and the other cannot

DISCUSSION QUESTIONS

1. If a patient cannot cooperate during the clinical bedside examination, what alternatives does

the clinician have to assess patient readiness to swallow

2. FEES and the modified barium swallow are both used in many hospitals and clinics. Discuss the main reasons for using one or the other in:
   A. A 67-year-old male who has been diagnosed with a brain stem CVA.
   B. A 35-year-old female who is grossly overweight and who is complaining of food "sticking" in her throat when she swallows.
   C. An 85-year-old otherwise healthy female who has been gradually losing weight over the past 3 months. She does not appear to have had a CVA but has mild slurring of her speech and some slowness to respond to questions.

Assume that both tests are available and there is someone competent to administer both tests.

REFERENCES

1. McHorney CA, Bricker E, Kramer AE, et al. The Swal-Qol outcomes tool for oropharyngeal dysphagia in adults 1. Conceptual foundation and item development. *Dysphagia*. 2000;15:115–121.
2. McHorney CA, Bricker E, Robbins JE, Kramer AE, Rosenbek JC, Chignell KA. The Swal-Qol outcomes tool for oropharyngeal dysphagia in adults II. Item reduction and preliminary scaling. *Dysphagia*. 2000;15:122–133.
3. McHorney CA, Robbins J, Lomax K, et al. The SWAL-QOL and SWAL-CARE outcomes tool for oropharyngeal dysphagia in adults: III. Documentation of reliability and validity. *Dysphagia*. 2002 Spring;17(2):97–114.
4. Khaldoun E, Woisard V, Verin, C. Validation in French of the Swal-Qol scale in patients with oropharyngeal dysphagia. *Gastroentérologie Clinique et Biologique*. 2009; 33;167–171.
5. Bogaardt HC, Grolman W, Fokkens WJ. The use of biofeedback in the treatment of chronic dysphagia in stroke patients. *Folia Phoniatr Logop*. 2009;61(4):200–205.
6. McHorney CA, Martin-Harris B, Robbins J, Rosenbek J. Clinical validity of the SWAL-QOL and SWAL-CARE outcome tools with respect to bolus flow measures. *Dysphagia*. 2006;21(3):141–148.
7. Bandeira AK, Azevedo EH, Vartanian JG, Nishimoto IN, Kowalski LP, Carrara-deAngelis E. Quality of life related to swallowing after tongue cancer treatment. *Dysphagia*. 2007;23(2):183–192.
8. Robbins J, Kays SA, Gagnon RE, et al. The effects of lingual exercise in stroke patients with dysphagia. *Arch Phys Med Rehab*. 2007;88(2):150–158.
9. Chen AY, Frankowski R, Bishop-Leone J, et al. The development and validation of a dysphagia-specific quality-of-life questionnaire for patients with head and neck cancer: the M. D. Anderson dysphagia inventory. *Arch Otolaryngol Head Neck Surg*. 2001 Jul;127(7):870–876.
10. Gillespie MB, Brodsky MB, Day TA, Lee FS, Martin-Harris B. Swallowing-related quality of life after head and neck cancer treatment. *Laryngoscope*. 2004 Aug;114(8): 1362–1367.
11. Schindler A, Borghi E, Giddia C, Ginocchio D, Felisati G, Ottaviani F. Adaptation and validation of the Italian MD Anderson Dysphagia Inventory (MDADI). *Rev Laryngol Otol Rhinol (Bord)*. 2008;129(2):97–100.
12. Belafsky PC, Mouadeb DA, Rees CJ, et al. Validity and reliability of the eating assessment tool (EAT-10). *Ann Otol Rhinol Laryngol*. 2008;117(12):919–924.
13. Belafsky PC, Postma GN, Koufman JA. Validity and reliability of the reflux symptom index (RSI). *J Voice*. 2002; 16:274–277.
14. Byrne SM, Allen KL, Dove ER, Watt FJ, Nathan PR. The reliability and validity of the dichotomous thinking and eating disorders scale. *Eat Behav*. 2008;9:154–162.
15. Wallace KL, Middleton S, Cook IJ. Development and validation of a self-report symptom inventory to assess the severity of oral-pharyngeal dysphagia. *Gastroenterology*. 2000;118:678–687.
16. DePippo KL, Holas MA, Redding MJ. The Burke dysphagia screening test: validation of its use in patients with stroke. *Arch Phys Med Rehab*. 1994;75(12);1284–1286.
17. Winklmaier U, Wüst K, Plinkert PK, Wallner F. The accuracy of the modified Evans blue dye test in detecting aspiration in head and neck cancer patients. *Eur Arch Otorhinolaryngol*. 2007 Sep;264(9):1059–1064.
18. Belafsky PC, Blumenfeld L, LePage A, Nahrstedt K. The accuracy of the modified Evan's blue dye test in predicting aspiration. *Laryngoscope*. 2003 Nov;113(11):1969–1972.
19. Daniels SK, Brailey K, Priestly DH, Herrington LR, Weisberg LA, Foundas AL. Aspiration in patients with acute stroke. *Arch Phys Med Rehab*. 1998;79:14–19.
20. Martina R, Silver F, Teasell R, et al. The Toronto bedside swallowing screening test (TOR-BSST): development and validation of a dysphagia screening tool for patients with stroke. *Stroke*. 2009;40:555–561.
21. McCullough GH, Wertz RT, Rosenbek JC. Sensitivity and specificity of clinical/bedside examination signs for detecting aspiration in adults subsequent to stroke. *J Commun Disord*. 2001;34:55–72.
22. Ramsey DJ, Smithard DG, Kalra L. Early assessments of dysphagia and aspiration risk in acute stroke patients. *Stroke*. 2003;34(5):1252–1257.
23. Peruzzi WT, Logemann JA, Currie D, Moen SG. Assessment of aspiration in patients with tracheotomies: comparison of the bedside colored dye assessment with

videofluoroscopic examination. *Respiratory Care*. 2001; 46(3):243–247.

24. Collins MJ, Bakheit Am. Does pulse oximetry reliably detect aspiration in dysphagic stroke patients? *Stroke*. 1997;28(9):1773–1775.
25. Smith HA, Lee SH, O'Neill PA, Connolly MJ. The combination of bedside swallowing assessment and oxygen saturation monitoring of swallowing in acute stroke: a safe and humane screening tool. *Age Ageing*. 2000;29:495–499.
26. Lim SH, Lieu PK, Phua SY, et al. Accuracy of bedside clinical methods compared with fiberoptic endoscopic examination of swallowing (FEES) in determining the risk of aspiration in acute stroke patients. *Dysphagia*. 2001;16:1–6.
27. Logemann JA. *Evaluation and Treatment of Swallowing Disorders*. San Diego, CA: College Hill Press; 1983:121.
28. Daniels SK, Meltam CP, Brailey K, Fundas AL. Clinical assessment of swallowing and prediction of dysphagia severity. *Am J Speech-Lang Pathol*. 1997;6:17–23.
29. Mann G. *MASA: The Mann Assessment of Swallowing Ability*. Clifton, NY: Thompson Learning; 2002.
30. Antonios N, Carnaby-Mann G, Crary M, et al. Analysis of a physician tool for evaluating dysphagia on an inpatient stroke unit: the Modified Mann Assessment of Swallowing Ability. *J Stroke Cerebrovasc Dis*. 2010;19(1):49–57.
31. Splaingard M, Hutchins B, Sultan L Chaudhuri G. Aspiration in rehabilitation patients: videofluoroscopic vs. bedside clinical assessment. *Arch Phys Med Rehab*. 1988; 69:637–640.
32. Aviv JE, Martin JH, Keen MS, Debell M, Blitzer, A. Air-pulse quantification of supraglottic and pharyngeal sensation: a new technique. *Ann Otol Rhinol Laryngol*. 1993; 102:777–780.
33. DePippo KL, Hitdas MH, Reding MJ. Validation of the 3 oz. water swallow test for aspiration following stroke. *Arch Neurol*. 1992;49:1259–1261.
34. Langmore SE, Schatz K, Olsen N. Fiber-optic endoscopic examination of swallowing safety: a new procedure. *Dysphagia*. 1988;2:216–219.
35. Aviv JE. Sensory discrimination in the larynx and hypopharynx. *Otolaryngol Head Neck Surg*. 1997;116:331–334.
36. Bastian RW. Videoendoscopic evaluation of patients with dysphagia: an adjunct to the modified barium swallow. *Otolaryngol Head Neck Surg*. 1991;104:339–350.
37. Jafari S, Prince RA, Kim DY, Paydarfar D. Sensory regulation of swallowing and airway protection: a role for the internal superior laryngeal nerve in humans. *J Physiol*. 2003;550:287–304.
38. Aviv JE, Liu H, Parides M, Kaplan ST, Close LG. Laryngopharyngeal sensory deficits in patients with laryngopharyngeal reflux and dysphagia. *Ann Otol Rhinol Laryngol*. 2000;109:1000–1006.
39. Aviv JE, Murry T. *FEESST Fiberpoptic Endoscopic Evaluation of Swallowing with Sensory Testing*. San Diego, CA: Plural Publishing; 2006.
40. Cohen MA, Setzen M, Perlman PW, Ditkoff M, Mattucci KF, Guss J. The safety of flexible endoscopic evaluation

of swallowing with sensory testing in an outpatient otolaryngology setting. *Laryngoscope*. 2003;113:21–24.
41. Aviv JE, Murry T, Cohen MS, Zschommler A, Gartner C. Flexible endoscopic evaluation of swallowing with sensory testing; patient characteristics and analysis of safety in 1340 consecutive examinations. *Ann Otol Rhinol Laryngol*. 2005;114(3):173–176.
42. Rosenbek JC, Robbins J, Roeker EB, Coyle JL, Woods JL. A penetration-aspiration scale. *Dysphagia*. 1996;11: 93–98.
43. Allen JE, White CJ, Leonard RJ, Belafsky PC. Prevalence of penetration and aspiration on videofluoroscopy in normal individuals without dysphagia. *Otolaryngol Head Neck Surg*. 2010 Feb;142(2):208–213.
44. Troche MS, Huebner I, Rosenbek JC, Okun MS, Sapienza CM. Respiratory-swallowing coordination and swallowing safety in patients with Parkinson's disease. *Dysphagia*. Epub 2010 Jul 11.
45. Martin-Harris B, Brodsky MB, Price CC, et al. MBS Measurement tool f swallow impairment: MBSImp: establishing a standard. *Dysphagia*. 2008;23:392–405.
46 Leder SB, Espinosa MS. Aspiration risk after acute stroke: comparison of clinical examination and fiberoptic endoscopic evaluation of swallowing. *Dysphagia*. 2002;17: 214–218.
47. Tabaee A, Johnson PE, Gartner CJ, Kalwerisky K, Desloge RB, Stewart MD. Patient-controlled comparison of flexible endoscopic evaluation of swallowing with sensory testing FEESST and videofluoroscopy. *Laryngoscope*. 2006;116:821–825.
48. Bulow M, Ollson R, Ekberg O. Videomanometric analysis of supraglottic swallow, effortful swallow and chin tuck in patients with pharyngeal dysfunction. *Dysphagia*. 2001;16:190–195.
49. Kawahara H, Kubota A, Okkkuyama H, Oue T, Tazuke Y, Okada A. The usefulness of videomanometry for studying pediatric esophageal motor disease. *J Pediatr Surg*. 2004;39(12):1754–1757.
50. Gracco VL, Tremblay P, Pike B. Imaging speech production using fMRI. *Neuroimage*. 2005;26(1):294–301.
51. Birn RM, Bandettini PA, Cox RW, Shaker R. Event-related fMRI of tasks involving brief motion. *Hum Brain Mapp*. 1999;7:106–114.
52. Galgano J. *A study of voice onset using functional magnetic resonance imaging*. Unpublished manuscript. Columbia University, 32005.
53. Smithard DG. Swallowing and stroke. Neurological effects and recovery. *Cerebrovasc Dis*. 2002;14:1–8.
54. Belafsky PC, Postma GN, Daniel E, Koufman JA. Transnasal esophagoscopy. *Otolaryngol Head Neck Surg*. 2001 Dec;125(6):588–589.
55. Postma GN, Cohen JT, Belafsky PC, et al. Transnasal esophagoscopy: revisited (over 700 consecutive cases). *Laryngoscope*. 2005 Feb;115(2):321–323.
56. Richter JE. Diagnostic tests for gastroesophageal reflux disease. *Am J Med Sci*. 2003;326:300–308.

57. Aviv JE. Prospective, randomized outcome study of endoscopy versus modified barium swallow in patients with dysphagia. *Laryngoscope.* 2000;110:563–574.

58. Botoman VA, Hanft KL, Breno SM, et al. Prospective controlled evaluation of pH testing, laryngoscopy and laryngopharyngeal sensory testing (LPST) shows a specific post inter-arytenoid neuropathy in proximal GERD (P-GERD). LPST improves laryngoscopy diagnostic yield in P-GERD. *Am J Gastroenterol.* 2002;97(9 suppl):S11–12.

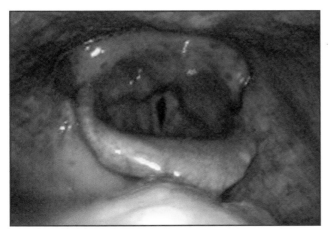

Figure 2–2. View from flexible endoscope showing the epiglottis and vocal folds shortly after the bolus has passed into the upper esophagus.

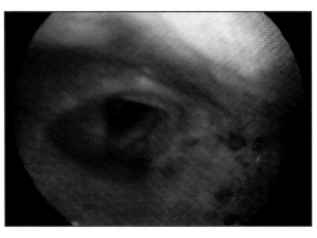

Figure 3–1. An example of penetration found during flexible endoscopy.

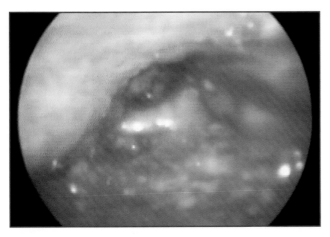

Figure 3–2. A portion of the food bolus is shown below the vocal folds before the patient expels it.

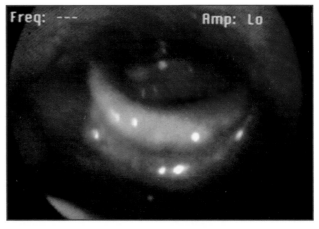

Figure 3–3. Mucous pooling (white matter) after the swallow in patient with Parkinson disease.

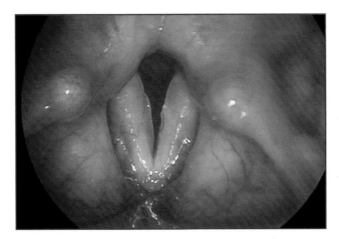

Figure 3–9. Patient with significant edema at the level of the larynx and vocal folds.

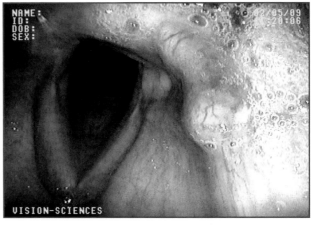

Figure 3–10. The larynx following radiation therapy (XRT) for laryngeal cancer.

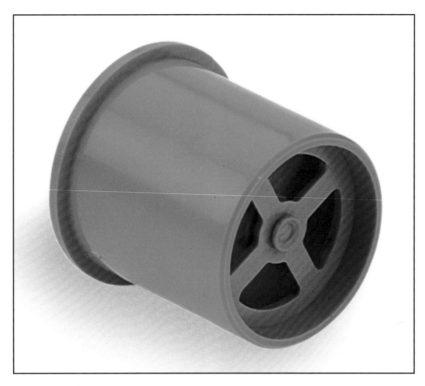

Figure 4–1. An expiratory speaking valve designed to fit over the open tracheostomy tube to restore subglottic air pressure during swallowing.

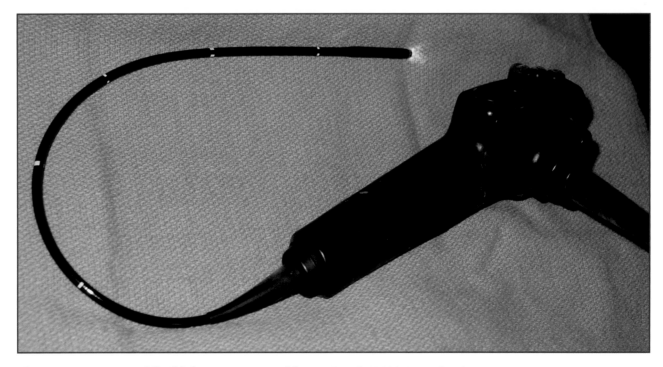

Figure 5–1. Transnasal flexible laryngoscope used for FEES and FEESST examinations.

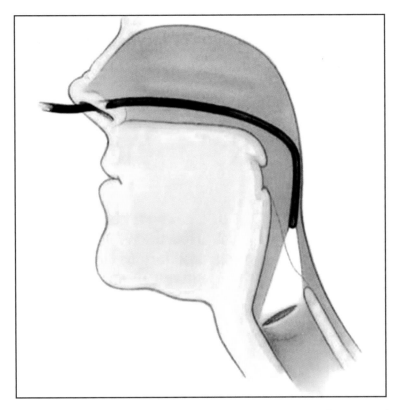

Figure 5–2. Drawing from lateral view showing proper placement of scope prior to feeding the patient. Note the scope is above the epiglottis.

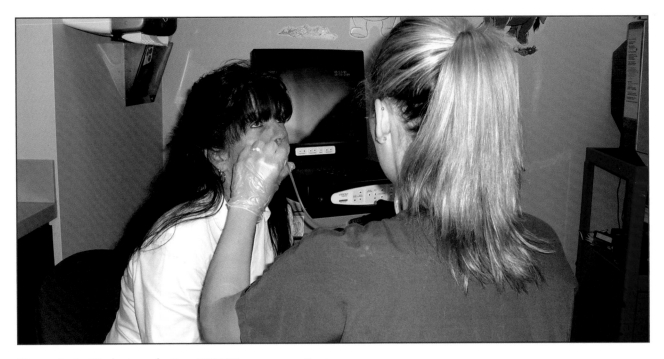

Figure 5–3. Student conducting FEESST exam on patient.

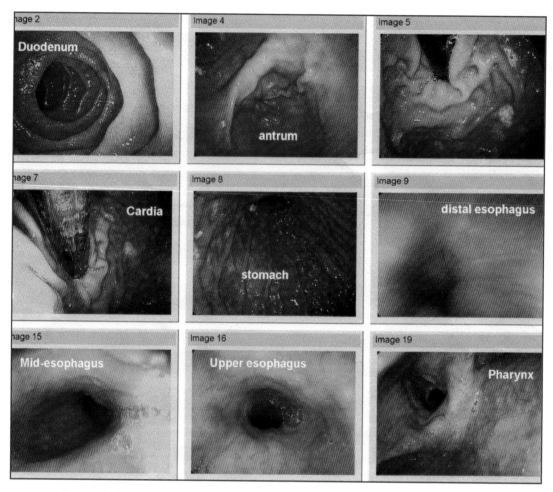

Figure 5–9. Lateral view of a barium swallow shows the impression of a prominent cricopharyngeus muscle (arrow) on the barium column. An osteophyte at C5-6 causes a smaller impression. Source: *Adapted from Weissman JL. Chapter 11. Carrau RL, Murry T, eds.* Comprehensive Management of Swallowing Disorders. *Singular Publishing; 1999:67, Figure 11–2.*

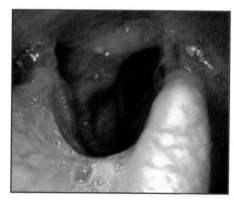

Figure 5–4. A large portion of the bolus remaining in the hypopharynx after patient attempted to swallow. View of larynx following swallow of liquid by a 58-year-old male with bilateral vocal fold paresis and atrophy.

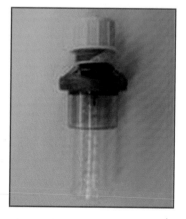

Figure 6–2A. Expiratory muscle strength training device used to improve force for various types of patients.

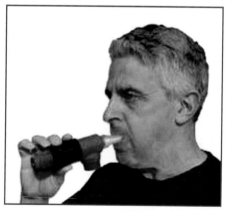

Figure 6–2B. Patient with EMST device in place.

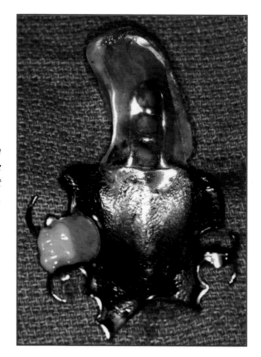

Figure 7–2. Soft palate prosthesis with obturator extending posteriorly into the pharyngeal area to improve contact during swallowing.

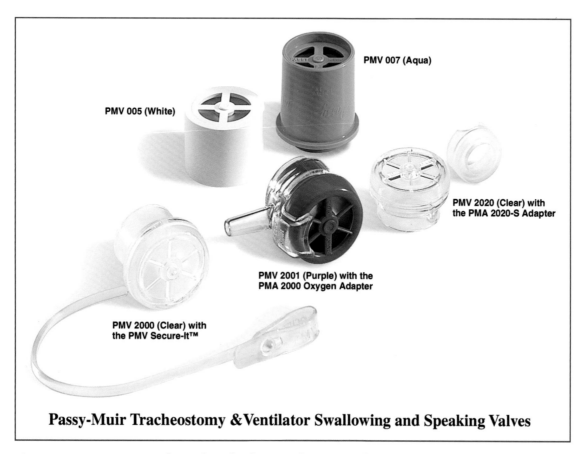

PMV 007 (Aqua)

PMV 005 (White)

PMV 2020 (Clear) with the PMA 2020-S Adapter

PMV 2001 (Purple) with the PMA 2000 Oxygen Adapter

PMV 2000 (Clear) with the PMV Secure-It™

Passy-Muir Tracheostomy & Ventilator Swallowing and Speaking Valves

Figure 7–3. Passy-Muir valves. The valve fits over the open tracheotomy tube to restore subglottic pressure when talking or swallowing.

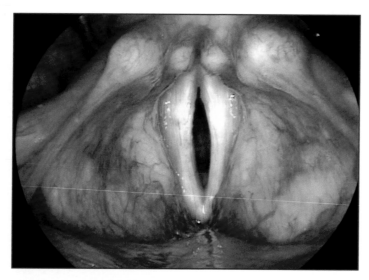

Figure 8–1. Vocal folds of patient with bilateral atrophy prior to undergoing vocal fold injection.

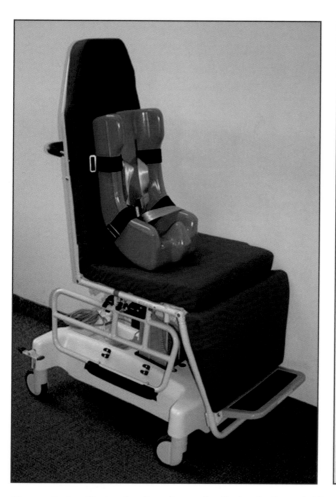

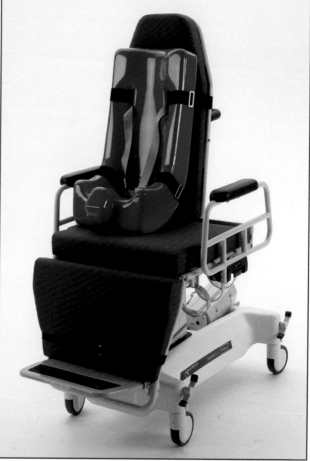

Figure 9–2. Chairs developed specifically for feeding children in a semi-upright position.

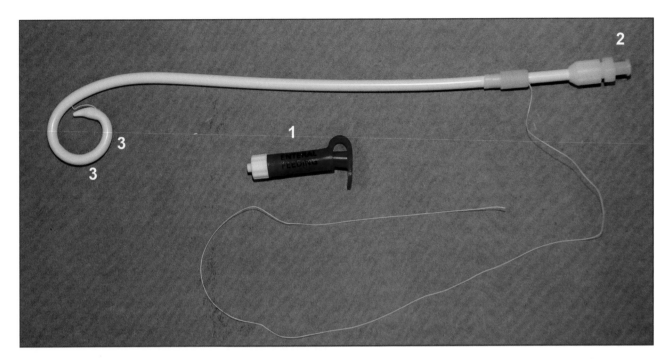

Figure 10–2. Deutsch Gastrostomy Catheter with AQ Hydrophilic Coating, 16-Fr., 25 cm long with Cook-Cope type locking loop. (1) Enteral feeding adapter with male Luer lock fitting, (2) Luer lock tube opening, and (3) exits ports. Source: *From Leonard R, Kendall K. Dysphagia Assessment and Treatment Planning: A Team Approach (2nd ed.), San Diego, CA: Plural, 153 (Figure 10–6).*

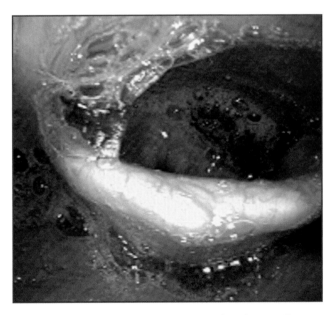

Figure 11–1. Patient with diagnosis of Parkinson disease. The examination photo was taken after eating a small piece of cracker coated with green food coloring. The patient noted that he swallowed it completely but coughed afterward.

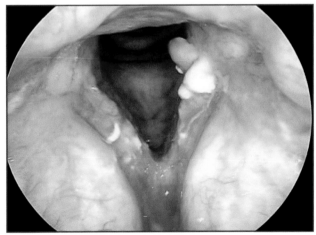

Figure 11–2. Vocal folds of a patient with left vocal fold granuloma. The white areas seen may be related to the extensive use of antibiotics, which were prescribed prior to his current examination.

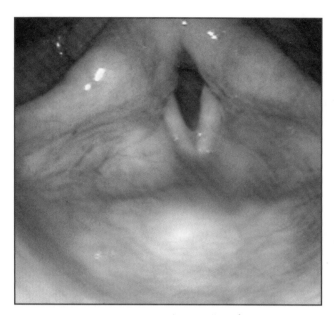

Figure 11–3. Patient with significant laryngopharyngeal reflux, vocal fold edema, and right vocal fold paresis. Note the food coloring down to the level of the vocal folds, indicating penetration of blue colored water.

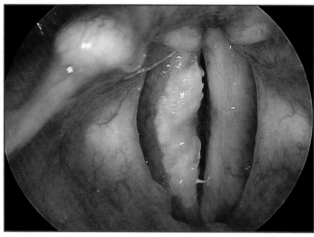

Figure 11–5. A 49-year-old male patient following biopsy of right true vocal fold. The diagnosis was T1 vocal fold cancer.

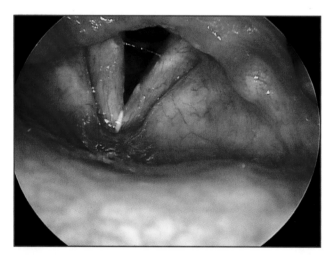

Figure 11–6. A 67-year-old male with a left vocal fold paralysis.

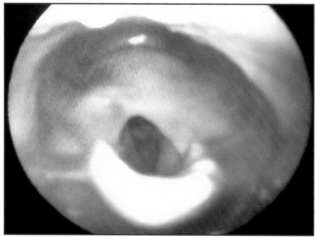

Figure 11–7. A 51-year-old male with late effects of radiation therapy toxicity.

VI

Nonsurgical Treatment of Swallowing Disorders

CHAPTER OUTLINE

I. INTRODUCTION
II. COMPENSATORY SWALLOWING THERAPY
    A. Introduction
    B. Oral Motor Exercises
    C. Shaker Exercise
    D. Thermal Tactile Oral Stimulation (TTOS)
    E. Expiratory Muscle Strength Training (EMST)
    F. Neuromuscular Electrical Stimulation (NMES)
III. REHABILITATIVE SWALLOWING THERAPY
    A. Introduction
    B. Swallowing Maneuvers
    C. Swallowing Postures
    D. Swallowing Therapy and Aspiration
IV. SUMMARY
V. STUDY QUESTIONS
VI. DISCUSSION QUESTIONS
VII. REFERENCES

INTRODUCTION

Once the evaluation of the swallowing disorder is completed, a treatment plan is developed and carried out by multiple members of the dysphagia team. As in the diagnostic process, the treatment process initially focuses on swallow safety, the prevention of aspiration through sensory awareness, and proper bolus transit. By maintaining the focus on safety, clinicians will find it necessary to rely on multiple approaches, beginning with oral care and hygiene.

The most common location of bacteria is in the mouth. Therefore, patients with swallowing disorders should brush their teeth, or someone should do it for them, three times per day. Mouth rinse is also suggested provided it does not lead to aspiration if swallowed accidently.

The major nonsurgical treatment modalities for swallowing disorders include compensatory swallowing therapy and rehabilitative swallowing therapy. A third treatment modality that combines these 2 modalities with prosthodontic management is covered in Chapter 7. The primary member of the swallowing team in the nonsurgical management of swallowing disorders is the speech-language pathologist (SLP). Other team members indirectly involved in these techniques include the occupational therapist, dietitian, nurse, and attending physician. Still others such as the radiologist, gerontologist, gastroenterologist, practical nurse, and family members may also be involved. Each person who participates in the patient's treatment either directly or indirectly, whether a professional or a family member, must be acutely aware of the need for swallow safety and prevention of aspiration and aspiration pneumonia.

> Treatment is a team process to ensure swallow safety, improve nutrition, and contribute to the overall rehabilitative effort.

As treatment implies change, clinicians must maintain a high degree of vigilance and monitor changes, both positive and negative. To do so requires accurate understanding of the disorder, acute observational skills, and knowledge of when to use instrumental assessments as part of the decision-making process during treatment. The instrumental assessments described in Chapter 5 are the basis for a treatment plan, which is developed by the treatment team and then presented to the patient and family members.

Changes in patients' swallowing resulting from treatment or simply with the passage of time may be observed through weight changes, speed of eating, types of foods being consumed, or by special scales to assess changes in quality of life brought about through improved swallowing. Such changes can occur throughout the swallowing rehabilitation period.[1] In this chapter, traditional and evolving nonsurgical treatments to enhance swallowing and maintain safety are described.

COMPENSATORY SWALLOWING THERAPY

Introduction

Compensatory swallowing therapy consists of oral motor or neuromotor exercises to strengthen and control the voluntary oral preparatory and oral phases of swallowing. In addition, this therapy includes methods to stimulate the pharyngeal swallow and increase protective valving at the level of the vocal folds to prevent aspiration.

> Compensatory swallowing therapy involves exercises for the organs of swallowing without requiring the patient to swallow foods or liquids.

Numerous studies have provided limited evidence that indirect techniques are useful in the management of dysphagia. However, it should be pointed out that most of the evidence to support the use of compensatory therapy to treat swallowing disorders was obtained from small groups and usually without the benefit of a control group. Moreover, in many of these treatment groups, improvement or recovery of part or all of the oral swallowing function could be expected, such as in patients with mild CVA.

Compensatory swallowing therapy should be done with patients who have:

A. Adequate cognitive skills to follow instruction
B. Motivation to improve
C. Willingness to practice independently
D. A need to increase muscle strength and range of motion
E. Deficits in sensory awareness as indicated by sensory testing.

Oral Motor Exercises

Oral motor exercises (OME) have long been suggested as a way to increase control over the swallowing event by increasing strength and volitional control over the movements of lips, tongue, and vocal folds. Many of these exercises have been derived from the speech and voice literature based on the treatment of dysarthria. Because dysarthric speech and voice generally improve when the patient controls the movements of the articulators, the rationale for use of oral motor exercises to treat swallowing disorders is to control the passage of the bolus, increase awareness of the bolus, and maximize the driving force of the bolus in transit to the oropharynx.

Table 6–1 lists the most common exercises for improving lip strength and awareness of the location of the bolus in the oral cavity. These exercises are derived from various articulation treatment protocols and may be applied in treatment plans for patients with swallowing disorders. It can be expected that patients with labial dysfunctions will have difficulty in the preparation of the bolus for transfer. It remains to be seen how these dysfunctions affect the entire coordination of the swallow.

Tongue control provides transmission of the bolus to the hypopharynx. In normal subjects, vocal fold closure is already happening, as the bolus is being propelled through the oral cavity. Lingual strength exercises may constitute a fundamental aspect of swallowing treatment because of the crucial role that the tongue plays in the oral preparatory, oral, and pharyngeal phases of swallowing. Lingual weakness may result from damage to cranial nerves VII, IX, or XII. Tongue strength exercises also aim to improve tongue elevation and lateralization. One

of the earliest studies to show the value of tongue strengthening exercises was reported by Lazarus and colleagues, using young normal subjects.[2] The subjects were asked to press a rubber bulb or a tongue blade against their hard palate. After a month, both groups showed improved tongue strength compared to a group that received no treatment. Robbins et al[3] found similar results with 8 healthy elderly volunteers and, more recently, Robbins and her group found lingual exercises to improve lingual strength and swallowing outcomes in 6 patients following CVA.[4]

Clark et al[5] reported that although oral motor exercises have long been used to improve articulation in patients with tongue weakness as well as rigidity, arguments have been made that these exercises offer few long-term benefits. They studied normal healthy individuals trained to increase lingual strength, protrusion, and lateralization over 9 weeks. They found improvement in the measures following training but suggested that the gains may diminish when training is stopped. Based on their study and the results of a previous study by Clark[6] and data from Robbins et al,[4] tongue strength exercises appear to be efficacious in the functional improvement of swallowing but must be maintained to retain the improvement.

The oral motor exercises shown in Table 6–1 target tongue strength, tongue lateralization, tongue protrusion, and tongue contact with other structures.[7] More recent data by Martin-Harris et al[8] suggest that the tongue may even play a role in the laryngeal phase of swallowing.

> Martin-Harris and colleagues[8] found that the oropharyngeal swallow consists of a synergistic mechanism in which there are overlapping events that reflect an interdependence with each other in order to properly propel the bolus through the swallow channels into the esophagus in a safe manner.

Table 6–2 summarizes exercises for the tongue and mandible. Exercises to increase mouth opening using a device such as the TheraBite allow the clinician and the patient to set goals and track progress. For those patients who can increase mouth opening,

Table 6–1. Labial Exercises to Improve Strength and Awareness of Control of the Swallowing Mechanism

1. Rapid labial opening and closing using the consonants /p, b/.
2. Extended lip squeeze followed by lip retraction.
3. Repeating the vowels /u, i/ with increased lip movement. Vocalization provides additional stimulation and awareness.
4. Thermal stimulation of the lips with ice. Movement of the ice may be medial-lateral or more focal if drooling on one side is prevalent.
5. Holding different objects between the lips such as a straw, tongue blade, plastic spoon, etc, to improve sensory awareness. Objects may be of different sizes, shapes, and weights.
6. Apply various foods to lips, such as yogurt and peanut butter, and encourage the patient to massage the lips together.
7. Use the index finger to apply a sudden or quick stretch to the edges of the upper and lower lips.
8. Practice humming. Cue patient to start and stop humming. When humming stops, the patient should open the lips, then close again.
9. Have patient close the lips. Ask him or her to keep them closed while you try to gently break the lip seal.
10. Practice a "facial squeeze" by squeezing lips together. While keeping lips closed, alternate bringing teeth together and separating them. This mimics chewing activity.
11. Practice inhaling and exhaling through the nose rather than mouth. the patient may want to watch this activity with a mirror.
12. Prior to swallowing, the patient should hold a glass or cup to the lips. Practice the timing of opening the lips once the cup is placed on the lower lip.
13. Hold small objects such as a button (connected to a string) and place it between the lips and teeth. The clinician can put a gentle pull on the string the improve lip strength.
14. Intraoral stimulation of cheeks with a brush, cold object, or fingers.
15. Resistive exercises. Example: have the patient push the upper lip down while the clinician resists the movement with a tongue blade. Have the patient push the tongue against the cheek while the clinician resists against the outside of the cheek.

Source: Adapted from Murry T. Chapter 35. Carrau RL, Murry T, eds. *Comprehensive Management of Swallowing Disorders.* San Diego, CA: Plural Publishing; 2006:244, Figure 35–1.

the placement of food may significantly increase successful swallowing, especially if surgery or radiation has caused an altering or removal of all or part of some organs.

Not all patients may respond positively to tongue strengthening exercises. Patients with severe cognitive impairments and patients who are susceptible to fatigue may show little or no improvement with tongue strengthening. Patients with myasthenia gravis will show fatigue with exercises that require continuous or repetitive muscle contractions; it remains to be seen in controlled studies what

Table 6–2. Exercises for Tongue and Mandible Strength and Movement

1. Tongue tip elevation. Place tongue tip on alveolar ridge. Hold it for 2 seconds.
2. Tongue tip sweep. After holding the tongue on the alveolar ridge, sweep posteriorly against the palate.
3. Use the phonemes /t, d/ for rapid contact and release of the tongue tip to the alveolar ridge.
4. Use the "ch" sound to improve tongue contact to the middle of the soft palate. Similarly, the sounds "s" and "sh" help with lateral contact of tongue to palate as well as help to groove the tongue.
5. The /k, g/ phonemes are used to increase posterior tongue to soft palate contact. Combining syllables into quick movements such as "ta-ka" or "cha-ka" is helpful to improve the sweeping motion of the tongue.
6. Range of motion exercises can be done by chewing on gauze initially, then adding small amounts of food when it is safe.

7. To improve sensory awareness, use pressure and temperature stimulation.
   a. A cold spoon may be placed on the tip, blade, or back of tongue. Light pressure is applied and the patient is asked to lift the spoon.
   b. The palate is touched with tongue blade or cotton and the patient is asked to touch the area with the tongue.
   c. Cold or sour materials are given to the patient. They may be frozen on a stick if the patient is not yet cleared to swallow.
   d. Various sizes and textures of bolus may be given to identify the size and texture most easily transported by the tongue.

8. Mandible movement. Patients with reduced mandible movement may want to use a device such as TheraBite to increase mouth opening.
9. Resistive exercises to the mandible such as lowering or closing the mandible against the pressure applied by the therapist on the chin.
10. Sucking exercises increase tongue palate contact and help the patient to manage saliva. Sucking may be done with the tongue tip against the alveolar ridge and lips and teeth slightly apart or with teeth closed using a "slurping" or "suctioning" pull of the tongue to the midpalate area. The patient should try to do this will as much sound as possible to increase sensory feedback.

Source: Adapted from Murry T. Chapter 35. Carrau RL, Murry T, eds. *Comprehensive Management of Swallowing Disorders.* San Diego, CA: Plural Publishing; 2006:245, Figure 35–2.

effect tongue strengthening exercises have on these patients or others who have autoimmune diseases that result in muscle fatigue.

Vocal fold closure becomes a significant factor in preventing aspiration. When the vocal folds fail to close, the risk of aspiration increases. Table 6–3 lists some of the common procedures to increase vocal fold closure. These exercises have been advanced primarily for patients with vocal fold paralysis. Clinicians have tried numerous ways to increase vocal fold closure, including turning the head to one side or the other depending on which side of the larynx has the weaker vocal fold. Of specific note is item 6 in Table 6–3. The **Lee Silverman Voice Treatment (LSVT)** was developed for treating speech intelligibility in Parkinson disease patients. Studies by

Table 6–3. Vocal Fold Closure and Laryngeal Elevation *Techniques*

1. Practice coughing.
2. Increase the loudness of the voice.
3. Initiate voice with a hard glottal onset.
4. Produce sustained phonation. Try to increase the duration while maintaining consistent voice quality.
5. Sustain phonation at various pitches. This helps with anterior vocal fold closure as well as laryngeal elevation.
6. An excellent program of laryngeal exercise has been developed by Ramig and her colleagues. This program is called Lee Silverman Voice Treatment (LSVT).[9] Although this program is designed primarily to increase vocal effectiveness, it also offers promise to those who require increased vocal fold closure to reduce the risk of aspiration.

Source: Adapted from Murry T. Chapter 35. Carrau RL, Murry T, eds. *Comprehensive Management of Swallowing Disorders.* San Diego, CA: Plural Publishing; 2006:246, Figure 35–3.

Ramig and her colleagues have validated the efficacy of these exercises.[9] The focus of this treatment is on increasing the valving ability of the vocal folds.

> Sharkawi et al[10] demonstrated that oral and pharyngeal transit times were reduced significantly following the use of LSVT with patients having oropharyngeal dysphagia.

Sharkawi's group[10] found a reduction of 51% in temporal measures of swallowing (oral transit time and pharyngeal transit time) in patients with Parkinson disease one month after completing the LSVT program. They also found a reduction in oral residue following treatment and an increase in vocal intensity for sustained vowel production and oral reading. A review of the LSVT procedure and outcomes can be found in Fox et al.[11] Additional information on treatment of swallowing disorders in patients with Parkinson disease is discussed in Chapter 11 in conjunction with a case presentation.

Specific impairments may benefit from repetition of specific tasks. Table 6–4 lists 13 common impairments or defects found after tissue loss or

neurological damage along with goals and tasks to reach each goal.[12] The clinician should use the information derived from the FEES or MBS to focus on 1 or 2 goals at a time. Documentation is important for tracking progress and maintaining patient motivation to continue treatment despite the fact that indirect therapy alone does not involve swallowing foods or liquids. Accurate tracking of progress becomes essential not only for continued patient motivation but also for determining when to conduct additional tests of swallowing in order to assess changes that might allow direct swallowing therapy and the onset of oral eating.

Tongue strengthening exercises such as those in Table 6–2 are useful for improving oral phase swallowing functions such as bolus manipulation, mastication, and bolus clearance in the oral cavity. From a review of the current literature, it appears that only limited empirical data are available to validate neuromotor or oral motor exercises for use in treating swallowing disorders. Factors such as the need to increase strength of lip seal, tongue pump, tongue range of motion, and endurance of lip/tongue/jaw coordination remain to be determined.[7] Nonetheless, once the clinician understands the underlying anatomy, physiology, and neural control of these muscle groups, he or she will have a better understanding of whether and when to use a specific exercise.

The Agency for Healthcare Research and Quality reported on 4 studies of noninvasive or indirect swallowing therapy that met their policy for review.[13] The studies, summarized in Table 6–5, suggest that there is limited evidence that oral motor and neuromotor therapy have significant effects on clinical outcomes (reduced pneumonia, weight gain) for patients with neurological disorders. Nonetheless, clinicians continue to treat swallowing disorders using methods that in many cases defy validation. The efficacious approach would be to try the methods after a baseline set of reliable objective or subject tests/assessments were obtained. Clinicians should make every attempt to document changes that are brought about by the therapeutic process. In that way, they will no longer rely only on clinical impressions that may be misleading but begin to gather evidence related to the exercises. Improvement in some cases may simply be related to time since onset of the condition that brought on the swallowing disorder.

Table 6–4. *Exercises for Specific Impairments*

Impairment	Goal	Tasks May Include
Limited control, agility, or neck rotation, extension, and flexion.	Range, control, agility adequate for needed task.	Obtain consult from physical therapy, depending on need, tasks may focus on development of agility of movement as well as control and range of motion (ROM).
Trismus—Inability of the jaw to open due to injury to the trigeminal nerve or muscular deficiency.	Adequate opening for feeding route (spoon, fork, cup, or biting), for denture of palatal prosthesis placement, and for oral hygiene.	Maintain mandible-maxilla alignment while increasing passive and active range of mandible opening. Movements should be made slowly. Maximum stretch should be maintained ≥15 seconds. The TheraBite is a more sophisticated device, especially useful for marked trismus or when alignment of mandible and maxilla is difficult to maintain.
Weakness or absence of mandibular support/control.	Symmetric mandible-maxilla approximation supportive of potentials for posture, oral nutrition/hydration, and speech.	Establish optimal alignment passively or actively and present exercises graded for endurance. Increase strength and control using graded resistance and biting, munching tasks to strengthen muscles of mandibular closure and opening.
Weakness or absence of buccal tone.	Increased buccal tone.	Isometric tightening of the buccal area or squeezing of soft objects between check and teeth/gums or from buccal sulcus to the molar surface.
Diminished labial opening.	Adequate labial opening size for eating. Adequate shaping for speech.	Passive stretching and exercises to increase range and strength of lateral commissure movement. Maintain mandible alignment throughout.
Unilateral partial or complete lingual weakness or missing lateral lingual tissue.	Posterior bolus retention-release control for airway protection. Bolus and airflow control (minimize lateral "leaks").	Maximize lingual symmetry at rest and in a variety of nonspeech and speech gestures. Squeezing and lingual manipulation tasks may be appropriate. Palatal prosthesis may facilitate therapy.
Bilateral lingual weakness.	Oral transit with minimum oral loss. Maximum coordination with initiation of swallow gestures.	Address sectionally, as above.
Absent tongue.	Development of compensatory mandibular, labial, and head/neck movement strategies.	Develop ROM and agility of movements needed for compensations that take advantage of gravity. Consider mandibular or maxillary shaping prosthesis.
Unilateral or complete weakness or missing tissue of the palate.	Adequate velopharyngeal closure if tissue is adequate. Effective obturation if tissue is inadequate.	Sustained blowing against resistance may strengthen closure. Endoscopic feedback may be helpful even with objurgation. Objurgation may actually recruit improved compensatory participation in closure from the lateral and posterior pharyngeal walls.
Unilateral, bilateral, or regional failure of pharyngeal constriction.	Improved bolus compression.	Maximum lingual retraction. Laryngeal elevation and supraglottic closure.
Incomplete glottic closure.	Improved glottic closure.	Attempt to establish conditions resulting in improved true vocal fold approximation using pitch, positional, compression, and respiratory support strategies while avoiding false vocal fold participation.

continued

Table 6–4. continued

Impairment	Goal	Tasks May Include
Incomplete supraglottic closure.	Improved supraglottic closure.	Habituate early and effortful laryngeal closure and elevation for swallow. The Mendelsohn maneuver may be used.
Inadequate PES opening for swallow.	Maximum PES opening.	Maximizing extent and timing of hyoid/laryngeal elevation and the effects of pharyngeal compression of the bolus.

Source: Adapted from Leonard R, Kendall K. Dysphagia Assessment and Treatment Planning: A Team Approach. San Diego, CA: Singular Publishing; 1998:187–191.

Table 6–5. Studies of Noninvasive Methods of Swallowing Therapy That Met the Agency for Healthcare Policy Standards

Study	N	Study Design	Care Setting	Mean Age	Primary Disease(s)	Treatment	Time Frame
Groher[55]	23	RCT	Home nursing	71.8	CVA with history of aspiration	Pureed diet, mechanically altered diet	6 months
Kasprisin et al[56]	48 13 8	Retro CT	Hospital	NR	Various	Swallow therapy	NR
Martens et al[57]	16	HPCS	Acute hospital unit	49.3 46.1	Brain injury, tumor, CVA	Various (diet, exercise, counseling) No specific dysphagia treatment	NR
Di Pippo et al[58]		RCT	Rehab unit	76 74.5 43	CVA	Diet and swallow technique recommendations, therapist-prescribed diet and swallow techniques. Therapist-prescribed diet and techniques reinforced	1 year

RCT = randomized controlled trial; CT = controlled trial; HPCS = historical prospective case series; NR = not reported.

For patients following head and neck cancer or neurological disorders, it appears that noninvasive exercises that do not require the patient to swallow may have value despite lack of extensive clinical trials. Studies by Logemann,[14] Lazarus et al,[15] Pauloski et al,[16] and Sonies[17] have shown that active participation in a series of neuromuscular swallowing exercises by patients following head and neck surgery improves swallow function.

The use of compensatory exercises such as those listed in Tables 6–1 and 6–2 should be based on anatomical and physiological findings from instrumental and clinical bedside assessments. These exercises may be coupled with prosthetic management and with direct therapies.

It remains to be seen how efficacious indirect treatment is as a unitary method. Controlled studies involving the withholding or limiting of treatment or the use of sham treatments are questionable ethical approaches. Moreover, finding control groups that do not have the same physical or anatomical deficiencies to assess an exercise technique is not generally an option. Severely disordered patients are usually assigned to nonoral feeding options for health, nutrition, and safety reasons. Patients with stroke tend to have some natural recovery of swallow function from the acute phases of the event. However, clinicians must guard against blindly treating patients with oral motor exercises unless they can specify a rationale for treatment and document changes related to treatment, swallow safety, quality of life, and/or weight gain. Whenever possible, indirect therapy should be combined with other treatment modalities.

Shaker Exercise

An important aspect of swallowing is the ability to open the upper esophageal sphincter (UES) to allow the passage of the bolus. Studies by Shaker and others have shown that the UES opening is reduced in the elderly compared to healthy young individuals.[18–20] Shaker and his colleagues developed a head lift exercise (HLE) to increase the opening of the UES and therefore decrease the hypopharyngeal intrabolus pressure. In 1997, they studied healthy elderly subjects using manometry and videofluoroscopy to measure intrabolus pressure prior to and following a program of HLEs.[18] The HLE consists of lying in a supine position and doing a series of head lifts while the shoulders remain on the floor or bed.

The HLE, or Shaker exercise, was developed to treat UES dysfunction by strengthening the suprahyoid muscles. This would be expected to lead to an increase in the anteroposterior deglutitive opening diameter and cross-sectional area of the upper esophageal sphincter. The goals of the Shaker exercise are to:

1. Strengthen the muscles that contribute to the opening of the UES, specifically, the geniohyoid, thyrohyoid, and digastric muscles.
2. Significantly decrease the hypopharyngeal bolus pressure as it enters the UES, thus permitting bolus passage with less resistance.

The Shaker exercise increases UES opening and thus may contribute to the elimination of aspiration in individuals with residue in the pharynx after a swallow due to poor UES opening.[21] Strengthening the suprahyoid muscles through the Shaker exercise should result in a more efficient UES opening.

The original Shaker exercise involves isometric and isokinetic neck exercises while the individual lies in a supine position.[22] The individual alternates between 3 isometric repetitions of sustained 1-minute head raisings and 1-minute rest periods. The individual must raise his or her head high enough to see his or her toes without lifting the shoulders off the ground. The second part of the exercise consists of 30 consecutive head lifts without holding. The shoulders must also be kept on the ground during this portion.[23] The instructions for the patient are shown in Table 6–6. If the patient cannot sustain the head lift for 1 minute, an alternate baseline time can be used at the start of the exercises. Figure 6–1 shows the extended posture for the Shaker exercise once the head is lifted off the ground.

Table 6–6. Shaker Exercise Protocol

Please perform this exercise 3 times per day for the next _____ weeks.

1. Lay flat on your back on the floor or bed.
2. Hold your head off of the floor looking at your feet for 1 minute. Relax with your head back down for 1 minute and repeat the sequence 2 more times.*
3. Raise your head 30 more times and look at your toes. Do not sustain these head lifts.*

*Do not lift your shoulders while performing this exercise.

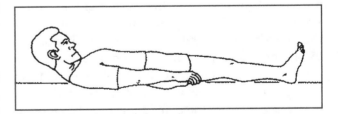

Figure 6–1. Depiction of the starting position for the Shaker exercise. Note the shoulders remain in contact with the floor surface.

Not only does the Shaker exercise strengthen the suprahyoid muscles, it also enhances shortening of the thyrohyoid muscle. According to Mepani et al,[24] the thyrohyoid muscle works in conjunction with the suprahyoid muscles to augment UES opening. In their recent study, they compared the effects of traditional dysphasia therapy (focusing on laryngeal and tongue range of motion exercises and swallowing maneuvers) and the Shaker exercise on thyrohyoid shortening across a course of 6 weeks. Thyrohyoid muscle shortening was measured before and after the 6-week period using videofluoroscopy to quantify any gains made in either group. Results from this study showed that the Shaker exercise proved significantly more effective in increasing thyrohyoid shortening compared to the traditional therapy. This would suggest that the Shaker exercise has a positive outcome on deglutition by enhancing UES opening.[24] Although Mepani et al[24] were unable to quantify the statistical significance of changes in thyrohyoid shortening compared to changes in deglutitive UES opening and clinical improvement due to small subject size, they noted a relationship between thyrohyoid muscle shortening and suprahyoid muscle contraction upon UES opening.

Several drawbacks exist with the Shaker exercise. In the Easterling et al[23] study, subjects needed repeated instruction, cueing, and encouragement to accurately perform the exercise. Subjects also reported neck muscle soreness and dizziness during the early weeks of the exercise program.[23] Fatigue may also be a factor for continuing the Shaker exercise. A study by White et al[21] found both positives and negatives for the Shaker exercise when looking at the relationship between the exercise and fatigue. Subjects performed the Shaker exercise with surface EMG electrodes positioned to evaluate the progression of fatigue in the suprahyoid muscles, infrahyoid muscles, and the sternocleidomastoid. After a 6-week training program, they found that the Shaker exercise fatigues the sternocleidomastoid, which may preclude the continuation of the exercise in some situations, especially with elderly subjects. This suggests that the Shaker exercise may not be appropriate for individuals prone to fatigue (ie, those with amyotrophic lateral sclerosis or other neuromuscular diseases).

It is important to note that the Shaker exercise cannot be used with individuals who have cervical spine deficits, reduced neck movement ability, and/or cognitive issues that may affect compliance. Unfortunately, these contraindications may eliminate a large group of individuals who would otherwise benefit from the Shaker exercise.

According to Burkhead, Sapienza, and Rosenbek,[25] the principles of exercise found to be effective in other areas such as physical rehabilitation and sports training also extends to exercise treatment of dysphagia. These principles include identifying the optimal volume and duration of the regimen, both of which are involved in the Shaker exercise. It has been shown that the Shaker exercise has been effective in treatment of swallowing dysfunction; however, the optimal volume and duration for the exercise needs further investigation. As reported by Burkhead et al,[25] exercises must place a load on the system, involve enough practice, and last for some duration to allow adaptation to the new behavior.

Further research is needed to refine the Shaker exercise, as well as other swallowing exercises to make it as effective as possible and to increase the likelihood of its continuation by patients. Although there are drawbacks in terms of patient populations and need for lengthy use, the Shaker exercise offers the patient whose problems are focused at the cricopharyngeal level an opportunity to improve swallow function.

Thermal Tactile Oral Stimulation (TTOS)

Thermal Tactile Oral Stimulation (TTOS) is defined as the stroking or rubbing of one or more of the organs of swallowing with a cold probe. The treatment is generally directed at the anterior faucial pillars. TTOS has long been an established method to treat patients with neurogenic damage, but more recently has also been utilized in patients with dysphagia, especially if the dysphagia is caused by sensory deficits. It has been hypothesized by Rosenbek and others that touch and cold stimulation provide heightened oral awareness and an alerting stimulus to the brain stem and brain, causing the pharyngeal swallow to trigger faster than it would without the stimulation.[26-28] Although these authors found slight improvements in the duration of stage transition and the total swallow duration, the amount of time needed varied and was generally extensive. In Sweden, Bove, Mansson, and Eliasson[29] found no significant differences in healthy individuals in swallowing durational measures following stimulation with a cold laryngeal mirror, but they did find that swallow times were shorter when swallowing cold water compared to swallowing body temperature water. Similar results of the effects of cold stimulation were reported by Sciortino et al.[28] They noted that whatever improvement in latency that was measured following stimulation was short-lived and generally limited to one swallow. To date, there is little research to support the extensive use of cold stimulation to the oral-pharyngeal mucosa to improve swallow function.

A study of tactile stimulation with a sour bolus by Logemann et al[30] found that there was an earlier onset of lingual activity to propel a bolus into the pharynx, triggering the pharyngeal motor response, and a shorter pharyngeal component of the swallow in patients following stroke or a mixed neurological disorder. Other studies of temperature, reported by Bisch et al,[31] and carbonation, reported by Bulow et al,[32] have been equivocal in showing changes in swallow function. However, it remains to be seen if there are cortical effects of these stimuli to alter swallow behavior.

Expiratory Muscle Strength Training (EMST)

In 2005, Kim and Sapienza[33] reported on a series of studies that demonstrated that expiratory muscle strength training (EMST) improves both ventilatory and nonventilatory functions such as with speech production, cough and swallow in normal healthy individuals, hypotonic children, and patients with multiple sclerosis. Since then, studies focusing specifically on swallow function have also shown that EMST may be a valuable adjunctive rehabilitative technique to use with patients who show muscular weakness resulting from neurological or neuromuscular diseases.

> EMST is a technique of respiratory muscle strengthening in which a device of some type is used to block the expiratory air flow until a sufficient expiratory pressure is produced.

Strength training of limb muscles has been shown effective for increasing muscle hypertrophy, suggesting that strength training of respiratory muscles may induce the same effect.[34,35]

Table 6–7 summarizes early work on EMST and suggests its use in swallowing rehabilitation. More recent studies have examined the impact of EMST on swallowing during specific assessments of swallowing. Wheeler-Hegland et al[36] studied hyoid movement using surface EMG under three conditions: the Mendelsohn maneuver, effortful swallow, and EMST. They found that EMST achieved higher maximum and average submental surface EMG activity versus normal swallowing. They suggested that the EMST training has the potential to induce strength gains to increase the activation speed in the submental musculature. Other studies reported in Table 6–7 have shown that there is evidence of improved swallowing following training with an expiratory muscle strength training device such as the one shown in Figure 6–2 for patients with Parkinson disease, multiple sclerosis, and sedentary elderly.

Neuromuscular Electrical Stimulation (NMES)

Neuromuscular electrical stimulation (NMES) is a technique that has been proposed to stimulate swallow function by applying electrical stimulation to the neck area as a means of stimulating laryngeal elevation. When electrical stimulation is applied to the skin (surface stimulation), it will activate sensory fibers in the skin and only those muscles immediately below the skin surface, if the right amount of intensity is applied. This procedure, also known as transcutaneous electrical stimulation (TES), is noninvasive and is now used by many to treat swallowing disorders.

Most applications for stimulating muscles use electrodes inserted into the muscles (intramuscular

Table 6–7. **Summary of Expiratory Muscle Strength Training (EMST) Studies**

Study	Subjects	N	Training Program	Training (wk)	Training Load	MEP Gain From Baseline (%)	Within Subject Significance Level	Functional Outcome
O'Kroy & Coast[59]	Healthy subjects	6	RT	4	32% of MEP	NS	NS	Not applicable
Suzuki et al[60]	Normal subjects	6	PT	4	30% of MEP	25	$p < 0.01$	Not applicable
Cerny et al[61]	Hypotonic children	9	RT	6	2.5 cm H_2O to 7.5 cm H_2O	69	$p = 0.0003$	Improvement of speech
Smeltzer et al[62]	Multiple sclerosis	10	PT	12	Not reported	37	No testing completed	Improvement of cough (subjective report)
Gosselink et al[63]	Multiple sclerosis	9	PT	12	60% of MEP	35	NS	Improvement of cough (subjective report)
Hoffman-Ruddy[64]	High-risk performers	8	PT	4	75% of MEP	84	No testing completed	Improvement in speech
Sapienza et al[65]	High school band students	26	PT	2	75% of MEP	47	$p = 0.000$	Not applicable
Baker[66]	Healthy young adults	32	PT	4 to 8	75% of MEP	50	$p = 0.000$	Improvement in speech and cough
Salem et al[67]	Parkinson patients	6	PT	4	75% of MEP	24 to 74	No testing completed	Improvement in speech, cough, and swallow

MEP = maximum expiratory pressure; N = number of subjects who were trained with EMST program; PT = pressure-threshold training; RT = resistance training; NS = not significant

Source: From Kim J, Sapienza CM. Implications of expiratory muscle strength training for rehabilitation of the elderly: tutorial. *J Rehab Res Dev.* 2005;42(2):211–224.

or IM) and an indwelling controller like a pacemaker to provide the stimulation either under patient or automatic control. Neuromuscular IM stimulation is used in rehabilitation of patients with spinal cord injury to control hand movements and bladder function, and is now being developed for sleep apnea and dysphagia.[37]

By stimulating the muscles in the neck via surface EMG, it has been hypothesized that the swallowing musculature will be strengthened or that the sensory pathways important for swallowing will have heightened awareness. A review of relevant studies of NMES in peer-reviewed literature was conducted in 2008 by Clark et al.[38] They reviewed 899 citations from 1960 to 2007 and found 14 articles that related to NMES. Of those, 10 were considered exploratory, with significant methodological limitations, according to the reviewers. From their review,

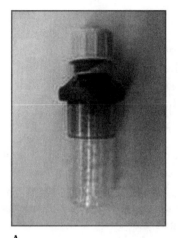
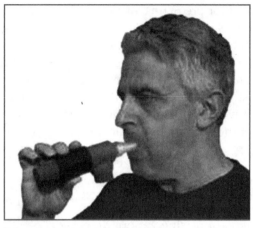

A   B

Figure 6–2. **A.** *Expiratory muscle strength training device used to improve force for various types of patients.* **B.** *Patient with EMST device in place.*

they concluded that there were few promising findings related to NMES for swallowing therapy and that there is a need for examining specific issues such as dosage, timing, surface versus intramuscular recording, and applications to specific populations. Moreover, the level of evidence for NMES was limited due to the lack of controlled studies, the lack of control groups, and the lack of sufficient outcome measures over a long period of time.

In contrast to surface stimulation, IM stimulation via hooked-wire electrodes are inserted into specific muscles or electrodes are more permanently implanted into the muscle to direct current locally to increase muscle activity and thus improve swallow function.

Ludlow[39] reviewed the evidence related to electrical stimulation. Her report, including data from up to 2009, suggests that electrical stimulation is most effective when the electrical stimulus is applied directly to the muscle (IM).

Intramuscular stimulation using electrodes inserted into these muscles has been shown to produce laryngeal elevation similar to that which occurs during normal swallowing.[40] However, electrical stimulation over the surface of the skin will provide stimulation of the skin but has not been shown to elicit movement to control laryngeal elevation.[41]

Only two well-controlled trials have compared traditional dysphagia therapy to NMES combined with therapy; one found no benefit of NMES over traditional therapy[42] in dysphagia poststroke, whereas the other found a greater improvement in the NMES group versus the sham group on only 1 of the 4 outcome measures in dysphagia secondary to head and neck cancer.[43] Therefore, the evidence reported through 2009 suggests only a very limited benefit, if any, of adding NMES to traditional therapy for the treatment of dysphagia.

REHABILITATIVE SWALLOWING THERAPY

Introduction

Rehabilitative swallow therapy combines the use of various consistencies of foods and liquids to practice swallowing maneuvers, postures, and compensatory exercises. Rehabilitative swallowing therapy, sometimes called direct swallowing therapy, is reserved for those patients who demonstrate, through instrumental studies or other means such as pulse oximetry, temperature monitoring, and so forth, that they can safely swallow small amounts of food or liquid. Although no diagnostic technique—instrumental or otherwise—is perfect for predicting swallow safety or the lack of it, the experienced clinician will be able to combine anatomical, physiological, psychological, and cognitive information derived from the bedside swallow evaluation, screening procedures, and instrumental studies to decide on the time to use direct rehabilitative procedures and the amounts and consistencies of the bolus to be swallowed.

Swallowing Maneuvers

The major maneuvers for placing various aspects of the pharyngeal swallow under the patient's control and for retaining control of the bolus during the pharyngeal swallow are:

1. Supraglottic swallow
2. Super-supraglottic swallow
3. Effortful swallow
4. Mendelsohn maneuver
5. Tongue hold maneuver

The **supraglottic swallow** is a 4-step maneuver: (1) inhale and hold breath, (2) place bolus in swallow position, (3) swallow while holding breath, and (4) cough after swallow before inhaling.

> The effects of the supraglottic swallow maneuver are to close the vocal folds (breath hold) during the swallow and then clear any residue that may have entered the laryngeal vestibule (cough) before breathing again.

This technique is often used with patients who have weak vocal folds, vocal fold paralysis, or laryngeal sensory deficits. This maneuver is considered a voluntary airway closure technique and, when done properly, closes the vocal folds prior to the swallow and keeps them closed during the swallow, thus preventing aspiration.

The **super-supraglottic swallow** is similar to the supraglottic swallow, with the addition of the instruction to bear down once the breath is being held. The effect of bearing down is to increase false vocal fold closure and assist in closing the posterior glottis. For both the supraglottic swallow and the super-supraglottic swallow, the patient is asked to "inhale and hold your breath very tightly." The super-supraglottic exercise adds "bearing down," "maintain the hold," "swallow," and then "cough." Although the airway may not be entirely closed, this maneuver offers a degree of protection by having the arytenoid cartilages tilt and possibly come into contact with the epiglottis or tongue base.[44]

The **effortful swallow** is simply a squeeze. The patient is told or shown to "squeeze hard with all of your muscles."

> The physiological goal is to increase retraction of the base of the tongue and pharyngeal pressure in order to improve bolus clearance from the valleculae.

This maneuver may be the easiest for patients who have trouble with multiple-stage commands, for children, or for those patients with significant sensory loss. The squeeze may help in propelling the bolus into the oropharynx due to weakness in the tongue. Lazarus reported that this maneuver produces high pharyngeal pressure and results in reduction or elimination of pharyngeal residue.[45] The effortful swallow maneuver should be used with caution if instrumental examination reveals oropharyngeal weakness or lack of vocal fold closure.

The **Mendelsohn maneuver** is a technique to open the UES by extending the duration of laryngeal elevation. In this maneuver, the patient initiates several dry swallows while trying to feel the thyroid prominence lift.[46] Then, the instruction is to "hold the thyroid up for several seconds."

> By keeping the larynx tilted and elevated, it is hypothesized that the UES relaxes to allow food to pass, leaving less residual material in the area.

The Mendelsohn maneuver is useful for treating patients who, for reasons of neurological injury or surgical treatment, cannot obtain adequate laryngeal excursion or elevation or who cannot coordinate the elevation motion with bolus passage.

The **tongue hold maneuver** (also referred to as the **Masako maneuver**) is used in an attempt to increase the pressures and time of contact of the tongue base to the pharyngeal wall. As pointed out by Lazarus and colleagues,[45] this technique is efficacious for patients with lingual weakness following surgery for oral cancer. Instructions to the patient are to "hold the tongue between your front teeth and swallow."

Recent evidence suggests that this maneuver may not actually benefit patients with increased pressure. Doeltgen et al[47] suggest that the tongue hold maneuver may potentially be contraindicated for individuals with generally decreased anterior hyoid movement. However, a beneficial effect, characterized by increased pharyngeal constrictor strength and ultimately increased pharyngeal pressure generation, may arise after regular training. Doeltgen et al[47] sug-

gest that the tongue hold maneuver may be useful when accompanied by the Shaker exercise.[18]

Pauloski[48] points out that as the maneuver may also result in increased pharyngeal residue, it may be best to do this exercise without food due to the risk of aspirating because of residue remaining as the result of delayed triggering of the pharyngeal swallow. Clearly, further investigation of this maneuver in various patient populations is required.

Table 6–8 summarizes the common swallow maneuvers, the problem for which they were designed, and the rationale. These maneuvers should be slowly explained to the patients, tried first without foods or liquids, and then ideally be examined during instrumental studies of swallow function before continuous therapy. They may be tried during the BSE on a limited basis as a method for determining the patient's ability to perform the tasks during instrumental examinations.

Table 6–8. Swallow Maneuvers and the Problems for Which They Were Designed

Swallow Maneuvers	Problem for Which Maneuver Was Designed	Rationale
Supraglottic swallow	Reduced or late vocal fold closure	Voluntary breath hold usually closes vocal folds before and during swallow.
	Delayed pharyngeal swallow	Closes vocal folds before and during delayed swallow
Super-supraglottic swallow	Reduced closure of airway entrance	Effortful breath hold tilts arytenoids forward, closing airway entrance before and during swallow.
Effortful swallow	Reduced posterior movement of the tongue base	Effort increases posterior tongue base movement.
Mendelsohn maneuver	Reduced laryngeal movement	Laryngeal movement opens the UES; prolonging laryngeal elevation prolongs UES opening.
	Discoordinated swallow	Normalizes timing of pharyngeal swallow events.
Tongue hold	Lack of posterior pharyngeal wall contact with tongue	Improve contact between tongue base and posterior pharyngeal wall.

Source: From Logemann JA. Therapy for oropharyngeal swallowing disorders. Perlman AL, Schulze-Delrieu K, eds. *Deglutition and Its Disorders.* San Diego, CA: Singular Publishing; 1997:451.

Swallowing Postures

Numerous individuals have demonstrated that by turning the head to one side, by tucking the chin down toward the chest, or by tilting the head back, swallowing can be facilitated or aspiration can be reduced or prevented.

> Postures used in swallow exercises can reduce aspiration, improve transit times (oral and pharyngeal), and decrease the amount of residue after the swallow compared to the amount of residue without a postural adjustment.

The most common swallow postures consist of:

1. Head back
2. Chin down
3. Head rotation
4. Head tilt

The **head back posture** relies on gravity to move the bolus out of the oral cavity. Patients with tongue paralysis or partial or total removal of the tongue due to oral cancer may benefit from this posture.

The **chin down posture** (also called the chin tuck or neck flexion posture) improves airway protection by moving the tongue base and epiglottis posterior toward the posterior pharyngeal wall. This, in turn, makes the airway entrance narrower and thus increases airway protection. The chin tuck posture is achieved by tilting the chin down toward the chest, holding that position until the bolus is swallowed. The chin tuck posture was found to be effective in patients with neurological and neuromuscular diseases[49] and in patients following pharyngectomy surgery for cancer.[50]

The **head rotation posture** is used to promote the flow of the bolus to the more normal side of the pharynx or larynx. Thus, the instruction to the patient is to rotate the head toward the weak or damaged side to attempt to close off that side. This posture is used in patients with unilateral pharyngeal or vocal fold weakness or impairment.

The **head tilt posture** (also called the lateral head tilt) is useful for patients who have unilateral oral or pharyngeal weakness. The instructions to the patient are to tilt the head to the stronger side so that gravity carries the bolus in that direction.

Table 6–9, adapted from Logemann,[14] reports the effects of postures during fluoroscopy and the rationale for using the postures. Especially notable is the chin tuck, which has been shown to significantly increase bolus propulsion through the UES in patients with excessive cricopharyngeal constriction. In addition to the studies reported in Table 6–8, Bulow and colleagues[51] found that the chin tuck did not reduce the number of misdirected swallows in patients with moderate to severe dysphagia but did reduce the depth of bolus penetration. However, Lewin et al[50] did find that the chin tuck eliminated 81% of aspiration when used with esophagectomy patients.

Additional information regarding the chin tuck was reported by Logemann and colleagues.[52] They found that although elderly patients preferred the chin tuck as a method of swallowing, bolus modification was actually more beneficial in preventing aspiration of penetration of the bolus.

> The importance of teaching the postures prior to the instrumental swallow evaluation is underscored here, as they may be tried during instrumental examinations.

The data demonstrating the efficacy of these postures has been primarily derived from small groups of patients with various neurological, neuromuscular, and head and neck cancer diagnoses. Each individual patient's ability to improve the speed of swallowing, reduce pooling, and control aspiration will dictate further treatment. Thus, although all of these techniques show variable results depending on the cause of the swallowing problem, the clinician must consider the information derived from the bedside swallow evaluation, the other team members, and the instrumental assessments to determine when to use the techniques when treating a patient with a swallowing disorder. Factors such as fatigue, attention to the task, and environmental distractions must also be taken into account to determine the length of sessions and the number of swallow trials.

Table 6–9. Postural Techniques to Reduce or Eliminate Aspiration or Residue

Disorder Observed on Fluoroscopy	Posture Applied	Rationale
Inefficient oral transit (reduced posterior propulsion of bolus by tongue)	Head back	Uses gravity to clear oral cavity
Delay in triggering the pharyngeal swallow (bolus past ramus of mandible but pharyngeal swallow is not triggered)	Chin down	Widens valleculae to prevent bolus entering airway; narrows airway entrance, reducing risk of aspiration
Reduced posterior motion of tongue base (residue in valleculae)	Chin down	Pushes tongue base backward toward pharyngeal wall
Unilateral vocal fold paralysis or surgical removal (aspiration during the swallow)	Head rotated to damaged side	Places extrinsic pressure on thyroid cartilage, improving vocal fold approximation, and directs bolus down stronger side
Reduced closure of laryngeal entrance and vocal folds (aspiration during the swallow)	Chin down; head rotated to damaged side	Puts epiglottis in more protective position; narrows laryngeal entrance; improves vocal fold closure by applying extrinsic pressure
Reduced pharyngeal contraction (residue spread throughout pharynx)	Lying down on one side	Eliminates gravitational effect on pharyngeal residue
Unilateral pharyngeal paresis (residue on one side of pharynx)	Head rotated to damaged side	Eliminates damaged side of pharynx from bolus path
Unilateral oral and pharyngeal weakness on same side (residue in mouth and pharynx on same side)	Head tilt to stronger side	Directs bolus down stronger side via gravity
Cricopharyngeal dysfunction (residue in piriform sinuses)	Head rotated	Pulls cricoid cartilage away from posterior pharyngeal wall, reducing resting pressure in cricopharyngeal sphincter

Source: From Logemann JA. Therapy for oropharyngeal swallowing disorders. Perlman AL, Schulze-Delrieu K, eds. *Deglutition and Its Disorders.* San Diego, CA: Singular Publishing; 1997:451.

Swallowing Therapy and Aspiration

It is to be expected that patients recovering from swallowing disorders will experience occasional aspiration. Using the compensatory swallow maneuvers and the postural techniques reviewed in this chapter can be efficacious in reducing aspiration events and preventing aspiration pneumonia. This may be a patient-by-patient experience, given that patients rarely present with a uniform case history and medical status. A summary of the nonsurgical methods to reduce or eliminate aspiration is shown in Table 6–10. Caution should be used by the clinician when applying these approaches.

Table 6–10. **Nonsurgical Methods for Controlling Aspiration**

1. *Oral motor exercises:*
   Lip seal
   Tongue retraction and elevation
   Tongue strengthening

2. *Head position maneuvers:*
   Chin tuck
   Head lift
   Rotating head to side of lesion in pharyngeal or vocal fold paresis

3. *Postural compensation techniques:*
   Sitting upright
   Lying on side

4. *Swallowing retraining:*
   Supraglottic swallow
   Super-supraglottic swallow
   Mendelsohn maneuver
   Multiple swallows
   Frequent throat clearing

5. *Diet modification:*
   Change in bolus size
   Change in food consistencies
   Changes in temperature and taste

6. *Nonoral diet (NPO)*

Source: Adapted and revised from Pou AM, Carrau RL. Chapter 23. Carrau RL, Murry T, eds. *Comprehensive Management of Swallowing Disorders.* San Diego, CA: Singular Publishing; 1999:157, Table 23–1.

A more comprehensive list summarizing the nonsurgical interventions for dysphagia is shown in Table 6–11. These data, taken from a recent public access manuscript by Pauloski,[48] offer range of motion, compensatory, and direct techniques for the management of various swallow-related disorders.

> Groher[53] reported that the variables that separate those who develop aspiration pneumonia from those who do not remain speculative.

To be sure, many more people, with or without swallowing problems, aspirate compared to those who develop aspiration pneumonia. Factors such as prior history of aspiration, mobility, age, state of consciousness, respiration status, upper airway reflexes, instrumental results of swallow evaluation, and the integrity of the lower airway protective mechanism all contribute to prevention of aspiration pneumonia. Prospective studies in which swallow safety is compromised in either postsurgical cases of head and neck cancer, post-CVA, or progressive neurological diseases are ethically questionable. Clinical judgment suggests that given a decreased medical condition and signs of aspiration, one may ultimately expect aspiration pneumonia and therefore should do everything possible to maintain swallow safety.

Table 6–11. **Swallowing Disorders Most Often Reported for Treated Head and Neck Cancer Patients Are Listed with Associated Postures, Maneuvers, Exercises, and Other Interventions That May Be Effective in Alleviating the Disorder or Reducing Its Negative Impact on Swallowing**

Swallow-Related Disorder	Possible Interventions
Reduced mouth opening	Jaw ROM exercises
Reduced tongue control/shaping	Chin down posture SSG swallow Tongue ROM exercises Bolus manipulation exercises Tongue strengthening exercises
Reduced vertical tongue movement	Tongue ROM exercises Maxillary reshaping prosthesis

Table 6–11. continued

Swallow-Related Disorder	Possible Interventions
Reduced anterior-posterior tongue movement	Head back posture Multiple swallows Alternate liquids and solids Tongue ROM exercises Bolus manipulation exercises Maxillary reshaping prosthesis
Reduced tongue strength	Effortful swallow Tongue strengthening exercises
Delayed pharyngeal swallow	Chin down posture Super-Supraglottic Swallow (SSG) Thermal/tactile stimulation
Reduced tongue base retraction	Chin down posture Effortful swallow SSG swallow Tongue hold maneuver Mendelsohn maneuver Tongue ROM exercises Gargle/yawn for tongue base retraction
Reduced laryngeal vestibule closure	Chin down posture SSG swallow Effortful swallow Mendelsohn maneuver Gargle/yawn for tongue base retraction
Reduced laryngeal elevation	Mendelsohn maneuver Chin down posture SSG swallow Effortful swallow Laryngeal ROM exercises Shaker exercise
Reduced glottic closure	Head rotation to weaker side SSG swallow Thickened liquids Vocal fold adduction exercises
Reduced pharyngeal constriction/clearance	Head rotation to weaker side Effortful swallow Mendelsohn maneuver Multiple swallows Alternate liquids and solids Gargle/yawn for tongue base retraction Tongue hold maneuver
Reduced/impaired cricopharyngeal opening	Head rotation to weaker side Mendelsohn maneuver Shaker exercise Effortful swallow

Source: From Pauloski B. *Rehabilitation of dysphagia following head and neck cancer.* NIH Public Access Manuscript. 2009 Nov 1; Table 1.

SUMMARY

Swallowing therapy is now commonly provided for acute and chronic swallowing disorders resulting from surgical excisions of tumors in the head and neck regions, neuromuscular disorders, neurological disorders, and debilitation associated with a cohort of aging conditions that affect the nerves and muscles involved in swallowing. Compensatory therapies continue to evolve and be tested in both normal subjects and in patients who can tolerate the various testing formats. Procedures such as LSVT and EMST, treatments that were developed for nonswallowing disorders, are now being explored in patients with swallowing disorders. The application of neuroplastic principles such as "use it or lose it," transference, repetition, and intensity in the treatment process offer an improved rationale for the nonsurgical treatment of swallowing. Such rationale may provide a basis for developing additional evidence for continued exploration of methods to improve swallow safety and quality of life in patients with dysphagia.

STUDY QUESTIONS

1. Exercises for patients with upper motor neuron injury might include:
   A. Lip strength
   B. Tongue strength
   C. Mendelsohn maneuver
   D. All of the above

2. Finger occlusion of the fenestrated tracheostomy tube:
   A. Prevents breathing
   B. Increases esophageal pressure
   C. Decreases esophageal pressure
   D. Prevents aspiration during swallowing

3. The use of the chin tuck during swallowing:
   A. Increases speed of bolus to the oropharynx
   B. Prevents aspiration and penetration
   C. Reduces the speed of bolus transit in the oral cavity
   D. Reduces the distance between the thyroid cartilage and hyoid bone

4. The primary outcome from studies using the Shaker exercise is:
   A. Significant increase in the anterior excursion of the larynx
   B. Reduced opening of the upper esophageal sphincter
   C. Increase in the speed of bolus transport to the upper esophageal sphincter
   D. No improvement in the types of liquid patients with UES difficulty could swallow

DISCUSSION QUESTIONS

1. Most swallowing exercises target a specific organ or posture. Martin-Harris[54] suggests that swallowing is a parallel process, with glottic closure beginning when the bolus has not yet reached the anterior facial arch. Write a rationale for studying one of the exercises in Table 6–1, 6–2, or 6–3. Discuss the exercise within the framework of parallel processing and suggest how that exercise can improve swallowing and how it will interact and improve the other phases of swallowing.

2. Muscle strength training is a relatively new method of treatment used by SLPs to improve various swallowing and communication conditions and disorders. Most of the studies to date have focused on strengthening the respiratory or phonatory systems. Design a muscle strength training protocol that might be useful for strengthening either the lips or tongue to improve oral phase swallowing disorders.

REFERENCES

1. McHorney CA, Robbins J, Lomax K, et al. The SWAL-QOL and SWOL-CARE outcomes tool for oropharyngeal dysphagia in adults. III. Documentation of reliability and validity. *Dysphagia*. 2002;17(2):97–114.
2. Lazarus CL, Logemann JA, Huang C, Rademaker AW. Effects of two types of tongue strengthening exercises in young normals. *Folia Phoniatri Logop*. 2003;55:199–205.

3. Robbins J, Gangnon RE, Theis SM, Kays SA, Hewitt AL, Hind JA. The effects of lingual exercise on swallowing in older adults. *J Am Geriatric Soc.* 2005;53:1483–1489.

4. Robbins J, Kays SA, Gangnon RE, et al. The effects of lingual exercise in stroke patients with dysphagia. *Arch Phys Med Rehab.* 2007 Feb;88(2):150–158.

5. Clark HM, O'Brien K, Calleja A, Newcomb CS. Effects of directional exercises on lingual strength. *J Speech Lang Hear Res.* 2009;52:1034–1047.

6. Clark HM. Clinical decision making and oral motor treatments. *ASHA Leader.* 2005 Aug 9;34–35.

7. Clark HM. Neuromuscular treatments for speech and swallowing: a tutorial. *Am J Speech-Lang Path.* 2003;12(4):400–415.

8. Martin-Harris B, Brodsky MB, Michel Y, Lee FS, Walters B. Delayed initiation of the pharyngeal swallow: normal variability in adult swallows. *J Speech Lang Hear Res.* 2007;50:585–594.

9. Ramig L, Shapiro S, Countryman S, et al. Intensive voice treatment (LSVT) for individuals with Parkinson's disease: a two-year follow up. *NCVS Status Report.* 1999;14:131–140.

10. Sharkawi AE, Ramig L, Logemann JA, et al. Swallowing and voice effects of Lee Silverman Voice Treatment (LSVT): a pilot study. *J Neurol Neurosurg Psychiatry.* 2002;72:31–36.

11. Fox CM, Ramig LO, Ciucci MR, Sapir S, McFarland DH, Farley BG. The science and practice of LSVT/LOUD: neural plasticity-principled approach to treating individuals with Parkinson disease and other neurological disorders. *Semin Speech Lang.* 2006 Nov;27(4):283–299.

12. Leonard R, Kendall K. *Dysphagia Assessment and Treatment Planning: A Team Approach.* San Diego, CA: Singular Publishing; 1988:187–191.

13. *Evidence Report/Technology Assessment No. 8: Diagnosis and Treatment of Swallowing Disorders (Dysphagia) in Acute Care Stroke Patients.* Rockville, MD: US Department of Health and Human Services, Agency for Healthcare Research and Quality; 1999 July. AHCPR Pub. 99-E024.

14. Logemann JA. Therapy for oropharyngeal swallowing disorders. In Perlman AL, Schulze-Delrieu K, eds. *Deglutition and Its Disorders.* San Diego, CA: Singular Publishing; 1997:451–455.

15. Lazarus C, Logemann JA, Song CW, Rademaker AW, Kahrilas PJ. Effects of voluntary maneuvers on tongue base function for swallowing. *Folia Phoniatri Logop.* 2002;54(4):171–176.

16. Pauloski BR, Rademaker AW, Logemann JA, et al. Surgical variables affecting swallowing in patients treated for oral/oropharyngeal cancer. *Head Neck.* 2004 Jul;26(7):625–636.

17. Sonies BC. Remediation challenges in treating dysphagia post head/neck cancer: a problem oriented approach. *Clin Commun Dis.* 1993;3:21–26.

18. Shaker R, Kern M, Bardan F, et al. Augmentation of deglutive upper esophageal sphincter opening of the elderly by exercise. *Am J Physiol.* 1997;272(6):1518–1522.

19. Shaker R, Easterling C, Kern M, et al. Rehabilitation of swallowing by exercise in tube-fed patients with pharyngeal dysphagia secondary to abnormal UES opening. *Gastroenterology.* 2002;122(5):1314–1321.

20. Medda BK, Kern M, Ren J, et al. Relative contribution of various protective mechanisms for prevention of aspiration during swallowing. *Am J Gastrointest Liver Physiolog.* 2003;284(6):933–939.

21. White K, Easterling C, Roberts N, Wertsch J, Shaker R. Fatigue analysis before and after Shaker exercise: physiologic tool for exercise design. *Dysphagia.* 2008;23:385–391.

22. Shaker R, Antonik S. The Shaker Exercise. *US Gastroenterology Review.* 2006;1:19–20.

23. Easterling C, Grande B, Kern M, Sears K, Shaker R. Attaining and maintaining isometric and isokinetic goals of the Shaker exercise. *Dysphagia.* 2005;20:133–138.

24. Mepani R, Antonik S, Massey B, et al. Augmentation of deglutitive thyrohyoid muscle shortening by the Shaker exercise. *Dysphagia.* 2009;24:26–31.

25. Burkhead L, Sapienza C, Rosenbek J. Strength-training exercise in dysphagia rehabilitation: principles, procedures, and directions for future research. *Dysphagia.* 2007;22:251–265.

26. Rosenbek JA, Robbins J, Willford WO, et al. Comparing treatment intensities of tactile-thermal application. *Dysphagia.* 1998;13:1–9.

27. Regan J, Walshe M, Tobin WO. Immediate effects of thermal tactile stimulation on timing of swallow in idiopathic Parkinson's disease. *Dysphagia.* 2010 Sep;25(3):207–215.

28. Sciortino K, Liss JM, Case JL, Gerritsen KG, Katz RC. Effects of mechanical, cold, gustatory and combined stimulation to the human anterior faucial arches. *Dysphagia.* 2003;18:16–26.

29. Bove M, Mansson I, Eliasson I. Thermal oral-pharyngeal stimulation and elicitation of swallowing. *Acta Otolaryngologica.* 1998;118:728–731.

30. Logemann JA, Pauloski BR, Colangelo L, Lazarus C, Fujiu M. The effects of sour bolus on oropharyngeal swallowing measures in patients with neurogenic dysphagia. *J Speech Hear Res.* 1995;38:556–563.

31. Bisch EM, Logemann JA, Rademaker AW, Kahrilas PJ, Lazarus CL. Pharyngeal effects of bolus volume, viscosity and temperature in patients with dysphagia resulting from neurologic impairment and in normal subjects. *J Speech Hear Res.* 1994;37:1041–1049.

32. Bulow M, Olsson R, Ekberg O. Videoradiographic analysis of how carbonated thin liquids and thickened liquids affect the physiology of swallowing in subjects with aspiration on thin liquids. *Acta Radiological.* 2003;44:366–372.

33. Kim J, Sapienza CM. Implications of expiratory muscle strength training for rehabilitation of the elderly. Tutorial. *J Rehab Res Dev.* 2005;42(2):211–224.

34. Baker S, Davenport P, Sapienza CM. Examination of strength training and detraining effects in expiratory muscles. *J Speech Hear Lang Res.* 2005;48:1325–1333.

35. Chiara T, Martin D, Sapienza CM. Expiratory muscle strength training: speech production outcomes in participants

with multiple sclerosis. *Neurohabil Neural Repair*. 2007;21: 239–249.

36. Wheeler-Hegland KM, Rosenbek JC, Sapienza CM. Submental EMG and hyoid movement during Mendelsohn maneuver, effort swallow and expiratory muscle strength training. *J Speech Lang Hear Res*. 2008;51:1072–1087.

37. Grill WM, Foreman R, Ludlow CL, Buller J. Emerging clinical applications: What wonders the future brings. *J Rehab Res Dev*. 2001;38:641–653.

38. Clark H, Lazarus C, Arvedson J, Schooling T, Frymark T. Evidenced-based systematic review: effects of neuromuscular electrical stimulation on swallowing and neural activation. *Am J Speech-Lang Path*. 2009;8:361–375.

39. Ludlow CL. Electrical neuromuscular stimulation in dysphagia: current status. *Curr Opin Otolaryngol Head Neck Surg*. 2010 Jun;18(3):159–164.

40. Burnett TA, Mann EA, Cornell SA, Ludlow CL. Laryngeal elevation achieved by neuromuscular stimulation at rest. *J Appl Physiol*. 2003;94:128–134.

41. Freed ML, Freed L, Chatburn RL, Christian M. Electrical stimulation for swallowing disorders caused by stroke. *Respiratory Care*. 2001;46:466–474.

42. Bulow M, Speyer R, Baijens L, et al. Neuromuscular electrical stimulation (NMES) in stroke patients with oral and pharyngeal dysfunction. *Dysphagia*. 2008;23:302–309.

43. Lin PH, Hsiao TY, Chang YC, et al. Effects of functional electrical stimulation on dysphagia caused by radiation therapy in patients with nasopharyngeal carcinoma. *Support Care Cancer*. 2011 Jan;19(1):91–99.

44. Ogura J, Kawasaki M, Takenouchi S. Neurophysiologic observations on the adaptive mechanism of deglutition. *Ann Otol Rhinol Laryngol*. 1964;73:1062–1081.

45. Lazarus CL, Logemann JA, Song CW, et al. Effects of voluntary' maneuvers on tongue base function for swallowing. *Folia Phoniatr Logop*. 2002;54:171–176.

46. Ding R, Larson CR, Logemann JA, Rademaker AW. Surface electromyographic and electroglottographic studies in normal subjects under two swallow conditions: normal and during the Mendelsohn maneuver. *Dysphagia*. 2002;17:1–12.

47. Doeltgen S, Witte U, Gumbley F, Huckabee M. Evaluation of manometric measures during tongue-hold swallows. *Am J Speech-Lang Path*. 2009;18:65–73.

48. Pauloski B. *Rehabilitation of dysphagia following head and neck cancer*. NIH Public Access Manuscript. 2009 Nov 1.

49. Logemann JA, Gensler G, Robbins J, et al. A randomized study of three interventions for aspiration of thin liquids in patients with dementia or Parkinson's disease. *J Speech Lang Hear Res*. 2009;51:173–183.

50. Lewin JS, Hebert TM, Putnam JB Jr, DuBrow RA. Experience with the chin tuck maneuver in postesophagectomy aspirators. *Dysphagia*. 2001;16(3):216–219.

51. Bulow M, Olsson R, Ekberg O. Videomanometric analysis of supraglottic swallow, effortful swallow and chin tuck in patients with pharyngeal dysfunction. *Dysphagia*. 2001; 16(3):190–195.

52. Logemann JA, Gensler G, Robbins J, et al. A randomised study of three interventions for aspiration of thin liquids in patients with dementia and Parkinson's disease. *J Speech Lang Hear Res*. 2008;51:173–183.

53. Groher M. Risks and benefits of oral feeding. *Dysphagia*. 1994;9:233–235.

54. Martin-Harris B, Michal Y, Castell DO. Physiologic model of oropharyngeal swallowing revisited. *Otolaryngol Head Neck Surg*. 2005;133:234–240.

55. Groher ME. Bolus management and aspiration pneumonia in patients with pseudo-bulbar dysphagia. *Dysphagia*. 1987;1:215–216.

56. Kasprison AT, Clumeck H, Nino-Morcia M. The efficacy of rehabilitative management of dysphagia. *Dysphagia*. 1989;4:48–52.

57. Martens L, Cameron T, Simonsen M. Effects of a multidisciplinary management program on neurologically impaired patients with dysphagia. *Dysphagia*. 1990;5:147–151.

58. DePippo KL, Holas MA, Reding MJ, Mandel FS, Lesser ML. Dysphagia therapy following stroke: a controlled trial. *Neurology*. 1994;44:1655–1660.

59. O'Kroy JA, Coast JR. Effects of flow and resistive training on respiratory muscle endurance and strength. *Respiration*. 1993;60(5):279–283.

60. Suzuki KS, Sato M, Okubo T. Expiratory muscle training and sensation of respiratory effort during exercise in normal subjects. *Thorax*. 1995;50(4):366–370.

61. Cerny FJ, Panzarella K, Stathopoulos ET. Expiratory muscles conditioning in hypotonic children with low vocal intensity levels. *J Med Speech Lang Pathol*. 1997;5:141–152.

62. Smeltzer SC, Lavietes MH, Cook SD. Expiratory training in multiple sclerosis. *Arch Phys Med Rehabil*. 1996;77(9): 909–912.

63. Gosselink R, Kovacs L, Ketelaer P, Carton H, Decramer M. Respiratory muscle weakness and respiratory muscle training in severely disabled multiple sclerosis patients. *Arch Phys Med Rehabil*. 2000;81(6):747–751.

64. Hoffman-Ruddy B. Expiratory pressure threshold training in high-risk performers [dissertation]. Gainesville (FL): University of Florida; 2003.

65. Sapienza CM, Davenport PW, Martin AD. Expiratory muscle training increases pressure support in high school band students. *J Voice*. 2002;16(4):495–501.

66. Baker SE. Expiratory muscle strength training and detraining: effects on speech and cough production [dissertation]. Gainesville (FL): University of Florida; 2003.

67. Salem AF, Rosenbek JC, Davenport P, Shrivastav R, Hoffman-Ruddy B, Okun MS, Sapienza CM. Expiratory muscle strength training in patients with idiopathic Parkinson's disease [poster session]. Conference on Motor Speech: Motor Speech Disorders; 2004 March 18–24; Albuquerque, New Mexico.

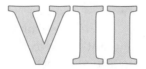

VII

Prosthetic Management of Swallowing Disorders

CHAPTER OUTLINE

    I. INTRODUCTION
    II. ORAL PROSTHODONTICS AND DENTURES
    III. PALATE LOWERING PROSTHESES
    IV. SOFT PALATE PROSTHESES
    V. LINGUAL PROSTHESES
    VI. SPEAKING VALVES
    VII. PHYSICAL AND ENVIRONMENTAL ADJUSTMENTS
    VIII. SUMMARY
    IX. STUDY QUESTIONS
    X. DISCUSSION QUESTION
    XI. REFERENCES

INTRODUCTION

Oral prosthodontics is the science of providing suitable substitutes for missing, lost, or removed structures in the oral cavity. Prostheses are used for two main etiological factors: (1) congenital defects and (2) acquired defects. Congenital oral defects include cleft lip, cleft palate, cleft mandible, and bifid uvula. Acquired oral defects are those primarily related to surgical treatment of diseases, traumas, pathologies, or burns.

> Oral prosthodontics takes into account direct swallowing management, including prosthetic management with dental, palatal, or tongue prostheses, medical therapy, and environmental adjustments such as proper types of utensils to improve and control feeding when a prosthesis is required.

As with other methods for treating dysphagia, bolus size, consistency, and viscosity must be considered in patients who are fitted with a prosthetic appliance after surgery or trauma to the head and neck organs. This chapter focuses on swallowing disorders related to acquired defects primarily as a result of surgery as opposed to congenital defects, which are discussed in Chapter 9.

Many acquired defects can be managed through surgery, but where surgical reconstruction is not feasible, prosthetic rehabilitation becomes the primary treatment. The prosthetics team is led by a **prosthodontist,** with input from the head and neck surgeon and often in conjunction with the speech-language pathologist (SLP).

> The role of the SLP is to assess function during and following fitting of the prosthesis.

Keep in mind that there may be several fittings, and the SLP may want to assess both speech and swallowing each time an adjustment to the prosthesis is made. Pressure measurement using the Iowa Oral Performance Instrument (IOPI) may be useful to select the ideal location and bulk of the prosthetic appliance to fit the patient's needs for both speech and swallowing. Once a device is fitted, the SLP may need to develop an exercise program for speech and swallowing to maximize the value of the prosthesis for both functions.

Prosthetic management in the oral cavity has long been advocated to improve speech intelligibility following limited or extensive surgery to the mandible, maxilla, tongue, or palate. Prosthetic appliances also serve to improve the oral preparatory and oral phases of swallowing through improvement of chewing, bolus formation, decreasing the tongue-palate distance, and increasing the propulsive pressure on the bolus.

> The incidence and severity of speech and swallowing problems following surgery is related to the size and location of the tumor, the structures involved in the surgery, radiation or chemotherapy and the amount of mobile tissue remaining.

Suarez-Conqueiro et al[1] reported that in large tumors (cancer stages III and IV), speech problems were reported in 64% and swallowing problems were reported in 75% of patients. As might be expected, quality of life changes significantly if there are both speech and swallowing problems associated with the cancer treatment. Following successful prosthetic management, both speech and swallowing functions can be expected to improve. Quality of life measures such as the SWAL-QOL suggest that oral cancer problems lead to significant quality of life changes, and as the tongue is one of the most important structures to manipulate and prepare the bolus for entrance into the esophagus, considerable effort should be made to manage the residual tongue in order to improve the swallow and thus the quality of life.[2]

ORAL PROSTHODONTICS AND DENTURES

Adequate dentition may be the difference between a liquid-only diet and a diet of liquids and food consistencies. Although many patients can manage more than liquid without normal dentition or a prosthetic dental appliance, a properly fitted dental prosthesis may speed up a meal or increase the number of food consistencies that a person can swallow safely. The **oral prosthesis** may consist of dentures only or may be a combined dental and palatal reshaping prosthesis. A **palatal reshaping prosthesis** like that shown in Figure 7–1 is used to create a new contour of the oral cavity, lower the palatal vault, and provide a framework for dentition. It creates a contact point or contact area with the tongue and, together, they provide the necessary propulsion for thickened liquids and foods. Dentures may be incorporated into the palatal reshaping prosthesis.

Dentures may also be fitted without a palatal shaping prosthesis, depending on whether major structures were removed during surgery. Dentures may be of 1 or 2 types: (1) fixed or implanted dentures or (2) movable dentures. Although the former are significantly more expensive, they offer greater stability than removable dentures, which eventually may not fit properly due to a change in tissue structure, damage to the denture, or atrophy of tissue that may occur after radiation therapy or chemotherapy. Implantable dentures, however, may not be an option in all patients due to surgical removal of tissue or bone associated with diseases.

The use of teeth to grind food to a bolus consistency is a major factor in increasing the types of food one can swallow. A full upper and lower dental arch ensures improved mastication even when oral

muscles are weak or partially missing following oral cancer surgery.

> Studies have shown that a proper denture aids in modifying diet consistencies, increases the rate of eating, and helps to improve the efficiency of tongue motion during swallowing.[3,4,5]

In general, the patients with more advanced cancers or those treated with surgery followed by adjuvant radiation therapy will undergo longer periods of rehabilitation and have more difficulty swallowing than those with early stage tumors or who do not undergo radiation treatment.

Dental implants have led to improved subjective assessments, such as appearance, followed by masticatory improvement and denture retention. However, functional impairment cannot be fully compensated by implant-supported prosthodontic reconstructions, but such treatment contributes essentially to general well-being and relief of disease-related social restrictions.[6]

The use of dental implants has been questioned by several authors,[7,8] suggesting that they may be a risk factor for developing cancer. Eguia del Valle et al[7] found presence of cancer cells in the inflamed tissue surrounding osseointegrated dental implants. Kwok et al[8] reported 3 cases of cancer in patients with dental implants.

Teoh et al[9] measured functional outcomes using 4 individual assessments (nutritional status, swallowing, masticatory performance, and speech) and 1 measure that combined the information from these assessments, the global measure of functional outcome (GMFO), in 2 groups of patients who had undergone mandibular resection and reconstruction for head and neck cancer with at least 6 months of postoperative convalescence. Statistical analyses were used to compare the baseline characteristics and functional outcomes between the group that had received prosthetic intervention and the group that did not. The group that received prosthetic intervention had significantly better GMFO scores than the comparison group. Use of a prosthesis was still associated with GMFO after controlling for other significant factors such as **xerostomia**,

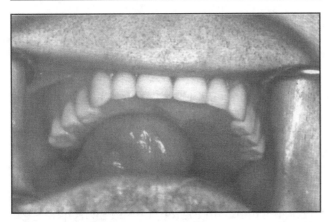

Figure 7–1. Prosthesis for palatal augmentation with anterior dental prosthesis attached to permanent dentition.

number of remaining mandibular teeth, number of tooth-to-tooth contacts, type of reconstruction, flap interference, and tongue defect. Patients who had fewer mandibular teeth and received a smaller prosthesis had better overall outcome than patients who received a larger prosthesis. Because the use of dental implants is relatively new, it might be expected that complications related to the implants such as necrosis and dislocation occur following radiation. Nonetheless, one might expect that quality of life remains a good reason to continue to use dental implants when chewing is not possible otherwise.

PALATE LOWERING PROSTHESES

Palate lowering prostheses are devices that help to complement the palatal vault. They are similar to palate reshaping prostheses, but generally do not include dentures. They are sometimes referred to as maxillary prostheses. They help to increase bolus transit to the posterior oral cavity and increase tongue palate contact pressures to propel the bolus into the oropharynx. The hard palate lowering prosthesis is designed by the maxillofacial prosthodontist along with the help of the SLP to maximize both speech and the oral preparatory and oral phases of swallowing.[10]

> Prosthetic restoration for swallowing disorders related to hard palate defects should begin early after surgery with a temporary obturating prosthesis, often inserted in the operating room or shortly thereafter.

The hard palate prosthesis is enhanced if the surgical device is created with the intention to fit a temporary obturator of this type. After 5 to 7 days, the surgical obturator is removed, remodeled, and finally constructed to fit the surgical defect. The obturator restores oronasal separation facilitation of oral feeding and usually improves speech intelligibility. Restoring the oronasal separation reduces the likelihood of wound infection from residual food particles collecting in spaces above the maxillary arch and helps to prevent food from being packed into the defect by separating the oral from the nasal cavity.

The temporary palatal prosthesis may be substituted by a permanent device several months after surgery. With adequate retention and stability, the prosthesis will provide important contouring to aid the tongue in oral phase manipulation of food boluses.

More recently, various types of materials have been advanced in the treatment of hard palate defects. **Polymethylmethacrylate** and other polymer-based obturators have been developed.[11] Titanium-based obturators have also been proposed and may offer less bacteria build up than older devices.[12]

SOFT PALATE PROSTHESES

Following proper fitting of a hard or soft palate prosthesis, it is expected that the oral preparatory and oral phases of swallowing will improve. Improvement is based on shaping the oral cavity to maintain maximal control of the bolus in the oral cavity without spillage, proper mastication of the bolus, directing the bolus to the posterior oral cavity, slowing down the transit of liquids, and increasing the force of propulsion.

> **Soft palate prostheses** are designed primarily to reduce the distance between the palate and posterior tongue.

If the defect is large, the prosthesis is extended into the pharyngeal region to facilitate the sphincteric action of the lateral and posterior pharyngeal wall, as shown in Figure 7–2. Exercises to complement prosthetic restoration are presented in Chapter 6.

Restoration of the soft palate for improved swallowing is recommended when there are large defects involving the posterior border of the soft palate, when there is a nonfunctional band of tissue posteriorly in the soft palate, or when lateral pharyngeal defects affect sphincteric action of the palate in conjunction with the tongue and pharynx.

The issue of velopharyngeal incompetence has typically been addressed using the soft palate

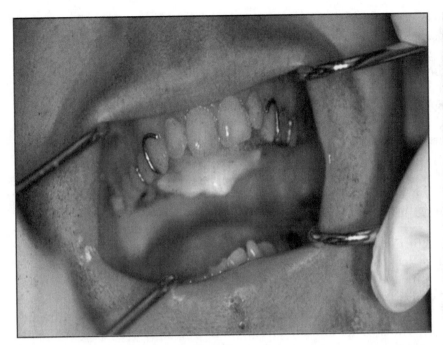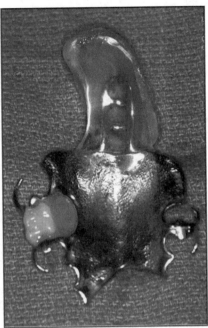

Figure 7–2. Soft palate prosthesis with obturator extending posteriorly into the pharyngeal area to improve contact during swallowing.

prosthesis. This prosthesis pushes or lifts the palate posteriorly to promote contact of the soft palate with the posterior and lateral pharyngeal walls. Use of this device requires adaptation by the patient, because initially they may feel discomfort or the prosthesis may stimulate the gag reflex. Shifman and colleagues[13] developed a speech and swallowing prosthesis for the management of velopharyngeal incompetence that relies on nasopharyngeal obturation instead of palatal elevation. Although the device was developed primarily for speech improvement, it may also aid in swallowing. Other newer devices have also been proposed, although they are mostly for improvement of speech. The nasal speaking valve (NSV) developed by Suwaki and colleagues[14,15] is a valve that is placed through the nose to reduce the air flow into the nose and increase oral pressure. Patients report that it is less unpleasant than oral obturators such as a palatal lift, and it provides improvement in nasal oral separation. The NSV can also be worn for a longer period of time. Because it is inserted into the nostrils (it relies on clips to hold it in place), this device can easily be used by edentulous patients.

A systematic review of speech and swallowing following surgical treatment of advanced oral and oropharyngeal carcinoma by Kreeft et al[16] found that the use of palatal obturators generally improved speech production to a level of intelligible speech in most settings, but swallowing deficits remain despite even the most advanced and customized devices.

LINGUAL PROSTHESES

The tongue is the primary means of transporting foods and liquids to the oropharynx. When the tongue is removed surgically, either partially or completely, the patient relies on dietary modifications (various liquid consistencies), modified postures (head tilted back), or, most often, a feeding tube to get the food into the stomach.

Partial or total surgery of the tongue (**glossectomy**) results in significant swallowing as well as speech disorders. Total glossectomy results in a large oral cavity where pooling of saliva and liquids can occur. This may ultimately cause postswallow aspiration. Leonard and Gillis[17] presented results of improved control of food bolus using a tongue prosthesis. Since then, several studies have shown that partial or total glossectomy results in moderate to severe articulation and swallowing disorders over a long period of time.[18,19,20] Although speech may be intelligible, articulation disorders persist and reflect the degree of tongue removed. Prosthethic treatment for the tongue may also improve swallowing, but problems often remain severe following surgery for oral and oropharyngeal cancer even with prosthetic management.

Table 7–1 lists the goals of prosthetic rehabilitation after total glossectomy. All of these factors play a role in recovery of swallowing function. A properly fitted tongue prosthesis reduces the oral cavity size, thus reducing the possibility of retained secretions that might later be aspirated. The SLP must help direct foods and liquids initially to gain the maximum benefit. This may require use of a syringe to place food posteriorly or may involve having the patient monitor placement by eating in front of a mirror.

Table 7–2 lists adjunctive techniques used to treat patients following partial glossectomy. The patient undergoing partial or total glossectomy will require management from many members of the treatment team, including those who can develop feeding devices to aid in the oral preparatory and oral phases of swallowing.

Table 7–1. Major Goals in Prosthetic Rehabilitation after Total Glossectomy

1. To reduce the size of the oral cavity, which will minimize the degree of pooling of saliva and improve resonance.
2. To develop surface contact with the surrounding structures during speech and swallowing.
3. To protect the underlying fragile mucosa.
4. To direct the food bolus into the oropharynx.
5. To improve appearance and psychosocial adjustment.

Source: Adapted from Zaki HS. Chapter 36. In: Carrau RL, Murry T, eds. *Comprehensive Management of Swallowing Disorders.* San Diego, CA: Plural Publishing. 2006:252.

SPEAKING VALVES

A valve that fits over a tracheotomy tube to improve speech articulation may also be considered a prosthetic device for swallowing. These valves, called **speaking valves**, have been in existence for well over 25 years, and were initially used to improve articulation in patients with a tracheotomy tube. The one-way valves open during inhalation but close during exhalation. In this way, air is directed past the vocal folds for voice production. One-way valves help the tracheotomized patient by providing a more natural approximation of the flow of air through the respiratory system.

It is well-known that decannulation or even tracheostomy tube occlusion using a finger will enhance the swallowing function in a patient with a tracheotomy. However, this is not feasible in all patients. For swallowing, the strategy is to place an expiratory speaking valve (Figure 7–3) on the open tracheotomy tube to restore the subglottic air pressure needed during swallowing.[19] The beneficial effect of a valve strengthens the theory that subglottic air pressure is

Table 7–2. Adjunctive Treatments to Improve Swallowing Following Partial Glossectomy

1. Tilt head posteriorly if anterior-posterior tongue movement is impaired. This increases the speed of oral transit.
2. Tilt head to the side least affected to control movement of bolus.
3. Thermal stimulation (see below) may assist in activating the pharyngeal swallow by increasing sensation near the anterior faucial pillars.
4. Tongue palate contact exercises with specific placement goals may strengthen the posterior tongue movement or increase the range of posterior tongue motion.
5. Chewing exercises manipulating wet gauze or chewing gum to practice manipulating the bolus.
6. Practicing speech sounds such as /d/, /t/, /g/, and /k/ to improve range of motion of remaining structures.

Source: Adapted and updated from Gross RD, Eibling DE. Chapter 37. In: Carrau RL, Murry T, eds. *Comprehensive Management of Swallowing Disorders.* San Diego, CA: Plural Publishing. 2006:258.

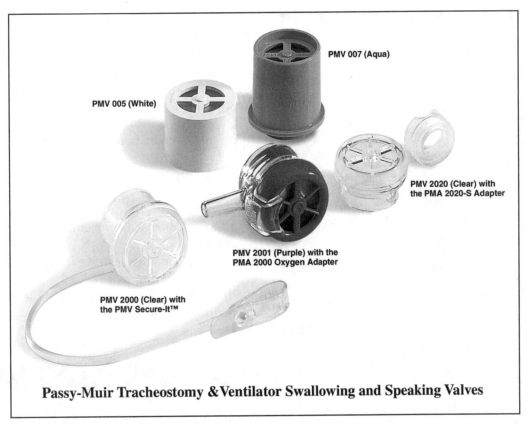

Passy-Muir Tracheostomy & Ventilator Swallowing and Speaking Valves

Figure 7–3. Passy-Muir valves. The valve fits over the open tracheotomy tube to restore subglottic pressure when talking or swallowing.

a critical factor in swallowing efficiency, probably through restoring proprioceptive cues.

A typical speaking valve allows air to enter the trachea. On expiration, the valve closes and the expired air is directed past the glottis.

> Subglottic air pressure increases, resulting in improved voice production and increased subglottic pressure for coughing and throat clearing following the swallow.

In general, speaking valves provide improvement in functional communication and swallowing.[21] However, there are contraindications that clinicians should follow when deciding on the use of a speaking valve. The major contraindications are listed in Table 7–3.

Occasionally, the SLP will encounter a patient with a tracheotomy tube in the hospital or rehabilitation center who does not have a diagnosis of dysphagia but is tracheotomized for conditions such as chronic obstructive pulmonary disease, respiratory failure following some type of surgery, or sleep apnea, to name a few. It should be remembered that even though the patient does not have a diagnosis of dysphagia, the presence of a tracheotomy may have an effect on his or her ability to swallow safely.[22,23] Data by Brady et al[24] suggest that in patients compromised for nondysphagic reasons such as chronic obstructive pulmonary disease (COPD), laryngeal penetration was a common finding but aspiration did not occur. Moreover, there was no difference in the durational measurements of swallow initiation or for the duration of the white-out phase of the swallow as observed through flexible endoscopy. Nonetheless, because penetration

Table 7–3. Contraindications for the Use of a Speaking Valve

1. Unconscious/comatose patients.
2. Severe behavior problems.
3. Severe medical instability, especially pulmonary failure.
4. Severe tracheal stenosis or edema.
5. Any airway obstruction above the tube that precludes expiration through the glottis.
6. Thick and copious secretions that persist after valve placement.
7. Foam-filled tracheotomy tube cuff (Bivona).
8. Total laryngectomy or laryngotracheal separation.
9. Insufficient passage for air around the tube, either with the cuff down or with a cuffless tube.
10. Inability to maintain adequate ventilation with cuff deflation in ventilator dependent patient.
11. Patients with cognitive disorders.
12. If valve is already placed, remove it if skin color changes.
13. Remove valve if the patient shows increased restlessness, stridor, grunting, head bobbing, or other signs of anxiousness.

was a common finding, nondysphagic patients with a tracheotomy should be considered "at risk" and their swallowing status should be assessed at regular intervals.

PHYSICAL AND ENVIRONMENTAL ADJUSTMENTS

Physical and occupational therapists play a significant role in the management of patients with swallowing disorders. Factors that may impede safe and successful nutritional management may be physical or environmental. Although the SLP does not generally manage the physical and environmental factors alone, it is incumbent on everyone who is involved with the patient's rehabilitation to see that feeding and eating are carried out in a way that ensures the patient's maximum benefit.

The following factors are of importance to achieving physical and environmental controls for the dysphagic patient:

a. Balance—chair height or proper positioning in bed
b. Head support
c. Tray positioning
d. Lighting
e. Adaptable utensils—specifically designed eating utensils
f. Hand rails in kitchen and eating areas
g. Adaptable syringes
h. Plates and bowls—not breakable, with deep retaining walls

SUMMARY

Prosthetic management offers an alternative to surgical management of defects following surgery, radiation, or chemotherapy for head and neck cancer. The goals of prosthetic management are to improve both speech and swallow function, restore esthetics to the head and neck areas, provide comfort in breathing, swallowing, and speaking, and improve the quality of life. New materials, the use of dental implants, and reduced time frames in prosthetic management all provide the clinician with tools that contribute to swallow safety. Computer-assisted models using 3-dimensional CT scans provide the maxillofacial prosthodontist with the ability to shape prostheses more accurately at the first fitting. Ultimately, preoperative modeling may allow the prosthesis to be fitted directly after surgery, thus speeding up the rehabilitation process and improving the quality of life. Although limited research exists on the materials used and on the long-term effects of preoperative prosthetic restoration modeling, there is an increased finding that with the proper assessment protocol, prosthetic restoration may be integrated into the early management of patients with head and neck cancer rather than being a delayed treatment.

STUDY QUESTIONS

1. Improvement in chewing can best be accomplished by a:
   A. Dental prosthesis
   B. Palatal prosthesis
   C. Nasal prosthesis
   D. Lingual prosthesis

2. To reduce the distance between the palate and the posterior tongue, the best prosthetic device would be a:
   A. Lingual prosthesis
   B. Hard palate prosthesis
   C. Surgical enlargement of the residual posterior tongue
   D. Soft palate prosthesis

3. Prosthetic restoration for swallowing purposes relies mainly on the:
   A. Team of head and neck surgeon and prosthodontist
   B. Team of head and neck surgeon and SLP
   C. Team of prosthodontist and SLP
   D. Team of prosthodontist and patient

4. Velopharyngeal incompetence following surgery to remove soft palate:
   A. Primarily affects speech
   B. Can be improved by nasal and palatal prostheses
   C. Cannot be improved regardless of the prosthetic device used
   D. Affects speech and swallowing and can be improved by prosthetic management

DISCUSSION QUESTION

Voice, speech, and swallowing are affected when there is major surgery for cancer in the oral cavity, oropharynx, or larynx. Discuss the differences in prioritizing management of the voice, speech, and swallowing problems in a relatively young adult (55 to 65 years old). Consider the need for a feeding tube, tracheostomy tube, and a prosthesis in this patient.

REFERENCES

1. Suarez-Conqueiro MM, Schramm A, Schoen R, et al. Speech and swallowing impairment after treatment for oral and oropharyngeal cancer. *Arch Otolaryngol Head Neck Surg.* 2008;134:1299–1304.
2. Costa-Bandeira AK, Azevedo EH, Vartanian JG, Nishimoto IN, Kowalski LP, Carrara-de Angelis E. Quality of life related to swallowing after tongue cancer treatment. *Dysphagia.* 2008;23:183–192.
3. Irish J, Sandhu N, Simpson C, et al. Quality of life in patients with maxillectomy prostheses. *Head Neck.* 2009; 31(6):813–821.
4. Liedberg B, Norten P, Owall B, Stoltze K. Masticatory and nutritional aspects of fixed and removeable partial dentures. *Clin Oral Invest.* 2004;8:11–17.
5. Hattori F. The relationship between wearing complete dentures and swallowing function in elderly individuals: a videofluorographic study. *Kokubyo Gakkai Zasshi.* 2004;71;102–111.
6. Muller F, Schadler M, Wahlmann U, Newton JP. The use of implant supported prostheses in the functional and psychosocial rehabilitation of tumor patients. *Int J Prosthodont.* 2004;17(5):512–517.
7. Eguia del Valle A, Martinez-Condo Llamosas R, López Vicente J, et al. Primary oral squamous cell carcinoma arising around dental osseointegrated implants mimicking peri-implantitis. *Med Oral Patol Oral Cir Bucal.* 2008;13:489–491.
8. Kwok J, Eyeson J, Thompson I, McGurk M. Dental implants and squamous cell carcinoma in the at risk patient: report of three cases. *Br Dent J.* 2008; 205: 543–545.
9. Teoh KH, Patel S, Hwang F, Huryn JM, Verbel D, Zlotolow IM. Prosthetic intervention in the era of microvascular reconstruction of the mandible—a retrospective analysis of functional outcome. *Int J Prosthodont.* 2005 Jan–Feb;18(1):42–54.
10. Wheeler R, Logemann JA, Rosen M. Maxillary reshaping prostheses: effectiveness in improving speech and swallowing of post surgical oral cancer patients. *J Prosthet Dent.* 1980; 43:313–319.
11. Ortegon SM, Martin JW, Lewin JS. A hollow delayed surgical obturtor for a bilateral subtotal maxillectomy patient: a clinical report. *J Prosthet Dent.* 2008;99:14–18.
12. Depprich RA, Handaschel JG, Meyer U, Meissner G. Comparison of prevalence of microorganisms on titanium and silicone/polyethyl methacrylate obturators used for rehabilitation of maxillary defects. *J Prosthet Dent.* 2008;99:400–405.
13. Shifman A, Finkelstein Y, Nachmani A, Ophir D. Speech-aid prostheses for neurogenic velopharyngeal incompetence. *J Prosthet Dent.* 2000;83(1):99–106.
14. Suwaki M, Nanba K, Ito E, Kumakkura I, Minagi S. The effect of nasal speaking valve on the speech under exper-

imental velopharyngeal incompetence condition. *J Oral Rehabil.* 2008;35(5):361–369.

15. Suwaki M, Nanba K, Ito E, Kumakkura I, Mingi S. Nasal speaking valve: a device for managing velopharyngeal incompetence. *J Oral Rehabil.* 2008 Jan;35(1):73–78.

16. Kreeft AM, Van der Molen L, Hilgers FJ, Balm AJ. Speech and swallowing after surgical treatment of advanced oral and oraopharyngeal carcinoma: a systematic review of the literature. *Eur Arch Otorhinolaryngol.* 2009;266:1687–1698.

17. Leonard R, Gillis R. Effects of a prosthetic tongue on vowel intelligibility and food management in a patient with total glossectomy. *J Speech Hear Dis.* 1982;47:25–32.

18. Reiger JM, Zalmanowitz JG, Li SY, et al. Functional outcomes after surgical reconstruction of the base of tongue using a radial forearm free flap in patients with oropharyngeal carcinoma. *Head Neck.* 2007;29:1024–1032.

19. Zuydam AC, Lowe D, Brown JS, Vaughan ED, Rogers SN. Predictors of speech and swallowing function following primary surgery for oral and oropharyngeal cancer. *Clin Otolaryngol.* 2007;30:428–437.

20. Furia CLB, Kowalski LP, Latoarre MD, et al. Speech intelligibility after glossectomy and speech rehabilitation. *Arch Otolaryngol Head Neck Surg.* 2001;127:877–883.

21. Eibling DE, Gross RD. Subglottic air pressure: a key component of swallowing efficiency. *Ann Otol Rhinol Laryngol.* 1996 Apr;105(4):253–258.

22. Logemann JA, Pauloski B, Colangelo L. Light digital occlusion of the tracheostomy tube: a pilot study of effects on aspiration and biomechanics of the swallow. *Head Neck.* 1998;20(1):52–57.

23. McCullough GH, Rosenbek JC, Wertz RT, Suiter D, McCoy SC. Defining swallowing function by age: promises and pitfalls of pigeonholing. *Top Geriatr Rehabil.* 2007;23:290–307.

24. Brady SL, Wesling M, Donzelli J. Pilot data on swallow function in nondysphagic patients requiring a tracheotomy tube. *Int J Otolaryngol.* 2009;2009. doi:10.1155/2009/610849

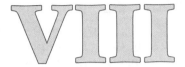

Surgical Treatment of Swallowing

CHAPTER OUTLINE

I. INTRODUCTION
II. VOCAL FOLD MEDIALIZATION
   A. Medialization of Vocal Fold Injection
   B. Laryngeal Framework Surgery
III. PALATOPEXY
IV. PHARYNGOESOPHAGEAL DILATATION
V. SURGICAL CLOSURE OF THE LARYNX
VI. GASTROSTOMY
VII. TRACHEOTOMY
VIII. TRACHEOSTOMY TUBES
   A. Expiratory Speaking Valve
   B. Fenestrated Tracheostomy Tube
   C. Decannulation
   D. Cricothyrotomy
IX. SWALLOWING FOLLOWING HEAD AND NECK CANCER
   A. Early Outcomes
   B. Late Outcomes
X. SUMMARY
XI. STUDY QUESTIONS
XII. DISCUSSION QUESTION
XIII. REFERENCES

INTRODUCTION

The goal of surgical treatment for swallowing disorders is to improve the sphincteric mechanisms of the velopalatine, glottic, or upper esophageal sphincters, or to reduce intraluminal or extraluminal obstruction. If nutritional adjustments and direct swallowing therapy fail to achieve a safe swallow, surgical therapy may be required to help the patient to compensate neuromuscular deficits by optimizing the remaining function.

> Surgical treatment for swallowing disorders upgrades dysfunctional valving mechanisms or expands the mechanical conduit of the swallowing passageway.

Enteric tubes such as a gastrostomy, jejunostomy, or gastrojejunostomy provide palliation to maintain hydration and nutrition for patients who are unable to maintain oral nutrition due to loss of organs or structures due to disease or injury. Surgical treatment of dysphagia aids swallowing rehabilitation and often results in a return to oral nutrition. Surgery should be used only as a last resort to maintain safe nutritional intake, but, if deemed necessary, the procedure should be performed expeditiously.

VOCAL FOLD MEDIALIZATION

Vocal fold medialization improves the closure of the glottis, thus improving swallowing efficiency and safety.[1,2] Medialization of the vocal fold(s) attempts to bring the vocal folds together to provide a secure closure of the vocal folds during the passage of the bolus and thus reduce the possibility of aspiration.

> It should be pointed out that vocal fold medialization may also improve phonation and thus offers the patient an opportunity to substantially improve his or her quality of life in both swallowing and vocalization.

Medialization of the vocal folds may be achieved by transendoscopic, transoral, or transcutaneous injection or by open transcervical laryngeal framework techniques.[1-9] Table 8–1 summarizes the current options for vocal fold medialization. Contraindications for medialization of a vocal fold include a compromised airway (eg, bilateral vocal fold paralysis) and/or lack of clear evidence that the dysphagia is secondary to a paralyzed vocal fold.

Medialization by Vocal Fold Injection

Vocal fold injection (VFI) is useful to medialize the vocal fold when the vocal folds are found to be atrophic, paretic, or immobile due to paralysis. There is

Table 8–1. Vocal Fold Medialization Procedures, Substances, and Origin of Substances

Injection:	
Gelfoam	Gelatin powder
Surgifoam	
Radiesse voice gel	Carbomethylcellulose
Cymetra	Cadaveric dermis
Teflon	Human engineered
Autologous tissue	
Fat	Human
Fascia	Human
Collagen	Human or animal
Hyaluronic acid gels (various)	Bacterial engineered
(GAG-polysaccharide)	Calcium hydroxyapetite
Radiesse	
Laryngeal Framework Surgery:	
Medialization laryngoplasty	
Silastic	Human engineered
Gore-Tex	Human engineered
Hydroxyapatite	Calcium hydroxyapatite
Cartilage	Human
Adjunctive procedure:	
Arytenoid adduction/ repositioning	

a good to fair prognosis of improvement or return of function following vocal fold injection. Vocal fold medialization by a lateral injection improves the glottic closure, thus improving swallowing efficiency and safety.[10–12] Figure 8–1 shows a patient with vocal fold atrophy who may be a suitable candidate for injection. The vocal folds show a transglottic gap (bowing) and thus do not approximate for phonation or swallowing.

Vocal fold injection has the advantage of avoiding open surgery, but, despite the ostensible simplicity of the procedure, it is technically demanding and may present complications such as those listed in Table 8–2.

> VFI is most effective when the arytenoid cartilage is not subluxated anteriorly and the vocal fold is in a paramedian position.

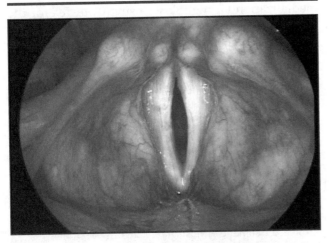

Figure 8–1. *Vocal folds of patient with bilateral atrophy prior to undergoing vocal fold injection.*

Table 8–2. Complications of Vocal Fold Injection

1. **Overinjection:** Improper vocal fold closure (early anterior contact); airway obstruction.
2. **Misplaced injection:** Inappropriate segmental glottis closure.
3. **Underinjection:** Lack of vocal fold closure.

However, when the paralyzed vocal fold is in the cadaveric position, VFI is not entirely effective in preventing aspiration. In such patients, a large posterior gap persists after VFI, even when there appears to be adequate closure of the anterior glottis. Contraindications for vocal fold injection include coagulation disorders or anticoagulation therapy, a compromised airway, and/or lack of evidence that the paralyzed vocal fold contributes to the dysphagia.

A paste made from a mixture of gelatin powder (eg, Gelfoam) and a buffered saline solution may be used as a temporary treatment of vocal fold paralysis. Injection of the vocal fold with the gelatin paste can result in improved glottic closure, and thus improved swallowing; therefore, it is an excellent, cost-effective option for the treatment of dysphagia due to vocal fold paralysis when recovery from the vocal fold paralysis is expected. **Hyaluronic acid** and acellular dermis are available in commercial preparations and are adequate, although more expensive, options. Reabsorbtion of these materials is variable, but overall they offer a medialization effect for 6 to 12 weeks.

Autologous fat injection has been used for treatment of both voice and swallowing disorders. Its reabsorbtion is extremely variable, thus making the final result unpredictable. In a typical injection, the vocal fold is overinjected, creating a convex vocal fold to account for the initial reabsorption of fat. However, the initial convexity causes early anterior contact and a posterior gap, which may increase the risk of aspiration as well as cause a temporary change in voice quality.

Teflon injection is effective in improving vocal function, particularly if the vocal fold is not too far from the midline. Teflon lost favor as an injectable material for the larynx due to the occurrence of Teflon (foreign body) granulomas. However, this is not a concern when treating patients with terminal diseases (eg, advanced lung cancer presenting with a vocal fold palsy). The complications and advantages of Teflon are shown in Table 8–3. Although Teflon injection may lead to an inflammatory foreign body reaction, it is not unique in this respect. This type of reaction can also occur with other injectable materials. Calcium hydroxyapatite is a newer injectable material that can be used as a "permanent" implant. The surgeon should be aware of an inflammatory reaction as well as the voice and airway consequences of overinjection.

Vocal fold injection has increased in popularity for correction of both voice and swallowing disorders due to the new and improved injectable materials, increased use of the procedure, and laryngological training to help in selecting the proper patients and the proper techniques for achieving maximum vocal fold approximation. Sulica et al[11] have recently outlined the current indications and complications of vocal fold injection. Although vocal fold injection augments the closure of the vocal folds, it alone may not be sufficient to curb aspiration.[13]

Laryngeal Framework Surgery

Laryngeal framework surgery should be considered the gold standard for the treatment of aspiration due to glottic insufficiency.

> Data suggest that more than 80% of patients with glottic insufficiency can be rehabilitated using these procedures and adjunct swallowing therapy.[1,2,3–8,12]

Table 8–3. **Intracordal Teflon Injection**

Problems and Complications
Difficult surgical exposure (eg, cervical spine limited range of motion)
Nonreversible
Technically challenging
Inconsistent postoperative vocal quality
Does not close posterior glottis gap
Teflon migration
Teflon granuloma
Advantages
Does not require surgery
May be performed in an office setting (selected cases)

Source: Adapted from Andrews RJ, Netterville JL, Mercati AL. Chapter 41. In: Carrau RL, Murry T, eds. *Comprehensive Management of Swallowing Disorders.* San Diego, CA: Plural Publishing; 2006:291, Table 41–1.

Medialization Laryngoplasty

Medialization laryngoplasty consists of inserting an implant, made from materials such as silicone, Gore-Tex, or calcium hydroxyapatite, between the ala of the thyroid cartilage and the vocal fold. The bulk of the implant medializes the vocal fold and, in selected cases, may even displace a subluxated arytenoid into a more anatomical position. Medialization laryngoplasty is adjustable to the patient's needs, reversible, and does not interfere with the neuromuscular recovery of the true vocal fold. With increased vocal fold closure, swallow safety is improved and diet can often be advanced. [6–8]

Table 8–4 lists the most common indications and contraindications for a medialization laryngoplasty. Table 8–5 reviews the advantages and disadvantages of medialization laryngoplasty. Table 8–6 summarizes the complications and limitations of medialization laryngoplasty. Figure 8–2 shows the typical position of the vocal fold silicone implant.

Hendricker et al[13] reported on the value of medialization laryngoplasty using Gore-Tex for the

Table 8–4. **Silastic Medialization Laryngoplasty**

Indications
Glottic incompetence secondary to unilateral vocal fold paralysis
Sacrifice of or injury to cranial nerve X during skull base surgery
Incomplete glottis closure secondary to vocal fold paresis or atrophy
Selected traumatic or postsurgical defects
Contraindications
Relative
Fibrosis resulting from laryngeal radiation
Loss of external framework (ie, vertical hemilaryngectomy)
Prior Teflon injection
Absolute
Impaired contralateral vocal fold abduction (ie, airway compromise)

Source: Andrews RJ, Netterville JL, Mercati AL. Chapter 41. In: Carrau RL, Murry T, eds. *Comprehensive Management of Swallowing Disorders.* San Diego, CA: Plural Publishing; 2006:292, Table 41–3.

Table 8–5. *Advantages of Medialization Laryngoplasty*

Advantages
Well tolerated under local anesthesia
Reversible and adjustable
Reproducible vocal results (does not interfere with mucosal wave)
Can be performed in conjunction with arytenoid adduction (closes posterior gap)
Implant does not migrate, change shape, or produce a foreign body reaction

Disadvantages
Learning curve
May extrude if ventricular mucosa is violated
Requires "open" transcervical approach
Unknown long-term effect

Source: Adapted from Andrews RJ, Netterville JL, Mercati AL. Chapter 41. In: Carrau RL, Murry T, eds. *Comprehensive Management of Swallowing Disorders.* San Diego, CA: Plural Publishing; 2006:292, Table 41–2.

Table 8–6. *Medialization Laryngoplasty: Complications and Limitations*

Undermedialization secondary to intraoperative vocal fold edema
Implant contamination from entry into the laryngeal ventricle
Intracordal hematoma
Transient stridor from postoperative edema
Overmedialization of anterior one-third of the true vocal fold resulting in a strained voice
Posterior glottis gap requiring addition of an arytenoid adduction for closure
Modest improvement with bilateral medialization for presbylaryngis

Source: Adapted from Andrews RJ, Netterville JL, Mercati AL. Chapter 41. In: Carrau RL, Murry T, eds. *Comprehensive Management of Swallowing Disorders.* San Diego, CA: Plural Publishing; 2006:294, Table 41–4.

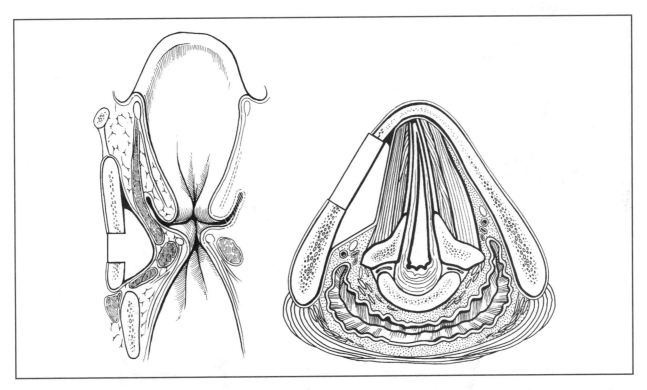

Figure 8–2. *The vocal fold silicone implant should have smooth contours that gently displace the entire paraglottic space as needed. The maximum plane of medialization can be placed at any level, either within the window or below the level of the window, as determined by the depth gauge. Here, the maximum plant of medialization is at the lower border of the window, with the implant tapered posterior to the window to prevent contact with the muscular process of the arytenoid.* Source: *Adapted from Andrews RJ, Netterville JL, Mercati AL. Chapter 41. In: Carrau RL, Murry T, eds.* Comprehensive Management of Swallowing Disorders. *San Diego, CA: Plural Publishing; 2006:294, Figure 41–2.*

treatment of aspiration. His group reviewed the results of 121 procedures for 113 patients. The main outcome measures were discontinuation of gastrostomy tubes (GTs), use or avoidance of GTs, and subjective improvement ratings. Their study included 20 patients with dysphagia who required GTs for alimentation. Eleven of 20 (55%) patients were able to discontinue G-tube use after Gore-Tex medialization laryngoplasty, and an additional 5 patients with aspiration were able to avoid need for GTs after medialization laryngoplasty. The patients with penetration also reported less penetration and improved swallow function.

Arytenoid Adduction and Medialization

Arytenoid adduction or **arytenoidopexy** are surgical procedures designed specifically to close the posterior glottis in patients with paralysis of the vocal fold.[6] The goal of the arytenoid adduction procedure is to place traction on the muscular process of the arytenoid, mimicking the activity of the lateral cricoarytenoid muscle.[4] The arytenoid is rotated internally, following an oblique axis, displacing the vocal process medially and caudally, thereby adducting the vocal fold.

In **arytenoid medialization** surgery, the body of the arytenoid is sutured in a medial position over the cricoid. Additionally, the arytenoid, which may be subluxated anteriorly (due to the paralysis of the posterior and lateral cricoarytenoid muscles that insert into its muscular process) may be pulled back and fixed in a more anatomical position. This corrects the vocal fold foreshortening and places the affected vocal fold at the same level as the "functioning" vocal fold, as shown in Figure 8–3.

Arytenoid repositioning helps address factors associated with an increased risk of aspiration, including a very wide glottal gap on maximum adduction, and helps compensate for deficits of the pharyngeal motor and sensory functions and lack of relaxation of the cricopharyngeus muscle.

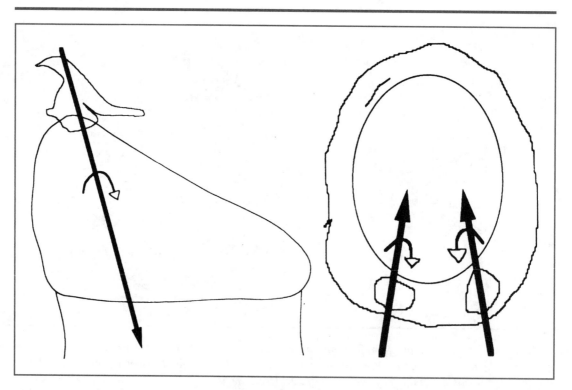

Figure 8–3. Axis of rotation in arytenoid adduction. Source: *Adapted from Newman TR, Hengesteg A, Lepage RP, Kaufman KR, Woodson GE. Three-dimensional motion of the arytenoid adduction procedure in cadaver larynges.* Ann Otol Rhinol Laryngol. *1994;103:269, with permission.*

Hypopharyngeal Pharyngoplasty

Hypopharyngeal pharyngoplasty involves the elimination of redundant piriform sinus mucosa, which is often associated with a paralyzed hypopharynx. The idea is to reduce the space and; therefore, reduce the retention of secretions in the sinus.

Cricopharyngeal Myotomy

Cricopharyngeal (CP) myotomy should be considered for patients with incomplete upper esophageal sphincter (UES) segment relaxation or abnormal muscular contractions during the relaxation period of the swallow. Common clinical scenarios include patients with laryngeal paralysis due to pathology of the central nervous system or proximal vagus nerve, which also produces pharyngeal motor or sensory deficits, or patients with Zenker diverticulum. Pharyngeal propulsion in patients presenting with a brain stem stroke or a high vagal paralysis (proximal lesion) is often inadequate to propel the bolus past a dysfunctional cricopharyngeal sphincter.[9,10] This leads to pharyngeal "pooling" of the swallowed material and spillage over the arytenoids/aryepiglottic folds into an insensate larynx ("post-swallow" aspiration). In such patients, restoration of glottic closure may not be sufficient to correct the dysphagia and aspiration.

Patients with Zenker diverticulum present with a dysfunctional opening of the UES and accumulation of secretions and food in the diverticulum.[14–16] These secretions can be regurgitated and aspirated. Transoral cricopharyngeal myotomy offers the advantage of avoiding a cervical scar and diminishing the possibility of injuring the RLN.[17]

CP myotomy is a useful adjunct to vocal fold medialization. Table 8–7 presents the common indications and Table 8–8 presents the pitfalls and complications of this procedure. CP myotomy is contraindicated in patients with significant gastropharyngeal reflux. In addition, patients with poor pharyngeal propulsion do not benefit from a CP myotomy.[18] Alternatively, a botulinum toxin injection (Botox) to the cricopharyngeus muscle may provide a "medical myotomy" and may confirm the diagnosis of CP spasm.[19,20]

Table 8–7. Cricopharyngeal Myotomy

Indications
Dysphagia secondary to
Central nervous system disorders
Peripheral nervous system disorders
Vagal injury (laryngeal/pharyngeal paralysis)
Diabetic/peripheral neuropathy
Muscular disease
Oculopharyngeal dystrophy
Steinert myotonic dystrophy
Polymyositis
Myasthenia gravis
Hyperthyroidism/hypothyroidism
Postsurgical
Total laryngectomy
Oral cavity/oropharyngeal resection
Zenker diverticulum
Cricopharyngeal achalasia
Contraindications
Severe weakness of the pharyngeal muscles (unable to propel bolus)
Severe/uncontrolled GERD
Pharyngeal varices
Post–bilateral neck injections
Thoracic outlet syndrome

Source: Adapted from Pou A. Chapter 43. In: Carrau RL, Murry T, eds. *Comprehensive Management of Swallowing Disorders.* San Diego, CA: Plural Publishing; 2006:300, Table 43–1.

Table 8–8. Cricopharyngeal Myotomy: Pitfalls and Complications

Patient Factors/Poor Patient Selection
Severe/uncontrolled GERD resulting in postoperative aspiration and pneumonia
Extreme pharyngeal muscle weakness with inability to propel bolus
Surgical Errors
Injury to the recurrent laryngeal nerve
Accidental pharyngotomy
Pharyngocutaneous fistule

Source: Adapted from Pou A. Chapter 43. In: Carrau RL, Murry T, eds. *Comprehensive Management of Swallowing Disorders.* San Diego, CA: Plural Publishing; 2006:308, Table 43–3.

PALATOPEXY

Acquired **velopalatine incompetence (VPI)** can result from partial or complete loss of the soft palate or neuromuscular dysfunction of the soft palate. Unilateral palatal adhesion (palatopexy) is indicated for patients with permanent unilateral palatal paral-ysis that does not respond to conservative measures. An adhesion is surgically created at the level of the Passavant ridge, a site of "normal" closure of the velopalatine valve.[17] Even patients with very mild liquid reflux often have a moderate to severe nasal quality to their speech that dramatically improves with palatal adhesion. Figure 8–4 shows the adhesion location.

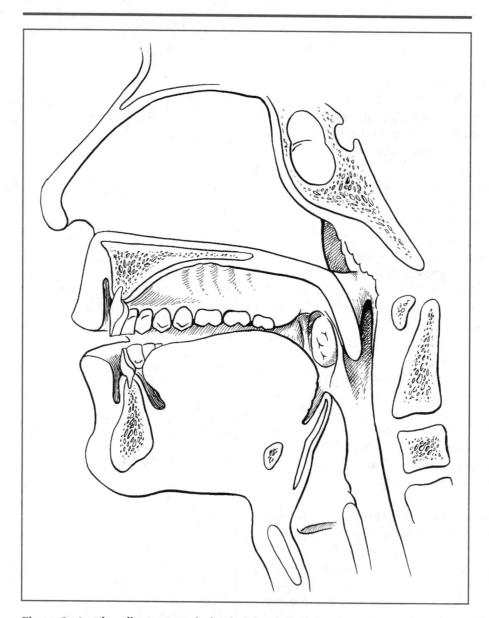

Figure 8–4. The adhesion is at the level of the Passavant ridge to allow closure of the contralateral normal velopharynx. Source: Adapted from Netterville JL. Chapter 44. In: Carrau RL, Murry T, eds. Comprehensive Management of Swallowing Disorders. San Diego, CA: Plural Publishing; 2006:311, Figure 44–3.

Dysfunction of the soft palate resulting in either unilateral or bilateral paralysis of the soft palate creates varying degrees of VPI. During the process of swallowing, VPI is manifested by the regurgitation of liquids and, rarely, solids into the nasopharynx and nasal cavity. Fifty percent of the patients with unilateral paralysis will improve over time, persisting with minimal complaints of swallowing dysfunction and voice. Older patients may not be as responsive and continue to have dysphagia, regurgitation, and excessive nasal speech.[21] Unilateral palatal adhesion (palatopexy) is indicated for patients with unilateral palatal paralysis. An adhesion is surgically created at the level of the Passavant ridge, a site of "normal" closure of the velopalatine valve. Even patients with very mild liquid reflux often have a moderate to severe nasal quality to their speech, which improves with a palatal adhesion.

PHARYNGOESOPHAGEAL DILATATION

Pharyngoesophageal dilatation is one of the oldest surgical procedures for the treatment of dysphagia. It involves the use of tapered bougie tubes of increasing diameter that are inserted sequentially to expand a stenotic segment, or the insertion of balloons that are inflated to a desired diameter, thus expanding the lumen. Its use is increasing due to the increased incidence of pharyngoesophageal stenosis associated with chemoradiation.[22,23]

SURGICAL CLOSURE OF THE LARYNX

When no other options are available due to intractable aspiration, a surgical separation of the airway from the food passageway provides palliation for individuals to continue oral nutrition. Patients who continue to aspirate despite the use of conservative measures and adjunctive surgical procedures may require surgical closure of the larynx. The most common diagnoses of patients requiring a laryngotracheal separation are neurological disorders such as cerebrovascular accidents (CVA) and amyotrophic lateral sclerosis (ALS). Laryngotracheal diversion, known as the standard Lindeman procedure, involves the creation of an anastomosis between the subglottic trachea and the esophagus, and a permanent stoma from the distal trachea. With laryngotracheal separation (the modified Lindeman procedure), the proximal subglottic trachea is closed as a blind pouch and a permanent stoma is created from the distal trachea, as shown in Figure 8–5. This latter technique best meets the desired criteria of simplicity, reliability, and reversibility, compared to other procedures (Table 8–9). The rare patient with intractable aspiration but who has a fair prognosis may benefit from a tracheotomy and the use of a laryngeal stent to close the proximal airway.[24,25]

GASTROSTOMY

Gastrostomy tubes (GTs) should be reserved for those patients in whom all other alternatives have been unsuccessful, and/or those patients with severe nutritional deficiencies who cannot meet their protein/caloric requirements with an oral diet. It should be noted, however, that GTs do not necessarily prevent aspiration, and in patients with diminished reflexes may even increase the risk of aspiration (ie, reflux aspiration). Thus, it appears that although GTs may benefit some dysphagic patients, such as stroke victims, they may not help and, indeed, may be a source of complications for other patient populations, such as those with dementia.[26–30] Jejunostomy or gastrojejunostomy tubes may be superior options and deserve study. Long-term monitoring of patients with GTs is mandatory,[31] as they may recover swallowing function even years after the primary event.

Percutaneous endoscopic gastrostomy (PEG) or open gastrostomy tubes provide an excellent route for feeding that can be temporary or permanent. These are discussed in Chapter 10. It should be noted, however, that PEG does not necessarily prevent aspiration.

TRACHEOTOMY

A tracheotomy does not enhance the ability of the patient to swallow, and in fact may result in greater swallowing dysfunction and aspiration. Thus,

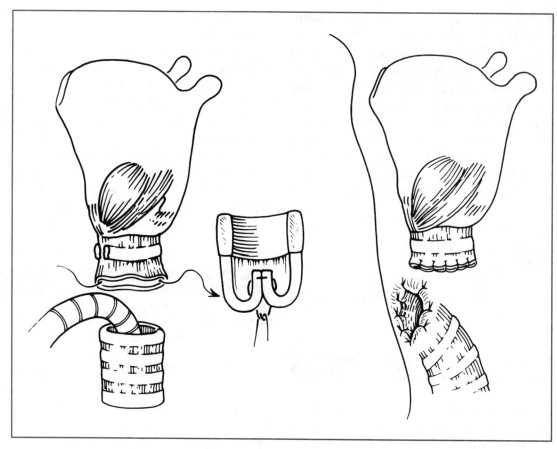

Figure 8–5. With laryngotracheal separation (modified Lindeman procedure), the proximal subglottic trachea is closed as a blind pouch and a permanent stoma is created from the distal trachea. Source: *Adapted from Snyderman CH. Chapter 45. In: Carrau RL, Murry T, eds.* Comprehensive Management of Swallowing Disorders. *San Diego, CA: Plural Publishing; 2006:314, Figure 45–1B.*

Table 8–9. Surgical Procedures Used to Separate Esophagus from Trachea

Procedure	Control of Aspiration	Preservation of Speech	Reversibility
Tracheostomy	−	+	+
Laryngeal stent	+/−	+/−	+
Laryngotracheal separation	+	−*	+
Total laryngectomy	+	−*	−

*Alaryngeal speech, either tracheoesophageal speech or esophageal speech, is possible.

Source: Adapted from Snyderman CH. Chapter 45. In: Carrau RL, Murry T, eds. *Comprehensive Management of Swallowing Disorders.* San Diego, CA: Plural Publishing; 2006:315, Table 45–3.

devices such as expiratory valves, fenestrated tubes, and decannulation are commonly advocated to aid swallowing in patients with a tracheotomy. Leder and Ross[32] challenged this concept, studying a small group of ventilator-dependent patients. Their study, although severely limited by the small number of patients included, suggests that these devices that act to build pressure may not always improve swallowing and reduce aspiration or penetration.

TRACHEOSTOMY TUBES

Tracheostomy is the placement of a tube into the trachea through a transcervical incision (Figure 8–6). The most common indication for the procedure is the need for prolonged mechanical ventilation. Other factors influencing a recommendation for tracheotomy are shown in Table 8–10. A tracheotomy

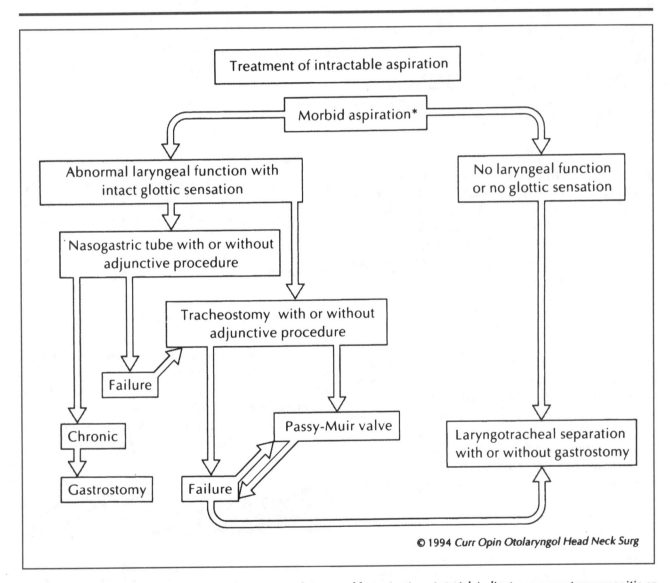

© 1994 *Curr Opin Otolaryngol Head Neck Surg*

Figure 8–6. Schematic for treatment of patients with intractable aspiration. Asterisk indicates recurrent pneumonitis or hypoxia. Source: *Adapted from Snyderman CD. Chapter 45. In: Carrau RL, Murry T, eds.* Comprehensive Management of Swallowing Disorders. *San Diego, CA: Plural Publishing; 2006:315, Figure 45–2.*

Table 8–10. *Factors Influencing the Recommendation for a Tracheotomy in Chronic Ventilator-Dependent Patients*

1. Need for prolonged mechanical ventilation
2. Primary diagnosis
3. Comorbidities
4. Nasal versus oral tube
5. Patient comfort
6. Ease of endotracheal suction
7. Expected duration of ventilator support
8. Effect of reducing "dead space"
9. Patient motion
10. Complications of endotracheal tube
11. Perceived risk of laryngeal complications

Source: Adapted from Eibling DE, Carrau RL. Chapter 38. In: Carrau RL, Murry T, eds. *Comprehensive Management of Swallowing Disorders.* San Diego, CA: Plural Publishing; 2006:260, Table 38–1.

Table 8–11. *Advantages of Expiratory Valve Use*

1. The patient can communicate verbally
2. Airflow provides proprioceptive cues during swallowing exercises and learning of maneuvers
3. True vocal fold adduction exercises will be minimized because of subglottic air pressure buildup
4. Improved pressure to aid in bolus propulsion

Source: Adapted from Gross RD, Eibling DE. Chapter 37. In: Carrau RL, Murry T, eds. *Comprehensive Management of Swallowing Disorders.* San Diego, CA: Plural Publishing; 2006:255.

provides an airway and permits suctioning of the aspirated secretions. The presence of a tracheotomy does not enhance the patient's ability to swallow; in fact, it may result in greater swallowing dysfunction and aspiration. Several maneuvers have been described to aid swallowing in patients with a tracheotomy, outlined next.

Expiratory Speaking Valve

An expiratory speaking valve is a removable, one-way valve that opens to permit inhalation but closes during expiration to divert the airflow through the larynx. The advantages of a speaking valve are shown in Table 8–11. The contraindications for the valve are shown in Table 7–3. It is important to monitor the patient when a speaking valve is first tried. Signs and symptoms of difficulty using a speaking valve are shown in Table 6–11.

Fenestrated Tracheostomy Tube

A fenestrated tracheostomy tube has an opening to permit air to pass into the upper airway and oral cavity. Long-term use of this tube is ill-advised, as the friction of the fenestra against the tracheal walls

produces exuberant granulation tissue, which has been associated with bleeding and/or life-threatening airway compromise. Figure 8–7 shows examples of fenestrated tracheostomy tubes.

Decannulation

The patient's ability to tolerate decannulation can be estimated by the amount of oral and tracheal secretions and by the patient's tolerance of tube capping. Decannulation is the most effective single intervention to enhance swallowing in patients with a tracheotomy.

Cricothyrotomy

Cricothyrotomy is an incision made through the skin and the cricothyroid membrane for relief of respiratory obstruction. It is used in lieu of tracheotomy in emergency situations and electively in selected patients undergoing surgery that requires a median sternotomy (eg, cardiac bypass surgery).

SWALLOWING FOLLOWING HEAD AND NECK CANCER

Early Outcomes

It is beyond the scope of this book to cover all of the surgeries for the treatment of head and neck cancers. Dysphagia is an early side effect or sequela of most

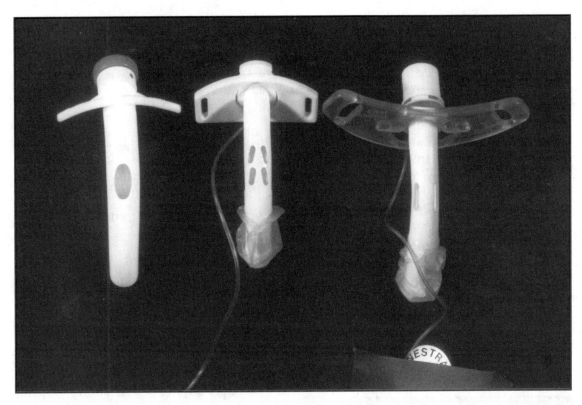

Figure 8–7. Examples of fenestrated tracheostomy tubes.

surgical procedures to treat head and neck cancer. As pointed out in Chapter 4, aggressive treatment following surgical removal of organs may reduce the time it takes to return to oral nutrition. Recent evidence has been presented to show that swallowing rehabilitation may even begin prior to surgery or chemoradiation[33,34] and can produce improvement in swallowing compared to patients who are not treated prior to their primary cancer treatments. Kulbersh et al[33] studied a group of patients who underwent swallowing exercises and found that the quality of life was significantly better in the group that started swallow exercises before cancer therapy compared to those who did not. Carroll et al[34] have shown in a pilot study that exercises including the Mendelsohn maneuver, tongue hold maneuver, effortful swallow, and Shaker exercise resulted in significant posttreatment swallow function in patients with advanced head and neck cancer who were given pretreatment exercises compared to those patients who did not receive pretreatment exercises.

Late Outcomes

Long-term outcomes of swallowing relate to the extent of surgery and the need for radiation or chemoradiation, as well as the adequacy of and compliance with the rehabilitation plan. In general, the more extensive the surgery, the longer it will take to regain oral nutrition and the more likely oral nutrition will result in some difficulties with swallow function. Using the SWAL-QOL, Bandeira et al[35] identified several factors that interfered with quality of life in patients treated for tongue cancer. These include:

A. Taking longer to eat than others
B. Difficulty chewing
C. Food sticking in the mouth
D. Drooling

Dworkin et al[36] examined patients with advanced stages laryngeal cancer before and after 1 year of treatment using FEES. All patients exhibited some degree of dysphagia, regardless of the time from the end of completed treatment, either less than one year or more than one year. Common long-term outcomes included persistent need for PEG feedings, texture modifications, slower than normal eating, and increased need to chew.

Although these studies examined effects mainly due to radiation or chemoradiation, it is apparent that loss of organ function, either as the result of surgery or nonsurgical treatments, has long-term effects on swallow function. Table 6–11 summarizes the swallowing disorders most often reported for treated head and neck cancer patients, with postures, maneuvers, and other interventions for treating the problems.[37] Little or no evidence exists to show that swallowing treatment prior to treatment of the head and neck disease is efficacious. However, for some patients, our clinical experience has shown that many of the maneuvers and postures clearly speed up the process from tube feedings to oral nutrition status.

SUMMARY

Surgical procedures are more commonly used as an adjunct to rehabilitative and compensatory therapy. They strive to improve the swallow by upgrading the function of the different valving mechanisms. In patients with severe swallowing disorders and/or malnutrition, they provide an avenue to maintain an adequate hydration and protein/caloric intake, as well as the means for tracheopulmonary toilette. A surgical separation of the airway and foodway is recommended for patients with intractable aspiration with a poor prognosis for recovery.

STUDY QUESTIONS

1. Surgical rehabilitation of swallowing disorders:
   A. Is contraindicated in patients with strokes
   B. Should precede swallowing rehabilitation
   C. Is adjunctive to swallowing rehabilitation
   D. B and C
   E. All of the above

2. A paralyzed vocal fold may lead to:
   A. Dysphonia
   B. Prandial aspiration
   C. Weak cough
   D. Atelectasis
   E. All of the above

3. Treatment of a paralyzed vocal fold may include:
   A. Vocal therapy
   B. Changes in neck rotation during swallowing
   C. Vocal fold medialization
   D. A and C
   E. All of the above

4. Reduction of prandial aspiration may be achieved by all *except*:
   A. Vocal fold medialization of a paralyzed vocal fold
   B. NPO
   C. Postural changes
   D. Super-supraglottic swallow
   E. Tracheotomy

5. Intractable aspiration is best treated by:
   A. Vocal fold medialization
   B. Tracheotomy
   C. Gastrostomy tube
   D. Cricopharyngeal myotomy
   E. Laryngotracheal separation

DISCUSSION QUESTION

Surgical repair of swallowing includes the need for surgery and the need for radiation therapy either before or following surgery. The speech-language pathologist (SLP) plays a vital role in the changing needs of the patient. Design a practical rehabilitation plan that could be used over the long term to assess recovery, change, and ongoing needs of the patient following surgery and radiation therapy for cancer of the oropharynx or an oral cancer of the tongue. Assume that the cancer was advanced and that the patient will undergo radiation therapy.

REFERENCES

1. Pou A, Carrau RL, Eibling DE, Murry T. Laryngeal framework surgery for the management of aspiration in high vagal lesions. *Am J Otolaryngol.* 1998;19:1–7.
2. Carrau RL, Pou A, Eibling DE, Murry T, Ferguson BJ. Laryngeal framework surgery for the management of aspiration. *Head Neck.* 1999;21:139–145.
3. Laccourreye O, Paczona R, Ageel M, et al. Intracordal autologous fat injection for aspiration after recurrent laryngeal nerve paralysis. *Eur Arch Otorhinolaryngol.* 1999;256:458–461.
4. Remacle M, Lawson G, Keghian J, Jamart J. Use of injectable autologous collagen for correcting glottic gaps: initial results. *J Voice.* 1999;13:280–288.
5. Zeitels SM, Hillman RE, Desloge RB, Bunting GA. Cricothyroid subluxation: a new innovation for enhancing the voice with laryngo plastic phonosurgery. *Ann Otol Rhinol Laryngol.* 1999;108:1126–1131.
6. Zeitels SM, Hochman I, Hillman RE. Adduction arytenopexy: a new procedure for paralytic dysphonia with implications for implant medialization. *Ann Otol Rhinol Laryngol Suppl.* 1998;173:2–24.
7. Maragos NE. The posterior thyroplasty window: anatomical considerations. *Laryngoscope.* 1999;109:1228–1231.
8. Link DT, Rutter MJ, Liu JH, Willgiung JP. Pediatric type I thyroplasty: an evolving procedure. *Ann Otol Rhinol Laryngol.* 1999;108:1105–1110.
9. Perie S, Coifier L, Laccourreye L, Hazebroucq. Swallowing disorders in paralysis of the lower cranial nerves: a functional analysis. *Ann Otol Rhinol Laryngol.* 1999;108: 606–611.
10. Shama L, Connor NP, Ciucci MR, McCulloch TM. Surgical treatment of dysphagia. *Phys Med Rehabil Clin N Am.* 2008 Nov;19(4):817–835, ix.
11. Sulica L, Rosen CA, Postma GN, et al. Current practice in injection augmentation of the vocal folds: indications, treatment principles, techniques, and complications. *Laryngoscope.* 2010 Feb;120(2):319–325.
12. Damrose EJ. Percutaneous injection laryngoplasty in the management of acute vocal fold paralysis. *Laryngoscope.* 2010 Aug;120(8):1582–1590.
13. Hendricker RM, deSilva BW, Forrest LA. Gore-Tex medialization laryngoplasty for treatment of dysphagia. *Otolaryngol Head Neck Surg.* 2010 Apr;142(4):536–539.
14. Ferreira LE, Simmons DT, Baron TH. Zenker's diverticula: pathophysiology, clinical presentation, and flexible endoscopic management. *Dis Esophagus.* 2008;21(1):1–8.
15. Oh TH, Brumfield KA, Hoskin TL, Kasperbauer JL, Basford JR. Dysphagia in inclusion body myositis: clinical features, management, and clinical outcome. *Am J Phys Med Rehabil.* 2008 Nov;87(11):883–889.
16. Lang RA, Spelsberg FW, Winter H, Jauch KW, Hüttl TP. Transoral diverticulostomy with a modified Endo-Gia stapler: results after 4 years of experience. *Surg Endosc.* 2007 Apr;21(4):532–536. Epub 2006 Dec 20.
17. Mok P, Woo P, Schaefer-Mojica J. Hypopharyngeal pharyngoplasty in the management of pharyngeal paralysis: a new procedure. *Ann Otol Rhinol Laryngol.* 2003 Oct; 112(10):844–852.
18. Jacobs JR, Logemann J, Pajak TF, Pauloski BR, Collins S, Casiano RR. Failure of cricopharyngeal myotomy to improve dysphagia following head and neck cancer surgery. *Arch Otolaryngol Head Neck Surg.* 1999;125:942–946.
19. Alberty J, Oelerich M, Ludwig K, Hartmann S, Stoll W. Efficacy of botulinum toxin A for treatment of upper esophageal sphincter dysfunction. *Laryngoscope.* 2000;110:1151–1156.
20. Ashan SE, Meleca RJ, Dworkin JP. Botulinum toxin injection of the cricopharyngeal muscle for the treatment of dysphagia. *Otolaryngol Head Neck Surg.* 2000;22:691–695.
21. Netterville JL. Palatal adhesion/pharyngeal flap. In Carrau RL, Murry T (eds): *Comprehensive Management of Swallowing Disorders.* San Diego, CA: Singular Publishing; 1999:309–312.
22. Tang SJ, Singh S, Truelson JM. Endotherapy for severe and complete pharyngo-esophageal post-radiation stenosis using wires, balloons and pharyngo-esophageal puncture (PEP) (with videos). *Surg Endosc.* 2010 Jan;24(1):210–214.
23. Nguyen NP, Smith HJ, Moltz CC, et al. Prevalence of pharyngeal and esophageal stenosis following radiation for head and neck cancer. *J Otolaryngol Head Neck Surg.* 2008 Apr;37(2):219–224.
24. Takano Y, Suga M, Sakamoto O, Sato K, et al. Satisfaction of patients treated surgically for intractable aspiration. *Chest.* 1999;116:1251–1256.
25. Qu SH, Li M, Liang JP, Su ZZ, Chen SQ, He XG. Laryngotracheal closure and cricopharyngeal myotomy for intractable aspiration and dysphagia secondary to cerebrovascular accident. *ORL J Otorhinolaryngol Relat Spec.* 2009;71(6):299–304. Epub 2009 Nov 24.
26. Klor BM, Milianti FJ. Rehabilitation of neurogenic dysphagia with percutaneous endoscopic gastrostomy. *Dysphagia.* 1999;14:162–164.
27. Nakajoh K, Nakagawa K, Sekizawa T, Arai MH, Sasaki H. Relation between incidence of pneumonia and protective reflexes in post-stroke patients with oral or tube feeding. *J Int Med.* 2000;247:19–42.
28. Finucane TE, Christmas C, Travis K. Tube feeding in patients with advanced dementia. A review of the evidence. *JAMA.* 1999;282:1365–1370.
29. McCann R. Lack of evidence about tube feeding—food for thought. *JAMA.* 1999;282(14):1380–1381.
30. James A, Kapur K, Hawthorne AB. Long-term outcome of percutaneous endoscopic gastrostomy feeding in patients with dysphagic stroke. *Age and Aging.* 1998;27:671–676.
31. Rehman HU, Knox J. There is a need for a regular review of swallowing ability in patients after PEG insertion to identify patients with delayed recovery of swallowing. Letter to the Editor. *Dysphagia.* 2000;15:48.

32. Leder SB, Ross DA. Investigation of the causal relationship between tracheotomy and aspiration in the acute care setting. *Laryngoscope.* 2000;110:641–644.

33. Kulbersh BD, Rosenthal EL, McGrew BM, et al. Pretreatment, preoperative swallowing exercises may improve dysphagia quality of life. *Laryngoscope.* 2006;116(6):883–886.

34. Carroll WR, Locher JL, Canon CL, Bohannon IA, McColloch NL, Magnuson JS. Pretreatment swallowing exercises improve swallow function after chemoradiation. *Laryngoscope.* 2007;118(1):39–43.

35. Bandeira AKC, Azevedo EH, Vartaiian JG, Nishimoto IN, Kawalski LP, Carrara-deAngelis E. Quality of life related to swallowing after tongue cancer treatment. *Dysphagia.* 2008;23:183–192.

36. Dworkin JP, Hill SL, Stachler RJ, Meleca RJ, Kewson D. Swallowing function outcomes following nonsurgical therapy for advanced stage laryngeal carcinoma. *Dysphagia.* 2006;21:66–74.

37. Pauloski BR. *Rehabilitation of dysphagia following head and neck cancer.* NIH Public Access pmr.2008.05.010.

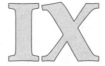

IX

Pediatric Swallowing and Feeding Disorders

CHAPTER OUTLINE

I. INTRODUCTION
II. INCIDENCE OF FEEDING AND SWALLOWING
   DISORDERS IN THE PEDIATRIC POPULATIONS
III. ANATOMY
IV. PHYSIOLOGY
   A. Neural Development
   B. Reflexes
   C. Apnea and Swallowing
   D. The Clinical Examination
   E. Oral Motor Examination
   F. Assessment of Early Reflexes
V. INSTRUMENTAL EXAMINATION
VI. RADIOLOGICAL EXAMINATION
VII. FEES AND FEESST EXAMINATIONS
VIII. TREATMENT OF FEEDING AND SWALLOWING
   DISORDERS
   A. Feeding and Swallowing Behaviors
   B. Treatment of Specific Disorders
IX. OPTIONS AND CONSIDERATIONS IN TREATMENT
   OF FEEDING DISORDERS IN INFANTS AND
   CHILDREN
   A. Oral Motor Interventions
   B. Nonnutritive Sucking
X. ADDITIONAL FACTORS IN INFANT FEEDING AND
   SWALLOWING
   A. Feeding Programs
XI. SUMMARY

XII.   STUDY QUESTIONS
XIII.   DISCUSSION QUESTIONS
XIV.   REFERENCES

INTRODUCTION

Pediatric swallowing and feeding disorders result from multiple medical problems developed before birth, at birth, or after birth and can lead to severe developmental problems for the infant should he or she survive. The increase in infant survival from conditions at birth or shortly thereafter requires specialized care to maximize survival and minimize long-term disorders that may result from pneumonia, aspiration, or other failure to thrive conditions. The methods employed to examine and assess swallowing in the newborn, infant, and pediatric populations must be specific to those populations.

> The clinician should not consider the issues in pediatric dysphagia as simply adult conditions on a smaller scale.

The study of pediatric swallowing disorders encompasses sucking, feeding, swallowing, and breathing and the sensory and motor controls that coordinate these functions. Disruption of normal swallowing in infants, as in adults, leads to food or liquids entering the airway. Children begin to choke, cough, and eventually avoid feeding, which in turn leads to failure to thrive, behavior problems at feeding time, and delay in normal physical development.

Feeding and swallowing disorders in the pediatric population may result from multiple conditions such as congenital or acquired neurological disorders and diseases, anatomical and physiological conditions, genetic disorders and syndromes, behavioral conditions, and systemic illnesses. These may be unitary conditions or, in the preterm infant, there may be several concurrent conditions or diseases that lead the clinician to work with an expanded team to manage the feeding and swallowing within the constraints of the infant's problems. Moreover, normal infant development means that the conditions are likely to change and those changes may occur rapidly. For example, a small amount of liquid in the lungs may be critical to an infant compared to an adult with a much larger pulmonary reservoir. Lack of developmental changes, however, is a sign of a disease or disorder and requires special attention.

This chapter reviews the clinical examination and objective tests for infants and young children with swallowing disorders and the feeding and treatment of children with swallowing disorders related to neurological, anatomical, and physiological conditions. In addition, this chapter addresses issues for feeding and treating children with common pediatric diseases and disorders.

INCIDENCE OF FEEDING AND SWALLOWING DISORDERS IN THE PEDIATRIC POPULATIONS

The incidence of swallowing disorders in the full-term newborn with normal birth weight is estimated to be extremely low. However, when a child is born prior to 37 weeks (full term), at low birth weight or without the normal prebirth medical care of the mother, the incidence of swallowing disorders may be very high. The incidence data on the most common feeding and swallowing problems in the newborn, infant, and pediatric populations range from a high of 85% in children born with cerebral palsy to 15% in children born with low birth weight. Table 9–1 presents a compilation of disorders of feeding and swallowing data for various conditions and diseases from various investigators over the past 25 years.

Table 9–1. *Incidence*

Medical Condition	Incidence	References
Head Trauma (TBI)	average 5.3%, 68% for severe TBI, 15% for moderate TBI, 1% for mild TBI	Morgan et al[45]
Neurological condition other than CP:		
Hemiplegia and diplegia	25–30%	Stallings, Charney, Davies, & Cronk[35]; Dahl et al[34]; Reilly et al[33]
	11.44%	Rommel et al[2]
Neurological	44%	Field et al[3]
	28% continuous drooling of saliva, 56% choked with food	Sullivan[46]
	56%	Newman et al[12]
Pierre Robin syndrome		
Cerebral palsy	32%	Field et al[3]
	57% sucking problems	Reilly et al[33]
	38% swallowing problems	Reilly et al[33]
	89% needed help with feeding	Reilly et al[33]
	27%	Waterman et al[47]
	Oral and pharyngeal abnormalities present in almost all patients 0	Day[48]
Spastic quadriplegia or extrapyramidal CP	50–75%	Stallings, Charney, Davies, & Cronk[35]; Dahl et al[34]; Reilly et al[33]
Gastric problems (reflux, constipation):		
Gastroesophageal reflux	56%	Field et al[3]
Gastrointestinal	14%	Field et al[3]
Gastrointestinal:		
Isolated gastrointestinal	42.45%	Rommel et al[2]
Gastrointestinal-neurological	6.14%	Rommel et al[2]
Gastrointestinal-genetic	1.66%	Rommel et al[2]
Gastrointestinal-ENT-orofacial	2.49%	Rommel et al[2]
Gastrointestinal-nephrological	1.66%	Rommel et al[2]
"Other combined medical pathologies"	18.57%	Rommel et al[2]
Low birth weight		
Developmental delays	74%	Burklow et al[26]

continues

Table 9–1. continued

Medical Condition	Incidence	References
Autism	24.4%	Field et al[3]
Down syndrome	39.9%	Field et al[3]
Anatomical anomalies:		
Cleft lip/cleft palate		
Velocardiofacial syndrome		
Prematurity	38%	Burklow et al[26]
	37%	Newman et al[12]
	40%	Hawdon et al[49]
	Prevalence and incidence estimates of feeding problems in extremely preterm infants are limited	Arvdeson et al[30]
Structural-neurological-behavioral	30%	Burklow et al[26]
Neurological-behavioral	27%	Burklow et al[26]
Structural-behavioral	9%	Burklow et al[26]
Structural-neurological	8%	Burklow et al[26]
Pneumonia	44%	Taniguchi and Moyer[50]
	49%	Newman et al[12]
Genetic	3.32%	Rommel et al[2]
Genetic: Infantile Pompe disease	100%	Jones et al[51]
Cardiological	2.82%	Rommel et al[2]
ENT — orofacial	3.32%	Rommel et al[2]
Metabolic	1.66%	Rommel et al[2]
Oncologic	2.49%	Rommel et al[2]
Nephrological	1.99%	Rommel et al[2]
Cardiopulmonary	35%	Field et al[3]
Anatomical anomalies	13%	Field et al[3]
Post–open heart surgery	18%	Kohr et al[52]
Apnea	23%	Newman et al[12]
Tube fed	21%	Newman et al[12]
Infants with oxygen-dependent chronic lung disease (CLD)	39.66%	Shaw et al[53]
CHARGE syndrome	90% on tube feeding at some point in time	Dobbelsteyn et al[54]

Although some infants and children have both feeding and swallowing problems, others may have only feeding problems (such as children with a cleft lip); others will have both feeding and swallowing problems (such as children with cleft lip and palate). Precise epidemiological data on the incidence of feeding and swallowing problems are further limited due to the problems of counting diseases rather than symptoms of the diseases, variations in the use of terminology (feeding vs swallowing), presence of multiple symptoms for one disease or several diseases accounting for various symptoms in the same child (for example, low birth weight and cleft palate), and the lack of a standardized test or test battery for classifying the problem.

In addition to being present in children born with low birth weight or premature births, swallowing and feeding disorders are prominent in children born with other neurological conditions and disorders such as **Pompe disease,**[1] gastroesophageal disorders,[2] and cardiopulmonary disorders.[3] It is not certain how low birth weight and premature births affect some of these ensuing conditions but it is safe to say that low birth weight infants must be carefully watched to avoid further conditions that lead to failure to thrive and develop.

> Although in past decades, those born with low birth weight and/or born prematurely did not survive, many of these children are now surviving and require the assistance of treatment teams, including the feeding and swallowing team members.

ANATOMY

The anatomy and physiology of swallowing has been described in Chapter 2. In the pediatric population, the anatomy is under constant change as a result of the growth and development of the child. The act of normal swallowing in the infant demands a highly coordinated and intact sensorimotor system with the reflexes integrated at the brain stem level. Unlike older children and adults, infants acquire nutrition by virtue of a suck-swallow-breathe sequence.

In the infant and young child, the differences in anatomy and physiology compared to those of the adult consist of the size and shape of the oral cavity, placement of the tongue, and the relationships among the locations of the velum, hyoid bone, epiglottis, and larynx. Figure 9–1 shows the outline of the infant head and chest at birth and at approximately 2 to 3 years of age. The size of the oral cavity is small in the infant in relationship to the overall size of the infant due to the small size and placement of the mandible.[4] More of the tongue is within the oral cavity. The hard palate has little or no arch compared to that of the older infant. Therefore, the tongue has very little space in which to move. In the newborn, a **suckling** motion is responsible for acquiring fluids. This is an anterior/posterior tongue motion. As the child develops, the suckling motion becomes a **sucking** motion (superior/inferior tongue motion) and the child is able to manipulate the tongue from side to side as well.

In the pharynx, the high position of the epiglottis appears attached to the tongue and contact is often made with the soft palate. This may cause the child to cough. In the infant, the larynx at rest is high in the neck at the level of C1–C3 vertebrae. The hyoid and larynx lie almost directly beneath the base of the tongue in the infant. This allows the tongue, velum, and epiglottis to approximate and separate the respiratory and digestive tracts. The anatomy of the infant may be a desirable arrangement for feeding because, if material lodges in the pharynx, it does not block the flow of air to the larynx as it would in the adult with the lower laryngeal position. In the infant, the small size of the oral cavity and mandible relative to the tongue position and the location of the buccal fat pads help to bring the cheeks, tongue, and lips in close proximity to allow suckling and, eventually, sucking to take place.

The buccal, laryngeal, and pharyngeal anatomy of the infant is continuously undergoing change with growth and development. At approximately 4 to 6 months, it has been hypothesized that respiratory instability may occur due to changes in the anatomical relationships of the mandible, tongue, and palate or due to the neuromuscular developments that increase the activity of the tongue.[5] As the hyoid, larynx, and base of the tongue descend and separate from the tongue and structures of the

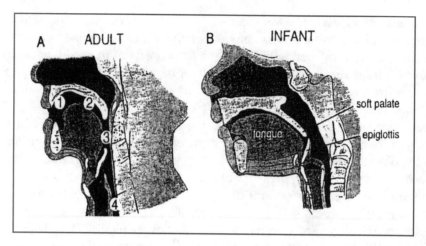

Figure 9–1. View showing the changes that take place in the anterior oral cavity (1), palate (2), pharynx (3), and esophagus (4) from infancy to adulthood. **Source:** *From Link DT, Willging JP, Cotton RT, Miller CK, Rudolf CD. Pediatric laryngopharyngeal sensory testing during flexible endoscopic evaluation of swallowing: feasible and correlative. Ann Otol Rhinol Laryngol. 2000;109(100):64–70.*

oral cavity, the coordination of swallowing activity becomes increasingly complex. By age 2 to 3, the respiratory and digestive pathways are functionally separated as a result of the descending structures. At this time in life, aspiration may occur if there are problems during oral control of the bolus, poor vocal fold closure, or coordination of glottis closure with the passage of the bolus.

PHYSIOLOGY

Neural Development

Chapter 2 describes the function of the swallowing mechanism. In the normal healthy adult, these structures undergo gradual changes as the adult ages. Other changes that do occur in the adult most often are brought about by injury and diseases. In infants and children, changes take place in the normal pediatric population as children develop and grow. The neurological maturity of the normal child keeps up with those changes. Early information on the neurology of infant swallowing has been hypothesized from animal studies for many years. More recently, the understanding of the neural coordination of swallowing has been obtained from careful evaluation of both healthy infants and those with neurological or anatomical disorders. Studies by Laitman et al,[6] Link et al,[7] Heuschkel et al,[8] Shaker and colleagues,[9,10] Arvedson,[11] and Newman et al[12] have focused on the developmental aspects of infant swallowing.

Neural control of swallowing primarily involves two areas of the medulla, the **nucleus of the tractus solitarius,** which is made up of the visceral afferent fibers of the CN VI, IX, and X as well as those of the superior laryngeal nerve (SLN—sensory from CN X) and the **nucleus ambiguus.** The nucleus of the tractus solitarius is the first synaptic relay for several different inputs that contribute to heart rate respiratory function as well as taste and deglutition. The nucleus of the tractus solitarius is the point of termination of the efferent fibers of the esophagus. The nucleus ambiguus leads to the brachial efferent motor fibers of the vagus nerve (CN X) as well as to the efferent motor fibers of the glossopharyngeal nerve (CN IX). These motor fibers terminate in various laryngeal, pharyngeal, and stylopharyngeal muscles. According to early studies on animals, the

CN X is not fully myelinated.[13] This may account for the lack of feedback to the tractus solitarius in the medulla, a relay for both respiration and swallowing.

Reflexes

The protective function in the normal infant begins early in life. For premature infants, or infants born with neurological or congenital disorders, the coordination of swallowing with the protective function of the laryngopharyngeal structures may not respond normally. The larynx is the major organ that responds to reflexes stimulated by the act of swallowing and, therefore, in the infant, it is the main organ that prevents pulmonary aspiration.

> The three important glottal closure mechanisms consist of the vocal fold closure reflex, also known as the **laryngeal adductor reflex (LAR)**, described in Chapter 2, the **esophagoglottal closure reflex (EGCR)**, and the **pharyngoglottal closure reflex (PGCR)**.[14]

To some degree, the glottal reflexes are dependent on the pressure and duration of the action of the pulmonary and laryngeal organs. The ability to produce a strong cough provides a response to materials in the pulmonary airway. Additional barriers to the prevention of aspiration at the laryngeal level are the contractions of the aryepiglottic folds and the dorsal/inferior motion of the epiglottis.

Aspiration into the pulmonary airway may also occur from regurgitation and vomiting, a common occurrence in the infant and pediatric populations due to the small stomach, the rapid rise in upper esophageal pressure with feeding, and the relatively high level of the larynx in the newborn and infant. The EGCR and the PGCR reflexes are responsible for reacting to the retrograde activity in the esophagus and pharynx respectively. Although these reflexes may exist in the premature infant, their response times are not well understood.[15]

The protective reflexes of the larynx, pharynx, and esophagus suggest a close relationship between the digestive and respiratory tracts during and after swallowing. The LAR is the most likely protective mechanism during the swallow, whereas the EGCR is the most likely protective mechanism during retrograde transit that occurs in belching, vomiting, and events associated with the regurgitation of acid, pepsin, or bile.

Apnea and Swallowing

Apnea is a significant part of the swallow activity. As in the adult, respiration ceases during swallowing in infants and children. Aspiration can result if there is inhalation during the swallow or if the upper esophageal sphincter fails to relax. In the infant, the respiration rate is high compared to that of the adult and the activity of vigorous sucking can lead to incoordination of the breathing-sucking-swallowing pattern. Swallowing apnea after birth is shorter for nutritive swallows than for nonnutritive swallows. Kelly et al[16] suggest that, in the infant swallow, the higher velocity of an ingested bolus may account for shorter nutritive swallow duration and subsequent shorter nutritive swallow apnea events.

The Clinical Examination

The evaluation of swallowing disorders in the pediatric population begins with a thorough history. The history should include birth-related information including the birth mother's general medical condition, the patient's medical history, including previous illnesses, medications, and eating and nutrition history, and especially incidents or events that occurred around the onset of the swallowing problem. The clinician should also inquire about swallowing problems in other children in the family and how those family members were treated.

After a complete history, the child should undergo a clinical examination, including a complete oral motor examination. The clinical examination begins by noting the child's overall awareness of their surroundings, social interaction, and responsiveness. The clinician should observe general motor ability, including head and trunk support, sitting posture, and the need for assistive devices for sitting or mobility. Awareness of neck flexion when the infant is touched on the neck should be identified, as lack of flexion may be a sign of neuromuscular weakness. The ability to suck, the response to placement of a pacifier on the tongue, and the presence of breathing through the mouth at rest should be noted. The cooperation of the child in the therapeutic program can be determined during the clinical assessment. Attention to the behavior and communication skills of the child may determine suitable future testing protocols. Table 9–2 lists the major reasons why children may refuse to eat.[11,12,15]

Oral Motor Examination

A thorough oral motor examination by the clinician should include an assessment of the structure, symmetry, tone, coordination, and function of the lips, tongue, palate, and jaw. Look inside the oral cavity to see that the uvula is not deviated to one side. Also, check the shape of the palate and see that the structures look normal. Assess strength of the lips, tongue, and cheeks. Assessment of the voice for appropriate pitch and loudness is also important. If the child has been eating, the clinician will want to know if the child is self-feeding, the kinds of foods he or she can and cannot tolerate, the types of utensils used, and if any adaptive feeding devices or postures are used when eating. If appropriate, trial samples of the types of food the child is eating may be tried. Attention to drooling, management of saliva, and residual food remaining in the mouth should be noted. Also, the behavior of the child should be noted: is he or she inattentive to the feeding/eating activity, is he or she fidgety or moving around or away from the food, and so forth.

Assessment of Early Reflexes

Feeding readiness changes rapidly during the first 3 years of life. Infant feeding and swallowing evaluation involves not only examining the oral mechanism but specifically assessing the child's developing reflexes.

Table 9–2. Major Reasons Why Children Refuse to Eat

Neurological/Neuromuscular
Cerebral palsy
Bulbar palsy
Myasthenia gravis
Arnold-Chiari malformation
Poliomyelitis
Muscular dystrophy
Tardive dyskinesia

Anatomic/Congenital
Cleft of palate, lip
Laryngomalacia
Subglottic stenosis
Tracheoesophageal fistula
Esophageal stricture
Foreign body sensation
Esophageal tumor
Pierre Robin syndrome
Tachypnea (respiration > 60 breaths/min)

Inflammatory
Laryngopharyngeal reflux
Gastroesophageal reflux
Caustic injection
Infections
Epiglotitis
Esophagitis
Adenotonsilitis

Behavioral
Depression
Taste aversion
Conditioned dysphagia

> The most rapidly changing oral reflexes occur during the first 12 months of life in the full-term infant. Reflexes may be absent or diminished in preterm infants.

In premature infants, feeding readiness can "catch up" to the full-term infant. However, Shadler et al[17] and Wiedmeier et al[18] note that a delay in normal feeding skills is common in children born prematurely. Others have noted that human milk feeding and the use of various supportive devices in case the child's muscle tone is not fully developed are important to consider in the feeding assessment.[19,20]

Oral Infant Reflexes

The common reflexes to assess vary with age. During the first 4 months of the infant's life, the **rooting reflex** is assessed by stroking the infant's cheek and observing the infant turning toward the sensation and opening the mouth. This early reflex eventually disappears around the fifth month. The **bite reflex** may be observed by the up-down motion of the jaw when a slight pressure is placed on the gums. The **suck reflex** can be assessed by placing the finger gently on the palate and feeling the pull toward the palate. The bite and suck reflexes usually disappear at about the sixth month of life. The tongue protrusion reflex can be assessed by placing a small amount of food or thickened liquid on the tongue. The tongue in the infant will move forward instead of backward. If the tongue protrusion lasts beyond 4 months, it is usually a sign that the child is not ready for solid foods.

The **gag reflex** is assessed by placing a small tongue blade on the tongue and then sliding it backward. The tongue generally will begin to elevate and may in fact cause the child to cough. The gag reflex may be absent and not interfere with swallowing. Unlike other infant reflexes, it may remain for the entire life.

The **swallow reflex** can be felt by placing a finger on the area of the cricoid cartilage and noting its upward movement when the infant is given some liquid to swallow. Verification of the swallow reflex may be necessary through an instrumental study if the child coughs or chokes when the liquid is presented and either a weak or absent upward motion at the level of the cricoid is noted.

Many of the infant reflexes disappear during the first 3 to 6 months of life. After the fifth month, the changes that take place involve the infant learning to control the motions in the oral cavity, manipulating the tongue to move food around, and assuming a more voluntary control of the swallowing activity. By 12 months of age, the early reflexes have subsided and the infant begins to self-feed. Observation of self-feeding may determine the presence of mild neurological disorders. The inability to manipulate utensils and occasional drooling, gagging, or choking during self-feeding may suggest the need for a more thorough assessment of the infant's ability to manage solids and liquids. Table 9–3 is a comprehensive summary of the feeding development along with the motor skills and language development from birth to 3 years of age.

The clinical examination offers the clinician a time to determine if an instrumental assessment is appropriate and how to adapt instrumental assessment to effectively obtain additional valid diagnostic information and treatment planning strategies.

INSTRUMENTAL EXAMINATION

The clinical assessment is the precursor to a more specific examination of the swallowing process. The clinician is encouraged to complete the clinical assessment as thoroughly as possible, as not all children will be cooperative enough to participate in an instrumental examination that can provide sufficient information to develop further treatment plans already identified in the clinical swallow examination.

Swallowing occurs rapidly. Ideally, a record of those rapid movements will aid in the diagnosis and treatment planning. Thus, whether the clinical team selects the modified barium swallow (MBS) or the flexible endoscopic evaluation of swallowing (FEES), videorecording is necessary to examine the details of the swallow activity.

Chapter 5 presented the methods used in the instrumental examination of swallowing. This chapter summarizes the reasons for advancing to an instrumental study after the clinical assessment and the advantages of the instrumental methods as they apply to infants and children.

Table 9–3. Feeding Development from Infants to Three Years of Age

Month	Feeding Skills	Oral Motor Skills	Food Type	Fine Motor Skills	Gross Motor Skills	Cognitive/Sensory Skills	Language: Expressive/Receptive Skills	Socioemotional Development Skills
1	Suck and swallow reflex. Starts interaction with caregivers.	Suck and swallow reflex, rooting reflex. Bite reflex.	Liquids (breast feeding, bottle).	Palmar grasp reflex.	Holds head up.	Visual fixation and tracking.	E = Coos R = Alert to sounds	Regulation of states. Interest in the world. Can be calm. Eye contact and mutual gaze.
2	Pushes food out when placed on tongue. Initial swallow involves posterior part of the tongue.	Suckling pattern. Extension and retraction movements of the tongue.			Holds chest up.		R = smiles when stroked or talked	
3	Anterior part of the tongue starts to be involved in initial swallow, facilitating the ingestion of semisolids.	Corners of mouth become active during sucking. Extends tongue in anticipation.		Unfisted grasp.		Recognition of parents.		Smile. Mother-child interaction.
4	Voluntarily grasps with both hands. Sits with support.	Transfers bolus from anterior tongue to pharynx. Rooting reflex disappears.	Pureed food. Fed by caregiver, taken passively from spoon.	Starts reaching for objects. Objects to midline.	Rolls front to back.	Anticipates feeding.	E = Laughs R = Orients to voice	Shows positive affect to caregivers. Displays negative affect. Responds with pleasure to social interactions.
5	Upright supported position for spoon feeding. Approximates lips to rims of the cup.	Sucking pattern		Transfers objects	Rolls back to front, sits with support.	Stereoscopic vision. Enjoys looking around environment.	E = Razzes, blows bubbles, "Ah-goo" R = Orients to bell/keys	
6	Initiation of finger feeding. Drinks from the cup.	Chewing pattern emerges. Closes lips around spoon. Biting reflex disappears.	Pureed foods and teething crackers. Cup introduced.	Unilateral reach, raking grasp.	Sits.	Visual interest in small objects. Oral exploration of objects.	E = Babbles	Referential look. Reciprocal vowel play.

continues

Month	Feeding Skills	Oral Motor Skills	Food Type	Fine Motor Skills	Gross Motor Skills	Cognitive/Sensory Skills	Language: Expressive/Receptive Skills	Socioemotional Development Skills
7	Able to eat crackers. Starts helping spoon find mouth.	Lips begin to move while chewing.		Radial grasp.			R = Localizes bell indirectly	
8	Begins use of cup.	Lip closure achieved.			Sits/crawls.	Object permanence.	E = Dadda (not specific)	Stranger anxiety.
9	Pincer approach to food. Holds bottle.	Tongue lateralization of food bolus emerges.	Ground and mashed table foods.	3-finger grasp.	Pull to stand/cruises.		R = Understands no/gesture games.	Plays pat-a-cake, peek-a-boo. Interacts in a purposeful manner. Initiates interactions.
10	Finger feeding.						E = Mama/Dada R = Orients to bell directly	
11	Drinks from cup (parent holds it).			Mature pincer.	Walks alone.		E = 1st word other than mama or dada R = 1-step command with gesture	
12	Reaches for food. Plays with food (throwing food, spoon, etc). Tries to keep spoon for self.	Munching with improved lateralization. Licks food from lower lip	Soft table foods (easily chewed).	Voluntarily release.		Help dressing. Imitates actions.	E = 2 words other than mama.	
15	Begins using cup.			Tower 2 blocks.	Runs, creeps up stairs.	Use of tolls.	E = Jargon/4–5 words R = Command no gesture	Comprehends, communicates, elaborates sequences of interactions.

Table 9–3. continued

Month	Feeding Skills	Oral Motor Skills	Food Type	Fine Motor Skills	Gross Motor Skills	Cognitive/ Sensory Skills	Language: Expressive/ Receptive Skills	Socioemotional Development Skills
18	Prefers to feed self over longer periods of time. Imitates others during feeding.	Mature chewing and drinking.		Turns pages.	Throws ball from standing.	Imitates parents in tasks.	E = Mature jargon R = Points to body parts	Imitates parents in tasks.
21	Eats with spoon, but spills. Holds glass with both hands.		Soft table foods (easily chewed).	Tower 5 blocks.	Goes up steps.	Asks for food or toilet.	2-word phrases.	
24	Correct use of spoon. Distinguishes between food and inedible materials.			Turns 1 page.	Up/down stairs alone.	Help with undressing.	E = 50 words. R = Follows 2-step commands	Pretend play (representational capacity of ideas).
30	Spear with fork.		Table food. Vegetables, meat.	Unbuttons.	Jumps.		E = Pronouns appropriately R = Concept of 1	
3 years	Straw drinking, can eat by himself, can serve cup.			Copies circle.	Rides tricycle, throws ball.	Undresses completely.	E = Plurals/250 words/3-word phrase R = Concept of 12	

Source: Data from Arvedson[11]; Rudolph[28]; Stevenson and Allaire[55]
Note: E = Expressive, R = Receptive.

Table 9–4 presents some of the most common reasons for referral for an instrumental swallowing examination. The clinician proceeds to the instrumental assessment after the physician reviews the findings and recommendations of the clinical swallow assessment.

> The goals in the instrumental examination are to obtain new information about the anatomy and physiology of the swallow mechanism and to contribute to the specifics of the diagnosis and treatment plan.

No studies should be done unless there is a reason to believe that the study will aid in reaching a diagnosis, alter the management strategies, or change the method of feeding.

RADIOLOGICAL EXAMINATION

The modified barium swallow (MBS) is generally conducted by a radiologist, a speech-language pathologist (SLP), and a technician. Prior to taking the child to the x-ray suite, parents and child (if applicable) should be given an explanation of what will go on during the test. Pictures of the x-ray

Table 9–4. Indications, Signs, and Symptoms for Referring a Child for an Instrumental Swallowing Examination

Failure to thrive: remains at or recedes to a low weight
Vomiting, regurgitation
Coughing, gagging or drooling
Voice quality changes during feeding
Known or suspected structural abnormalities
Refusal to eat
One or more episodes of pneumonia
Lack of coordination in oral structures
Positive chest x-ray (infiltrates)
Lack of or reduced sensation noted in clinical examination
Suspected structural disorders (TE fistula, vocal fold paralysis)

chair and equipment in the room may be helpful. For infants and young children, special chairs are usually used to aid in proper positioning during the examination, such as in Figure 9–2. For children who may be averse to swallowing anything, withholding food for a few hours prior to the exam may induce them to want to swallow something. Because radiation exposure to children has some degree of risk, the planning of what consistencies to swallow and how many swallows are necessary should be decided before the child reaches the x-ray suite. A time frame of 30 to 120 seconds is usually sufficient to gather the necessary data when the study is planned appropriately and the child is cooperative. Newman et al[12] examined 43 children using MBS and found that it was necessary to obtain 4 to 5 specific swallows to make a diagnosis. The time frame was kept to less than 2 minutes by turning the fluorography unit on over 15 to 30 seconds to visualize the swallows.

It is important to remember that movements of the child during the exam may limit the amount of information obtained from the examination. Using an infant chair is helpful and having all necessary items ready when the child comes in for the exam will limit the amount of time in the chair as well as the time for the entire examination.

FEES AND FEESST EXAMINATIONS

The FEES and FEESST are ideal tests to use in the pediatric population because they do not require the child to be exposed to radiation, nor do they require the child to be fully cooperative (although the sensory testing portion does require the child to be somewhat cooperative). The fiberoptic endoscopic evaluation of swallowing (FEES) was developed by Langmore and is now a well-established method for evaluating the adult swallow mechanism and its functions.[21] The flexible endoscopic evaluation of swallowing with sensory testing (FEESST) was developed by Aviv and colleagues.[22,23] This test combines the FEES test with a test to quantify the laryngeal adductor reflex (LAR) response by delivering a calibrated air pulse to the mucosa innervated by the superior laryngeal nerve and observing the reflexive response. Stimulation to the area at the aryepiglottic

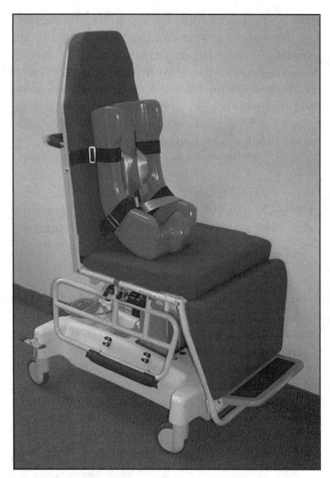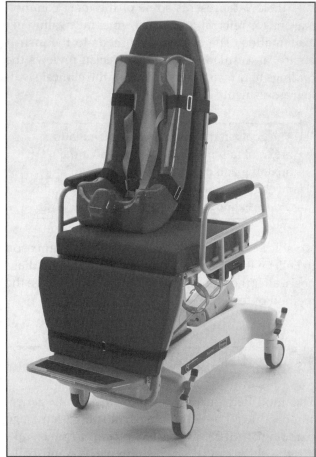

Figure 9–2. Chairs developed specifically for examining and feeding children in a semi-upright position.

fold induces the involuntary LAR. This test has been found to be useful in determining the laryngopharyngeal sensory deficits that relate to aspiration in patients following stroke or other injuries that may affect the superior laryngeal nerve.

The advantages of the FEES and FEESST were summarized in Chapter 5. In addition, it should be noted that for children, the parent may be present and help with the infant or child and offer observations that may not be apparent during the testing. Also, this test allows the examiner to use foods and liquids that the child is accustomed to swallowing. The work of Thompson and colleagues has demonstrated the use of the FEESST in infants and children from age one month to adulthood.[24]

The pediatric FEES/FEESST procedures require special equipment. A pediatric endoscope is ideal for the study. In some infants, there may be difficulty in passing a scope with a sensory channel; however, Link demonstrated successful sensory testing in 78 out of 100 children with multiple medical diagnoses.[7] Prior to testing, a topical anesthesia is directed to the middle meatus to avoid anesthetizing the hypopharynx. If anesthesia is required, it should be done under direct medical supervision. The use of the endoscope for conducting the test, however, does not require direct medical supervision. The child is tested in the upright position. Young children and infants may be held by the caregiver. With patient cooperation, the test lasts only a few minutes and both sensation and swallow function can be assessed. The beginning clinician may want to undergo specific training in the use of the pediatric endoscope as well as training in administering the air pulse.

Regardless of the examination that the clinician chooses, three factors are important to consider:

1. Will the examination give me additional information needed to plan a comprehensive treatment protocol?
2. Will the infant cooperate sufficiently to provide new information that was not obtained in the case history during the clinical bedside evaluation?
3. Is the examination team fully competent to provide the examination for the child, especially the child with special needs?

Once these three questions are answered in the affirmative and the examination room is prepared properly, the instrumental examination may be arranged. The primary goal in each instrumental examination is to plan for safe swallowing, either orally or via alternative routes in order to develop the plan of treatment.

TREATMENT OF FEEDING AND SWALLOWING DISORDERS

In the adult patient with dysphagia, the majority of treatment is directed to safe swallowing. In the child, feeding and swallowing are two aspects that must be considered. It is not uncommon for an infant to have feeding problems without swallowing problems or vice versa. In this section, the principles and guidelines for feeding and swallowing are reviewed with attention to individual groups of patients most commonly seen by the swallowing team.

Feeding disorders may be grouped into stages or phases related to function. Rudolph and Link[15] categorized these feeding phases in the following way:

Preoral Phase

Oral Phase

Pharyngeal Phase

Esophageal Phase

Gastroesophageal Phase

These phases are reviewed in detail in Chapter 2 and the caveats related to think of these as discrete phases has been discussed. However, the phases as they relate to infants and children, especially the preoral and oral phases, deserve additional consideration. It is the preoral and oral stages that are relatively different in infants and children compared to adults.

The preoral stage involves the child's alertness, the selection of appropriate food, and the proper manner of introducing food into the oral cavity. Children are sensitive to various aspects of their environment, their food selection, and states of wakefulness and sleep. Thus, as the child may not be able to communicate this information to the caregiver, feeding success may fluctuate unrelated to the underlying cause. Lack of proper behavior during feeding may also be related to smell of the food/liquid, not only to the feeding/swallowing disorder itself.

The oral phase of feeding consists of sucking or chewing and transfer. In the normal infant, sucking and mouthing motion may be normal, and it is not until some type of bolus is presented that the transfer aspect of this phase can be observed. Children with poor oral motor function may have difficulty in each part of this phase with the result being poorly controlled management of the bolus after the transfer.

In the pharyngeal phase, respiration ceases, the larynx elevates, the vocal folds close, and the upper esophageal sphincter opens. This phase of swallowing is involuntary and in the normal child is triggered by the bolus in contact with the tonsillar pillars. Once the bolus clears the upper esophagus, respiration resumes. Because this phase is involuntary, coordination with the oral phase is important to prevent aspiration.

The esophageal phase consists of esophageal transit and lower esophageal sphincter relaxation and opening. The upper esophageal sphincter relaxes in anticipation of the bolus reaching the esophagus. The lower esophagus relaxes to allow the bolus to enter the stomach. Various disorders of the esophagus may disrupt this activity and the contents of the bolus may be regurgitated if not allowed into the stomach. The gastrointestinal phase involves the delivery of the bolus to the stomach and moving it to the small intestine for digestion.

Arvedson[25] stressed the importance of each stage of feeding, noting that the preparatory feeding and oral stages, when not addressed carefully, may lead to refusal to eat due to the adverse sensations the infant may develop in the presence of foods or liquids. Further complexity of pediatric feeding was outlined by Burklow et al[26] who noted that, in addition to the structural-medical-neurological status of the child, a behavioral component is often present. In their evaluation of 103 children, the structural-neurological-behavioral paradigm was found to be the most common classification of children with feeding problems. They concluded that complex feeding problems must be addressed as biobehavioral feeding disorders in order to achieve normal feeding.

Feeding and Swallowing Behaviors

Feeding behavior is learned from the time the child begins the suck-swallow response to the need for nutrition. The complex interaction of the pulmonary, gastrointestinal, laryngeal, and oral systems along with the awareness of the caregiver helps to ensure that normal feeding progresses as the child increases his or her demand for more and varied foods. Table 9–5[27–29] shows the major systems that are required for normal feeding to progress. Although it

Table 9–5. Physiological and Behavioral Systems Involved in Normal Feeding

Systems	Required For
Oral motor function	Sucking, munching, chewing, and movement of the bolus; also needed for speech
Respiratory system	Maintaining normal oxygen exchange, coordinating suck and swallow, coughing to protect airways
Cardiovascular system	Maintaining normal blood pressure and oxygenation of the tissues
Pharyngeal coordination	Coordinating swallowing and breathing, safely transporting the bolus to the esophagus
Gastrointestinal system	Esophageal transporting of the bolus to the stomach and lower esophageal sphincter to avoid reflux. Gastric emptying to the duodenum and transporting throughout the bowel
Gross motor	Maintaining head in midline and upright position, sitting stability on the chair
Fine motor	Finger feeding, using a spoon, holding a cup
Expressive language	Asking for more or saying no
Nonverbal communication games	Pointing for food, opening mouth to receive food, gesturing, playing
Receptive language	Comprehension of the meaning of words "food, bottle," understanding of commands
Hypothalamus	Controlling hunger and satiety
Cognitive	Recognizing foods by color, appearance, taste, and so on; learning the associations related to feeding (ie, sound of the bottle = food is coming); learning to self-serve food
Social	Giving positive feedback to the caregiver, eye contact
Caregiver (socioeconomic)	Providing appropriate amount and type of food
Caregiver (emotional)	Funneling positive emotional support of a child during the learning process, setting rules and limits

Source: Data from Thomas[27]; Rudolph[28]; Arvedson and Rogers[29]

is generally accepted that the full-term birth healthy infant will begin feeding naturally, it is also possible that a preterm infant will also feed naturally.

When the child is immature, the feeding ability may be difficult and cause physiological distress, exhibited in many ways such as heart rate variations (bradycardia), changes in respiratory patterns (apnea), nasal flaring, or hypoxemia. Behavioral reactions to adverse feeding effects include fatigue, agitation, and disorganization. Arvedson et al[30] reviewed the evidence on the effects of oral motor interventions in preterm infants. They found that nonnutritive sucking (NNS) consistently was associated with significant positive changes on measures of swallowing physiology and reduced the number of days to reach total oral feeding in preterm infants. Oral stimulation alone was not found to have significant positive effects.

The importance of the initial feeding, whether by breast or bottle, sets the pattern for future feeding development. Van der Meer et al[31] studied the coordination of sucking, swallowing, and breathing in healthy newborns and concluded that normal sucking precedes normal feeding and that when there is no normal sucking pattern, a neurological reason must be identified. Table 9–6 summarizes their data related to the coordination of sucking, swallowing, and breathing in newborns.

In the child born with structural or neurological problems, the issue of feeding and the development of normal feeding may progress without significant

swallowing disorders but the length of time at each stage of development may exceed the normal durations, as described in Table 9–3.

The medical conditions that can affect the normal transition from sucking to swallowing and normal feeding may be grouped under 4 broad categories, as shown in Table 9–7.

Developmental delay can come from a number of conditions related to mental retardation. Children born with genetic syndromes may experience delay or inability to feed and progress to normal self-feeding depending on the syndrome and the accompanying issues. For example, a child with **Prader-Willi syndrome** (mental retardation and hypotonia) may reach normal status in his self-feeding but at a slower rate than a normal child. Conversely, a child born with **Down syndrome** (trisomy 21) will continue to experience feeding and swallowing problems into adulthood.

Table 9–7. Conditions That Can Affect the Transition to Normal Feeding and Swallowing in Infants

Condition	Possible Etiology
Developmental Delay	Mental Retardation
	Hypotonia
Neurogenic Diseases/ Disorders	Cerebral Palsy
	Arnold-Chiari Malformation
	Rett Syndrome
	Fetal Alcohol Syndrome (FAS)
	Mobius Syndrome
	Acquired Immune Deficiency Syndrome (AIDS)
Autism	Abnormal Social Development
	Abnormal Communicative Skills
	Resistive Behaviors
	Sensory Integrative Disorder
Oral-Mechanical	Understimulation due to Long-Term Gastrostomy
	Multiple Sensory Deficits
	Pierre Robin Syndrome
	Tracheoesophageal Fistula
	Cleft Lip or Palate

Table 9–6. A Review of a Normal Coordinate Feeding Pattern Developed from the Onset of Sucking

1. A well-coordinated feeding pattern is characterized by coordination of sucking, swallowing, and breathing, where maximum sucking pressure is coordinated with breathing out, and swallowing takes place just before the onset of the next suck and between breathing out and breathing in.
2. An efficient sucking pattern is characterized by a relatively lower sucking pressure and longer duration of each suck.
3. When the coordination breaks down, breathing is typically the bottleneck, with infants being unable to maintain adequate ventilation while sucking and swallowing during nutritive feeding.

Mental retardation is a global condition associated with swallowing. Table 9–8, modified from RightDiagnostics.com,[32] lists 40 conditions that contribute to swallowing disorders. Although treatment for each of these may involve individual treatments, the clinician must remember that three factors are important in the management of all infants and children with an underlying diagnosis of mental retardation:

1. Feeding and eating must be controlled based on the case history and clinical examination to avoid excessive rate of feeding/eating, inappropriate foods that may lead to choking or aspiration, and the need for environmental adaptation to maximize feeding without distraction.

2. The clinician may need to structure the feeding schedule around the medication schedule to maximize alertness of the child.

3. Children with some aspect of mental retardation may experience aberrant behavior in certain conditions. They may be averse to eating due to discomfort associated with gastroesophageal reflux, poor bowel movement, or other conditions, even fatigue.

The caregiver must be aware that feeding and eating may vary from time to time based on these conditions.

Table 9–8. *Causes of Mental Retardation and Swallowing Difficulty*

1. Absent patellae	18. Lissencephaly syndrome type 1
2. Adducted thumb syndrome recessive form	19. MRXS-Christianson
3. Adducted thumbs — arthrogryposis, Christian type	20. Macrogyria, pseudobulbar palsy
4. Adrenoleukodystrophy	21. Microcephaly, epilepsy; and ataxia syndrome
5. Alexander syndrome	22. Microcephaly brain defect spasticity hypernatremia
6. Angelman-like syndrome, X-linked	23. Mobius syndrome
7. Athabaskan brainstem dysgenesis	24. Duchenne muscular dystrophy
8. BBB syndrome, X-linked	25. Myopathy
9. Chromosome diseases	26. Myotonic dystrophy
Chromosome 1	27. Niemann-Pick disease
1p36 deletion syndrome	28. Opitz syndromes (G, G/BBB, Type 1, X-linked, autosomal dominant)
Chromosome 22 ring	29. Perisylvian syndrome
Chromosome 22 trisomy mosaic	30. Progeroid syndrome, neonatal
Chromosome 22q duplication syndrome	31. Pseudoadrenoleukodystrophy
Monosomy	32. Skeletal dysplasia associated with mental retardation
10. Diabetes insipidus, diabetes mellitus, optic atrophy	33. Southwestern Athabaskan genetic diseases
11. Epileptic encephalopathy, early infantile, 1	34. Striatonigral degeneration infantile
12. Franek-Bocker-Kahlen syndrome	35. Stuve-Wiedemann dysplasia
13. Gaucher disease	36. Stuve-Wiedemann syndrome
14. Glycogenosis type 2	37. Tay-Sachs
15. Hypertelorism with esophageal abnormality and hypospadias	38. Tetrahydrobiopterin deficiency
16. Hypospadias	39. Wolfram syndrome 2
17. Lead poisoning	40. Zellweger syndrome

Source: Modified from RightDiagnosis.com, September 7, 2011.

Treatment of Specific Disorders

Cerebral Palsy

Sucking and swallowing problems are common in the first 12 months of life for the cerebral palsy (CP) child due primarily to oral motor dysfunction.[33] CP children may have spastic, ataxic, or hypotonic neuromuscular conditions and the problem may be focused to one side (hemiplegia) or may be bilateral. CP children have a variety of oral motor problems, including abnormal bite, poor lip closure, weak sucking ability, and poor coordination of sucking with tongue movement. The need for oral motor development in these children has been emphasized in programs that involve occupational therapists, physical therapists, and SLPs. Eating and swallowing problems may extend into the teenage years. Dahl et al[34] reported that at least 60% of CP children remain undernourished and at nutritional risk at 8 years of age. Stallings et al[35] reported that approximately 30% of CP children remain undernourished and with stunted growth even into their late teenage years.

Treatment of the CP child focuses on the individual needs of the child identified in clinical and instrumental assessments. These children may require extensive oral motor exercises, dietary modification, sensory stimulation with thermal or sour stimuli, brushing or stroking the oral structures to improve lip closure, and bolus movement in the oral cavity.

Down Syndrome

Down syndrome is a genetic disorder that causes mental retardation and physical defects. It is caused by the presence of an extra copy of chromosome number 21. This condition is called trisomy 21. Children with Down syndrome are living longer than ever before. Many of these children have physical and mental challenges that require the child and the caregiver to pay close attention to their swallowing and eating behaviors long after childhood due to their limitations in motor control. Nonetheless, they can live independent and productive lives well into adulthood, although their swallowing problems may limit their ability to eat a regular diet in the normal time frame. Most children with Down syndrome have a large tongue with tongue protrusion, and a small mouth that predisposes them to feeding and swallowing problems. One of the most common problems for infants with Down syndrome who are learning to feed is their low muscle tone. In addition, these children are predisposed to cardiac, respiratory, and gastrointestinal problems. Furthermore, it is estimated that up to 10% of children with Down syndrome also have celiac disease.[36] Swallowing behaviors seen in a child with Down syndrome include:

Difficulty sucking or latching on.

Taking longer than 30 minutes to feed required amount of breast milk or formula.

Spitting out everything you try to spoon feed.

Not eating anything but baby food or refusing different textures beyond the appropriate age.

Coughing frequently on thin liquids.

The general treatments for dysphagia in the Down syndrome child are oral motor exercises and stimulation, diet modification, such as maintaining thickened foods and liquids to reduce aspiration, and arrangement of positional feeding postures, as shown in Figure 9–3.

Pierre Robin Syndrome

Pierre Robin syndrome (PRS) is a craniofacial anomaly that exists as an isolated condition characterized by cleft palate, micro/retrognathia, and glossoptosis, the latter being responsible for pharyngeal obstruction. Children with PRS are at high risk for respiratory insufficiency and prolonged hypoxia, which, left unrecognized, lead to impaired mental status. PRS may be part of other syndromes such as **velocardiofacial syndrome**, **Treacher Collins syndrome**, and **Beckwith-Wiedemann syndrome**. Because of the anomalies in the oral and pharyngeal cavities, the severity of airway obstruction is of high priority in these children. Dysphagia treatment in these children involves positioning the child to maintain a forward tongue, placing a nasopharyngeal tube to open the pharynx, or more extensive surgical procedures to improve the airway status.

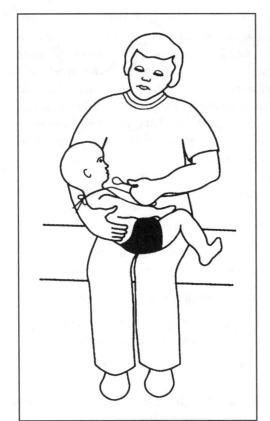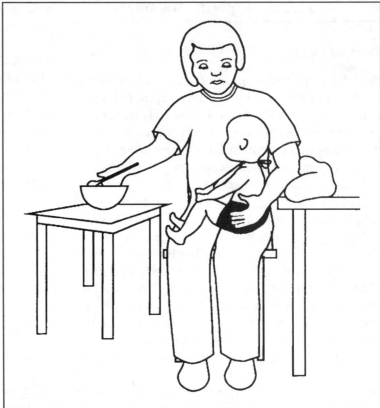

Figure 9–3. Two postures for managing children during feeding.

Feeding the young child may involve having him or her lie on his side for oral feeding. Also, children may require supportive nasogastric feeding at early ages. Eventually, when the issue of airway safety is no longer a problem, these children become self-feeders and learn to eat a regular diet.

Autism Spectrum Disorders

The spectrum of autism with regard to feeding and swallowing disorders is a collision between behavioral patterns and feeding difficulties. Social and cognitive issues coupled with oral motor and gastroesophageal disorders form a 4-part challenge to the swallowing rehabilitation team. To separate these 4 aspects of the autistic child's presentation is difficult because they interact with each other in feeding and swallowing as in other behaviors.

Treatment emphasizes structuring the feeding and swallowing activities through a focused sched- ule. This means removing distractions from the feeding area, limiting the utensils to those that are needed, presenting food based on previous food selectivity choices, using feeding "breaks" in the meal to prevent "shoveling, gulping, and stuffing," and selecting proper feeding times based on other behavioral patterns of sleep and wakefulness. The use of charts and pictures to aid in the development of eating habits may be helpful. Such charts and pictures can be found at the following websites: **TEACCH,** Treatment and Education of Autistic and Related Communication Handicapped Children (http://www.teacch.com) and **PECS,** Picture Exchange Communication System (http://www. pecs-usa.com).

Fetal Alcohol Syndrome

Fetal alcohol syndrome (FAS) results when the pregnant mother uses alcohol during pregnancy.

Alcohol poses extra risks to the fetus during pregnancy, especially during the first 3 months of pregnancy. When a pregnant woman drinks alcohol, it passes easily across the placenta to the fetus. Therefore, drinking alcohol can harm the baby's development. Currently, there is no safe level of alcohol use during pregnancy.

The child born with FAS generally has multiple physical and mental anomalies, many of which are seen in the head and neck. In addition, the cardiovascular and nervous systems are at risk because alcohol reduces the oxygen that passes through the placenta to the developing child. A baby with fetal alcohol syndrome can be expected to have poor growth while in the womb and after birth, decreased muscle tone, poor coordination resulting in sucking difficulty and tongue manipulation, and delayed development in cognitive skills, oral motor control, speech, and movement. Structural deficits include narrow eyes, small head, small maxilla, and poor lip development.

The child at birth may be of low birth weight, have difficulty sucking, fatigue easily, and need supportive nutrition through nasogastric feeding. The FAS child may progress to an all oral diet but this may take more than 1 year to accomplish. Moreover, the mental status of the child may limit his or her ability to learn feeding skills long after birth.

Rett Syndrome

Rett syndrome is a neurodevelopmental disorder that affects females almost exclusively. It is characterized by normal early growth and development followed by a slowing of development, loss of purposeful use of the hands, distinctive hand movements, slowed brain and head growth, problems with walking, seizures, and intellectual disability. The disorder was identified by Dr. Andreas Rett, an Austrian physician who first described it in a journal article in 1966. It was not until after a second article about the disorder, published in 1983 by Swedish researcher Dr. Bengt Hagberg, that the disorder was generally recognized. Apraxia is perhaps the most severely disabling feature of Rett syndrome, interfering with every body movement, including swallowing, eye gaze, and speech.[37]

Management of Rett syndrome is multidisciplinary in order to maximize all development skills

that emerge in the child. Because this disorder is progressive in nature, it may not be diagnosed at birth but requires clinical diagnosis with features similar to autism. Immature chewing patterns, weakness, and lack of control in the oral phase of swallowing and poor hand control (causing self-feeding problems) are present in children with Rett syndrome.[38] Despite this, many have voracious appetites, yet have poor weight gain and poor nutrition. Many require antireflux medications as well as seizure medications.

OPTIONS AND CONSIDERATIONS IN TREATMENT OF FEEDING DISORDERS IN INFANTS AND CHILDREN

After careful assessments of the infant, the clinical team should be ready to manage the conditions observed and documented. Children may refuse to eat for many reasons, including behavioral problems not readily identified during the case history and objective assessments but only during the feeding activity. Therefore, the clinician and the caregiver must be acutely aware of behavioral changes that do not correlate with the findings during the assessment.

Oral Motor Interventions

Because feeding efficiency in the infant involves the strength and maintenance of sucking during the meal, the importance of oral motor strength and coordination are of prime importance in infant feeding.[30] Without the coordination of the suck-swallow-breathe sequence, aspiration, poor nutrition, and failure to thrive will occur. Thus, the focus on oral motor strength and coordination begins in the neonatal care or intensive care unit following birth. Nonnutritive sucking and various forms of oral stimulation (brushing, thermal stimulation, and isometric stimulation) have become common as part of the treatment team's strategies. Many devices to aid in this process are now available and a list of suppliers is found in Table 9–9.

Although outcomes assessment of oral motor strategies is limited due to the clinical nature of

Table 9–9. Sources for Modified Feeding and Eating Utensils and Supplies

http://www.onestepahead.com/home.jsp **(key word: feeding utensils)**   flexible feeding utensils, suction bowls
http://www.landofnod.com **(key word: feeding)**
http://www.meijer.com/s/baby-toddler-baby-toddler-feeding-dishes-cups-utensils/_/N-5hn?cmpid = CASEM   multiple spoons, storage containers
http://www.alimed.com/alimed/rehabilitation/dining-aids/   broad list of bottles, utensils, serving trays, color coded supplies
http://www.equipmentshop.com/   bowls, cups, seating support
Enfamil: http://www.infamil.com/   pacifiers, nipples, feeding materials, parent information, formulas
http://www.philips-store.com/avent   bottles, sterilizers
Bionix Inc   http://www.bionixmed.com/MED_Pages/NutritionFeeding   bottles, nipples, enteral feeding equipment, safe straws, infant drinking cups

the treatment and the number of people who may be involved in the treatments, clinical observation suggests that oral motor intervention is essential in treating the developing infant with feeding difficulties. Nonnutritive sucking appears to improve digestion of enteric feeding, may reduce the length of stay in the hospital, and help to establish maturity in the sucking pattern.[39,40] Although the majority of studies of oral motor intervention have been done with preterm infants, these same strategies can be used with full-term infants when the clinician suspects short feeding times, refusal to eat, or other behaviors that cause the child to stop eating.

Oral motor interventions consist of techniques to create alertness and awareness of the need to swallow. These techniques consist of various types of brushing of the lips, tongue, or palate, icing placed on various oral structures, pressure massage, stim-ulation of the stretch reflexes by tapping with a pointed instrument, and stimulation with a vibrator. The value of these will depend on the individual to produce a response (for example, the tongue should respond to a quick tap with a pointed instrument). A complete program of oral motor intervention can be found at http://www.Beckman.com. This program is applicable to the entire team working with preterm infants.

Nonnutritive Sucking

The goal of nonnutritive sucking is to improve the strength and coordination of sucking in the preterm infant who is on gavage feeding or a feeding tube. Sucking during gavage feeding is thought to further the development of the sucking reflex, stimulate sucking behavior in children who are lethargic in feeding, and improve digestion. Others have found that nonnutritive sucking helps to calm infants who are hyperactive during the gavage feeding times. A recent study by Pinelli and Symington[41] found evidence that hospital costs decreased, children were less defensive when eating, and transition to bottle feeding was improved in children who were subjected to nonnutritive sucking activities.

ADDITIONAL FACTORS IN INFANT FEEDING AND SWALLOWING

Feeding in infants and children can be addressed in a number of ways. Postural adjustments using chairs such as those shown in Figure 9–2 and seating arrangements such as shown in Figure 9–3 are helpful because they offer support for the child, adjust the child to the proper position for swallowing, and prevent distractions by limiting movement.

Types of foods and fluids that the infant swallows may also improve the nutritive aspect of feeding and swallowing. Feeding premature infants with human milk has the advantages of speeding up gastrointestinal maturation, reducing the duration of hospitalization, and reducing the development of later metabolic syndromes that have been associated with formula feeds.[42]

In previous chapters, the swallowing maneuvers and postures were discussed. These interventions should not be ignored in infants when appropriate. Although the maneuvers and postures require infant cooperation, applying a maneuver "game" with young children, especially autistic children, may lead to improved nutrition.

The use of properly modified utensils and cups are now available from a number of sources, as shown in Table 9–9. Children with cleft palate, CHARGE syndrome, and Down syndrome may require modified bottle nipples in early infancy, and later will need modified utensils, cups, and plates long after infancy to facilitate the easy manipulation of the food from plate to spoon/fork and from spoon/fork to mouth. Although many infants and children can adapt to a common nipple, premature children need a nipple that can match the size of the oral cavity opening and also one that may require an improved seal to prevent leakage around the sides of the mouth in case the child has poor muscle tone.

Bottles for feeding come in various shapes and hardness. A hard plastic bottle may be sufficient for most children and parents can maintain a better grip on a hard bottle. However, a soft bottle offers the feeder an opportunity to squeeze the bottle to keep the feeding going.

Feeding Programs

Over the past 15 years, several individuals have developed specific feeding programs that encompass the work of the SLP, the occupational therapist, and other developmental specialists. The Beckman program mentioned above focuses on oral motor training for infants and children with limitations in their ability to manage the fine motor control needed to feed and eat independently.

The feeding program developed by Toomey,[43] called the Sequential Oral Sensory Approach (SOS), integrates feeding training into a program for children with limitations in growth and development. This program focuses on the acquisition of feeding skills based on the acquisition of other motor skills. In addition, the program focuses on desensitizing the child who will not eat using touch, smell, and taste. This popular program has yet to be tested rigorously but those who follow the guidelines of the program speak highly of it.

Feeding programs have become multidisciplinary over the years and the combined approaches of the SLP, the occupational therapist, and the dietician have shown that clinically, improvement in feeding in low birth weight children, premature children, or children with neurological diseases occurs when the parent has help to support the feeding program.

Early work on the use of expiratory muscle strength training (EMST) in adults for the treatment of swallowing may have implications for infants and children. Troche et al[44] have shown that the use of expiratory muscle strength training may help restore functional swallowing behavior in those patients with Parkinson disease. They explained that the reason for improvement in a group of Parkinson disease patients was due to improved hypolaryngeal activity. Future work may find that for patients with poor motor control, EMST may offer additional improvement to swallowing in infants and children than current oral motor exercises.

SUMMARY

Children must not be considered "little adults." Normal children are in a constant state of neurological, neuromuscular, and behavioral development. They progress through the stages of feeding and swallowing as their bodies develop. When communication is normal, children understand the feeding and eating processes.

When developmental delays, prematurity, or diseases and disorders are seen in the newborn, a comprehensive program to address the developmental aspects of the child must include feeding and swallowing. Dysphagia in the infant is simply not a matter of preventing aspiration; rather, it is a program to ensure that the infant is getting enough nutrition to grow and overcome the issues of prematurity and low birth weight as well as a program to stimulate oral motor control of the muscles needed to achieve safe self-feeding. Although not all children can reach that stage, aggressive management of the child may ultimately allow him or her to reach a safe oral feeding behavior that provides proper nutrition to maximize physical development and growth.

STUDY QUESTIONS

1. The condition that has been shown to be the primary basis for feeding disorders in newborn infants is:
   A. Neurological disorders
   B. Prematurity
   C. Parental feeding skills
   D. Birth weight

2. A child born at full birth weight and at full term is likely to have:
   A. Minor swallowing disorders
   B. Normal feeding and swallowing
   C. Weak oral motor control for liquids
   D. 25–30% probability of aspiration at birth

3. The true incidence of feeding and swallowing problems in premature infants:
   A. Is about 25%
   B. Can be found at the Centers for Disease Control and Prevention
   C. Remains relatively unknown due to the problems of counting diseases versus symptoms
   D. Is recorded at the National Institutes of Health

4. The infant tongue is rather large compared to the oral cavity space. Therefore:
   A. The tongue motion is limited in newborn infants
   B. The tongue can move only from side to side in the newborn
   C. The proximity of the tongue to the cheeks and lips helps in suckling and sucking
   D. The tongue is less important in the infant than in the older child for swallowing purposes

5. Glottal closure reflexes in the infant are dependent on:
   A. The ability to produce a strong cough
   B. Normal sensory stimulation of a bolus
   C. Normal function of the pulmonary system
   D. All of the above

DISCUSSION QUESTIONS

1. Look at the conditions in Table 9–7. Identify specific feeding strategies that could be used to treat the disorders outlined in that table.

2. Search the literature and review the work of the occupational therapists that treat infants with swallowing disorders. In what ways do you see an overlap in their activities and the activities of SLPs? How does this overlap benefit the child?

REFERENCES

1. Jones HN, Muller CW, Lin M, et al. Oropharyngeal dysphagia in infants and children with infantile Pompe disease. *Dysphagia*. 2010;25(4):277–283.
2. Rommel N, DeMeyer AM, Feenstra L, Veereman-Wauters G. The complexity of feeding problems in 700 infants and young children presenting to a tertiary care institution. *J Pediatr Gasroenterol Nutr.* 2003;37:75–84.
3. Field D, Garland M, Williams K. Correlates of specific childhood feeding problems. *J Pediatr Child Health.* 2003; 39(4):289–304.
4. Crelin E. *Functional Anatomy of the Newborn.* New Haven, CT: Yale University Press; 1973.
5. Laitman JT, Reidenberg JS. Specializations of the human upper respiratory and upper digestive systems as seen through comparative and developmental anatomy. *Dysphagia.* 1993;8:318–325.
6. Laitman JT, Reidenberg JS. The evolution of the human larynx: nature's great experiment. In: Fried MP, Ferlito A, eds. *The Larynx.* 3rd ed. San Diego, CA: Plural Publishing; 2009:19–38.
7. Link DT, Willging JP, Cotton RT, Miller CK, Rudolf CD. Pediatric laryngopharyngeal sensory testing during flexible endoscopic evaluation of swallowing: feasible and correlative. *Ann Otol Rhinol Laryngol.* 2000;109(100):64–70.
8. Heuschkel RB, Fletcher K, Hill A, Buonomo C, Bousvaros A, Nurko S. Isolated neonatal swallowing dysfunction: a

case series and review of the literature. *Dig Dis Sci.* 2003; 48(1)30–35.

9. Jadcherla SR, Duong HQ, Hoffmann RG, Shaker R. Characteristics of upper esophageal sphincter and esophageal body during maturation in healthy human neonates compared with adults. *Neurogastrenterol Motil.* 2005;17:663–670.

10. Jadcherla SR, Gupta A, Coley BD, Fernandez S, Shaker R. Esophagoglottal closure reflex in human infants: a novel reflex elicited with concurrent manometry and ultrasonography. *Am J Gastroenterol.* 2007;102:2286–2293.

11. Arvedson J. Anatomy, embryology, and physiology. In: Arvedson JC, Brodsky L, eds. *Pediatric Swallowing and Feeding: Assessment and Management.* San Diego, CA: Singular Publishing; 1993:37–45.

12. Newman LA, Keckley C, Petersen MC, Hammer A. Swallowing function and medical diagnoses in infants suspected of dysphagia. *Pediatrics.* 2001;108, e106.

13. Miller A. Deglutition. *Physiol Rev.* 1982;62:129–184.

14. Jadcherla SR, Hogan WJ, Shaker R. Physiology and pathophysiology of glottis reflexes and pulmonary aspiration from neonates to adults. *Semin Respir Crit Care Med.* 2010;31:554–560.

15. Rudolf CD, Link DT. Feeding disorders in infants and children. *Pediatr Clin North Am.* 2002;49:97–112.

16. Kelly BN, Huckabee ML, Jones RD, Frampton CMA. Nutritive and non-nutritive swallowing apnea duration in term infants: implications for neural control mechanisms. *Respir Physiol Neurobiol.* 2006;154(3):372–378.

17. Shadler G, Suss-Burghart H, Toschke AM. Feeding disorders in ex-prematures: causes-response to therapy-long term outcomes. *Eur J Pediatr.* 2007;166:803.

18. Wiedmeier JE, Joss-Moore LA, Land RH, Neu J. Early postnatal nutrition and programming of the preterm neonate. *Nutrition Rev.* 2011;69(2):76–82.

19. Shanler RJ. Outcomes of human milk-fed premature infants. *Semin Perinatol.* 2011;35(1):29–33.

20. Hwang YS, Lin CH, Coster WJ, Bigsby R, Vergara E. Effectiveness of cheek and jaw support to improve feeding performance of preterm infants. *Am J Occup Ther.* 2010;64(6):886–894.

21. Langmore SE, Schatz K, Olsen N. Fiberoptic endoscopic examination of swallowing safety: a new procedure. *Dysphagia.* 1988;2:216–219.

22. Aviv JE, Kim T, Thompson JE, Sunshine S, Kaplan S, Close LG. Fiberoptic endoscopic evaluation of swallowing with sensory testing (FEESST) in healthy controls. *Dysphagia.* 1998;13:87–92.

23. Aviv JE, Martin JH, Keen MS, Debell M, Blitzer A. Air pulse quantification of supraglottic and pharyngeal sensation: a new technique. *Ann Otol Rhinol Laryngol.* 1993;102:777–780.

24. Thompson DM. Laryngopharyngeal sensory testing and assessment of air way protection inpediatric patients. *Am J Med.* 2003;115(suppl 3A):166S–168S.

25. Arvedson J. Management of swallowing problems. In: Arvedson JC, Brodsky L, eds. *Pediatric Swallowing and Feeding: Assessment and Management.* San Diego, CA: Singular Publishing; 1993:348–373.

26. Burklow KA, Phelps AN, Schultz JR, McConnell K, Rudolph C. Classifying complex pediatric feeding disorders. *J Pediatr Gastroenterol Nutr.* 1998;27(2):143–147.

27. Thomas JA. Guidelines for bottle feeding your premature baby. *Adv Neonatal Care.* 2007 Dec;7(6):311–318.

28. Rudolph CD. Feeding disorders in infants and children. *J Pediatr.* 1994;125:5116–5124.

29. Arvedson JC, Rogers BT. Pediatric feeding and swallowing disorder. *J Med Speech-Lang Pathol.* 1993;1:202–203.

30. Arvedson J, Clark H, Lazarus C, Schooling T, Frymark T. Evidence-based systematic review: effects or oral motor interventions on feeding and swallowing in preterm infants. *Am J Speech-Lang Pathol.* 2010;19(4):321–340.

31. van der Meer A, Holden G, van der Weel R. Coordination of sucking, swallowing and breathing in healthy newborns. *J Pediatr Neonatol.* 2005;2(2):NT69–72.

32. Rightdiagnostics.com, Sept 7, 2011.

33. Reilly S, Skuse D, Poblete X. Prevalence of feeding problems and oral motor dysfunction in children with cerebral palsy: a community survey. *J Pediatr.* 1996;129(6):877–882.

34. Dahl, M. Thommessen, M. Rasmussen, M. Seiberg, T. Feeding and nutritional characteristics in children with moderate or severe cerebral palsy. *Acta Paediatica.* 1996;85:697–701.

35. Stallings VA, Charney EB, Davies JC, Cronk CE. Nutritional status and growth of children with diplegic or hemiplegic cerebral palsy. *Dev Med Child Neurol.* 1993; 35(11):997–1006.

36. Cooper-Brown L, Copeland S, Dailey S, Downey D, Petersen MC, Stimson C, VanDyke DC. Feeding and swallowing dysfunction in genetic syndromes. *Dev Disabil Res Rev.* 2008;14:147–157.

37. Neul JL, Zoghbi HY. Rett syndrome: a prototypical neurodevelopmental disorder. *Neuroscientist.* 2004 Apr; 10(2):118–128.

38. Weaving LS, Ellaway CJ, Gecz J, Christodoulou J. Rett syndrome: clinical review and genetic update. *J Med Genet.* 2005;42:1–7.

39. Fucile S, Gisel E, Lau C. Effect of an oral stimulation program on sucking skill maturation in preterm infants. *Dev Med Child Neurol.* 2005;47:158–162.

40. Bernbaum JC, Pereira GR, Watkins JB, Peckham GJ. Nonnutritive sucking during gavage feeding enhances growth and maturation in premature infants. *Pediatrics.* 1983;71:41–45.

41. Pinelli J, Symington AJ. Non-nutritive sucking for promoting physiologic stability and nutrition in preterm infants. *Cochrane Database Syst Rev.* 2005;4.

42. Schanler RJ. Outcomes of human milk-fed premature infants. *Semin Perinatol.* 2011;35(1):29–33.

43. Toomey K.The Sequential Oral Sensory (SOS) Approach to Feeding Program of the Children's Hospital Oral Feeding Clinic, Denver, CO. 2001.

44. Troche MS, Okun MS, Rosenbek JC, et al. Aspiration and swallowing in Parkinson disease and rehabilitation with

EMST: a randomized trial. *Neurology.* 2010 Nov 23;75(21): 1912–1919.

45. Morgan AT, Mageandran SD, Mei C. Incidence and clinical presentation of dysarthria and dysphagia in the acute setting following paediatric traumatic brain injury. *Child Care Health Dev.* 2010 Jan;36(1):44–53. Epub 2009 Mar 23. PMID:19320903

46. Sullivan PB. Gastrointestinal disorders in children with neurodevelopmental disabilities. *Dev Disabil Res Rev.* 2008;14(2):128–136.

47. Waterman ET, Koltai PJ, Downey JC, Cacace AT. Swallowing disorders in a population of children with cerebral palsy. *Int J Pediatr Otorhinolaryngol.* 1992 Jul;24(1): 63–71.

48. Day SM. Do we know what the prevalence of cerebral palsy is? *Dev Med Child Neurol.* 2011 Oct;53(10):876–877.

49. Hawdon JM, Beauregard N, Slattery J, Kennedy G. Identification of neonates at risk of developing feeding problems in infancy. *Dev Med Child Neurol.* 2000 Apr; 42(4):235–239.

50. Taniguchi MH, Moyer RS. Assessment of risk factors for pneumonia in dysphagic children: significance of video-fluoroscopic swallowing evaluation. *Dev Med Child Neurol.* 1994 Jun;36(6):495–502.

51. Jones HN, Muller CW, Lin M, et al. Oropharyngeal dysphagia in infants and children with infantile Pompe disease. *Dysphagia.* 2010 Dec;25(4):277–283.

52. Kohr LM, Dargan M, Hague A, et al. The incidence of dysphagia in pediatric patients after open heart procedures with transesophageal echocardiography. *Ann Thorac Surg.* 2003 Nov;76(5):1450–1456.

53. Shah SS, Ohlsson A, Halliday H, Shah VS. Inhaled versus systemic corticosteroids for the treatment of chronic lung disease in ventilated very low birth weight preterm infants. *Cochrane Database Syst Rev.* 2003;(2):CD002057. Update in: *Cochrane Database Syst Rev.* 2007;(4):CD002057. PMID:12804423.

54. Dobbelsteyn C, Peacocke SD, Blake K, Crist W, Rashid M. Feeding difficulties in children with CHARGE syndrome: prevalence, risk factors, and prognosis. *Dysphagia.* 2008 Jun;23(2):127–135. Epub 2007 Nov 20.PMID:18027028.

55. Stevenson RD, Allaire JH. The development of normal feeding and swallowing. *Pediatr Clin North Am.* 1991 Dec; 38(6):1439–1453.

X

Nutrition and Diets

CHAPTER OUTLINE

I. INTRODUCTION

II. PROPERTIES OF LIQUIDS AND FOODS
   A. Rheology Terminology
   B. Applications of Rheology
   C. Textures

III. ORAL NUTRITION AND DYSPHAGIA DIETS
   A. National Dysphagia Diet
   B. American Dietetic Association Diet
   C. Diets and Consistencies

IV. NONORAL DIETS
   A. Introduction
   B. Nasogastric, Nasoduodenal, and Nasojejunal Tubes
   C. Gastrostomy tubes

V. MALNUTRITION AND DEHYDRATION
   A. Stroke
   B. Head and Neck Cancer

VI. NUTRITION IN THE AGING POPULATION

VII. SUMMARY

VIII. STUDY QUESTIONS

IX. DISCUSSION QUESTION

X. REFERENCES

INTRODUCTION

The importance of proper nutrition cannot be overestimated in the management of swallowing disorders. Nutritional status can have a significant impact on recovery from disease and swallowing rehabilitation, especially those factors related to self-esteem, psychosocial concomitants of oral eating, and overall quality of life.

> The highest priority in the management of the dysphagic patient is swallow safety. The dysphagia team must also ensure that, no matter how the dysphagic patient is managed, he or she must receive adequate nourishment, measured by the amount of calories received, the content of the calories, and the degree of satisfaction when eating or drinking those calories.

Failure to achieve proper nutrition, whether it is via an oral or nonoral pathway, will result in **malnutrition**, a major complication in the recovery process.

In this chapter, the properties of liquids and foods are examined in relationship to the safety and nutrition of the dysphagic patient. Oral diets and nonoral feeding alternatives are reviewed. Malnutrition and its consequences as they relate to dysphagia are considered. Nutrition and its importance in the recovery from sickness, injury, or surgery are extensive topics and have far-reaching implications. Comprehensive reviews of nutrition including enteral feeding requirements and calorie intake calculation are summarized and references are provided for those who need specific patient requirements.

Proper nutrition can be achieved through oral or nonoral diets or from a combination of the two. In the recovery process from cancer of the organs in the head and neck, nutrition usually begins with a nonoral diet, often a nasogastric tube, and then proceeds to a combined oral and nonoral diet and finally an oral diet in most cases. Stroke recovery is similar; however, with the stroke patient, the patient's cognitive status, degree of alertness, and understanding of the nutritional process must also be taken into account. For these reasons, the nutritional status of the stroke patient must be managed carefully.

A comprehensive dysphagia treatment program makes extensive use of the nutritionist/dietitian (the term **"dietitian"** is used in this chapter in reference to **"registered dietitian"**) in order to prevent malnutrition, maintain or increase strength, and maintain immune status.

> The dietitian is a trained professional who selects the proper calorie and nutrition content of the diet and monitors the nutritional status and continuing needs of the patient.

As such, it is important for the speech-language pathologist (SLP) and dietitian to work together, as nutritional needs will change with changing medical status. The dietitian may elect to perform a comprehensive nutrition assessment, as seen in Table 10–1, or may limit the assessment to the specific needs of the patient at treatment modification stages. The dietitian also works closely with other rehabilitation team members to select foods or supplements for oral feeding that provide proper nourishment while at the same time maximize proper oral control, transit, and timing of swallowing. If nutrition is nonoral, the dietitian monitors selection amounts and timing of enteral feeding to assure proper energy requirements and to ensure that the foods/supplements selected do not interfere with other conditions such as cardiac disease and diabetes. A comprehensive review of the roles of the dietitian may be found in the publications of the American Dietetic Association.[1,2]

PROPERTIES OF LIQUIDS AND FOODS

Rheology is the study of fluids and their properties. The need to use the proper thickeners in treating patients with dysphagia has influenced the recent development of this science specific to swallowing disorders.

> Advances in rheology have formed the basis for the development of stable consistencies in nutrition.

Table 10–1. Comprehensive Examination in Conjunction with a Nutritional Assessment by a Dietitian

Medical History
Primary diagnosis
Planned medical procedures
Medical comorbidities
Current cognitive status
Gastrointestinal history
History of pneumonia
Neurological status
Review of medications
Review results of previous swallow studies
Physical Assessments
Current weight and recent weight change
Coordination skills
Dentition
Edema
Handedness and recent change in handedness
Feeding skills
Living status
Nutritional History
Diet history
Recent diet changes
Tolerances to foods
Use of nutritional supplements
Medical restrictions to types of foods
Vitamin supplements
History of anorexia
Alcohol Intake
Recent Biochemical Data
Albumin, Transferrin, Prealbumin Glucose
Electrolytes Hemoglobin/Hemocrit
BUN/Creatinine

Source: Adapted and revised from Molseed L. Clinical evaluation of swallowing: the nutritionist's perspective. In: Murry T, Carrau RL, eds. *Clinical Management of Swallowing Disorders.* San Diego, CA. Singular; 2001, p.150.

Although standards are not completely established for all consistencies, an attempt has been made to establish standards for fluid consistencies.[3] Fluids are categorized according to their rheological properties. To understand this analysis completely goes beyond the scope of most members of the dysphagia team. However, a basic knowledge of rheology and how it relates to dysphagia is important to the clinician.

Rheology Terminology

Although their clinical significance is not completely determined, the rheological properties of food may be useful for the study and development of standard dysphagia diets and feeding protocols. More importantly, by obtaining a set of standards for different food and liquid consistencies, instrumental testing (whether it is the modified barium swallow, FEES, or other instrumental testing) can also approach standardization. The most common terms relating to the study of fluid flow properties are the following:

Constitutive equation: An equation relating to stress with strain and sometimes other variables, including time, temperature, and concentration.

Creep test: A test to determine the deformation of a material exposed to a constant stress. These are like relaxation tests, but a constant stress is applied, rather than a constant strain. The simplest creep test would be to apply a weight on top of a sample and record the change in shape (strain) over time; for example, placing a book on a cake and measuring the deformation over time.

Density: The compactness of a substance; the ratio of its mass to its volume measured in grams per milliliter (g/ml) or kilograms per milliliter (kg/ml).

Homogeneous: Well mixed and compositionally similar regardless of location.

Incompressible: Material that shows no change in density when a constant stress is applied (eg, water).

Isotropic: The material response is not a function of location or direction.

Kinematic viscosity: Viscosity divided by the density of the material.

Laminar flow: Nonturbulent flow.

Linear viscoelasticity: Viscoelasticity within the region where stress and strain are linearly related.

Newtonian fluid: A fluid with a linear relationship between shear stress and shear rate with a yield stress. The fluid viscosity of a newtonian fluid does not vary with shear rate.

Non-newtonian fluid: Any fluid deviating from newtonian behavior, for example, fluids that are suspensions. The attractive force between suspended particles weakens as shear rate increases.

Rheogram: A graph showing rheological relationships.

Rheology: The study of properties of fluids. Rheological models are mathematical expressions providing a "flow fingerprint" for fluid foods.

Rheometer: An instrument used for measuring rheological properties. This device is used in creep tests.

Shear (strain) rate: Change in strain with respect to time.

Strain: Relative deformation.

Viscoelastic: A material having both viscous and elastic properties.

Viscosity: Resistance to flow or alteration of shape by a substance as a result of molecular cohesion. This is perhaps the most important property when planning a diet for someone with a swallowing disorder. **Newton's postulate** reasons that if the shear stress is doubled, the velocity gradient (shear strain rate) within the fluid is doubled. For fluids, strain is measured in terms of shear rate, and the shear stress may be expressed as some function of shear rate and viscosity. For

newtonian fluids, the viscosity function is constant and called the coefficient of viscosity or **newtonian viscosity**.

Viscometer: A device used to measure the resistance of a material to flowing.

Applications of Rheology

Viscosity is a prime variable in the study of newtonian fluids.

> For simplicity, the clinician may view the viscosity of a fluid as being **proportional** to the **force** required to move it through.

A bolus that is twice as viscous requires roughly twice as much power from the swallow musculature to transport the bolus. Viscosity sheer rate profiles are shown in Table 10–2. As can be seen, standard barium is a non-newtonian fluid with a density greater than thin barium or a cordial fluid.[4] Thus, when studying swallow patterns with the modified barium swallow, the clinician should note the type and consistency of the barium. Where regular MBS studies are done, premixed barium consistencies should be available to the clinician so that when a report is generated, the treatment team will know the conditions under which the patient was evaluated.

An instrumental assessment of swallowing provides an indication of acceptable viscosities for maximum safe swallowing once it has been shown that the patient has normal sensation. It is important that the entire team understands the viscosities and use consistent mixtures during the treatment. Table 10–3 lists common agents that may be used to alter the viscosity of fluids. Ideally, these agents should be mixed with predetermined amounts of barium to provide consistent references to the dysphagia treatment. Some commercial products that list the density and the coefficient of viscosity are now available.

Testing of various materials to thicken foods is a relatively new area in relation to dysphagia. The **National Dysphagia Diet (NDD)** recommends thickeners in relation to the categories of food in the

Table 10–2. Viscosity-Shear Rate Profiles and Density Measurements of Various Fluids

Fluid	Newtonian or Non-Newtonian	Density (kg/ml)	Viscosity Range
Fluid 1: Thin cordial	newtonian	980	Constant cP = 2 cP*
Fluid 2: Thickened cordial	non-newtonian	1,000	Range of cP 100,000–300 cP from 1 to 100 l/s, "shear thinning"
Fluid 3: Standard barium (nectar)	non-newtonian	2,800	Range of cP 4,000–200 cP from 1 to 100 l/s, "shear thinning" + "plateau"
Fluid 4: Thin barium	newtonian	2,300	Constant cP = 26 cP, "Poor resolution at low rates"
Fluid 5: Thickened barium	non-newtonian	2,500	Range of cP 30,000–900 cP from 1 to 100 l/s, "shear thinning"

Source: From Cichero JA, Jackson O, Halley PJ, Murdoch BE. *J Med Speech Lang Pathol.* 1997;5:210.
*cP = centipoise: a measure of dynamic visocity.

Table 10–3. **Common Agents Used to Alter the Viscosity of Foods and Fluids**

Thinning Agents/Blenderizing Agents
Milk
Gravy
Juice
Tomato juice
Thickening Agents
Cornstarch
Baby cereal (or other dehydrated baby food)
Mashed potato flakes
Instant pudding
Unflavored gelatin

Source: Adapted from Molseed L. Chapter 34 In: Carrau RL, Murry T, eds. *Comprehensive Management of Swallowing Disorders.* San Diego, CA: Plural; 2006, p. 239 (Tables 34–5 and 34–6).

diet. Strowd et al[5] published a summary of various dysphagia diet foods (DDF) that are available for thickening. They found that the viscosity of honey-thick DDF was consistent with the NDD but other products were not. In general, they found that there was a poor relationship between the viscosity of DDF and barium test foods. Factors such as temperature, shaking up the substances, flavor selection,

and stability over time were all capable of changing the viscosity, as outlined in the NDD.

Payne et al[6] also found that there was a large range of viscosities over a number of commercially available starch products used in thickening liquids in Great Britain. They noted that the physical properties of the materials changed after opening, despite correct storage procedures.

> Of concern is the fact that starch-based thickeners may not be a stable product when it comes from the manufacturer.

Although there has been a significant increase in the number of thickeners available, there remains a need to identify the rheological properties as they relate to viscosity, because viscosity plays a major role in the consistency of the fluid swallowed.

An additional issue with thickeners involves the preparation of the thickeners by the health care team member responsible for the dietary consistency. Ideally, a liquid should be thickened to the consistency of the NDD recommendations. Most manufacturers list those instructions on their thickening products. Garcia et al[7] found that in a study of 42 health care providers, the range of thickened materials did not compare favorably to the published findings of laboratory viscosity measures or to the ranges of the NDD. Final thickened products were either too thick or too thin in their relationship to the target values. Reasons for this may be as simple as not following the guidelines on the product or perhaps may be related to the actual range in the makeup of the thickener itself.

Density also plays a role in the analysis of liquids. Density can be affected by temperature and the thickening agent. As the compactness of a substance changes, its flow will also change. Thus, the density may decrease as the compactness decreases. Moreover, if a product stays in the oral cavity for any length of time, its denseness may change, leading to misinterpretation of the type of fluid a patient can or cannot swallow.

> When a patient retains food in the oral cavity for lengthy periods of time, the density is no longer the same as when it was prepared.

The same may be said for density when it is left to stand in an overly warm or cold room or simply left to stand for a long period of time.

Textures

Texture refers to the composition of foods. The goal of normal swallowing is oral intake of all foods, liquids as well as solids. The intake of solid foods is related to the severity of impairment, adequate dentition for chewing, and muscular strength and coordination for bolus transit and control.

The management of oral feeding requires an understanding of liquid viscosities and food textures. According to Bourne,[8] there are 5 characteristics for defining food texture. These characteristics and examples of the textures related to these characteristics are shown in Table 10–4.

Common texture terminology includes thin liquids, thick liquids, slippery puree, and puree. These terms are purely perceptual in nature, as even common terms such as puree or nectar can have a wide range of viscosities and densities. Table 10–5, from Leonard and Kendall,[9] summarizes the terms that remain in use in many clinical settings. The textures range from thin liquids to foods requiring mastication.

Table 10–6 provides information showing the relationship between solid textures and swallowing

Table 10–4. *Characteristics of Food Textures as Outlined by Bourne[8] and the 8 Most Common Textures That Have a Significant Role in Dysphagia Diets, According to the American Dietetic Association*

Characteristics of Food Texture

1. It is a group of physical properties that derive from the structure of the food.

2. It consists of a group of properties, not a single property

3. It is sensed by touch, usually in the mouth but hands may also be used.

4. It is not related to chemical senses of taste or odor.

5. It can be measured objectively by means of mass, distance, and time.

8 Textures Most Significant in Dysphagia Diets and Treatments

1. *Adhesiveness* — The work required to overcome the attractive forces between the surface of a food and another surface to which it has contact. EX: amount of work required to remove peanut butter from the palate.

2. *Cohesiveness* — The degree to which the food deforms. EX: when a moist bolus of cracker is compressed between tongue and palate.

3. *Firmness* — The force required to compress a semisolid food. EX: Compressing pudding between the tongue and palate.

4. *Fracturability ("Biteability")* — The force that causes a solid food to break. EX: Biting peanut brittle with the incisors.

5. *Hardness* — The force required to compress a solid food to attain a certain deformation. EX: Chewing a hot dog just prior to when it begins to shear.

6. *Springiness* — The degree or rate that a sample returns to its original shape after being compressed. EX: Marshmallows.

7. *Viscosity* — The rate of flow per unit force. EX: The rate at which a milkshake or nectar is drawn through a straw.

8. *Yield Stress* — The minimum amount of shear stress that must be applied to food before it begins to flow. EX: Force required to get ketchup to flow from a bottle.

severity, as reported by Cherney et al.[10] The table provides examples of each texture and their properties along the viscosity continuum. Because the terms are somewhat general, the clinician must be aware of the instrumental test results along with the medical history and cognitive status of the patient when interpreting impairment level and food texture.

Table 10–5. Continuum of Viscosities and Textures

		Texture or Viscosity Continuum			
		Places stress on agility of airway closure for swallow but facilitates bolus transfer ⟷ Relieves demands on agility of airway closure and facilitates bolus transfer ⟷ Places stress on oral preparation and oral and pharyngeal transfer competence			
	Thin Liquids	**Thick Liquids**	**Slippery Puree**	**Puree**	**Foods Requiring Mastication (in order of descending difficulty)**
Example	(assumed to be at body temperature) Apple juice, cranberry juice, non, low-fat, and whole milk, fruit, ice, sherbet, jello, soft drinks	(assumed to be at body temperature) Tomato juice, nectar, apple juice with thickener, instant breakfast, > 1.5 cal/cc commercial supplement	(assumed to be at body temperature) Pudding, custard, puree fruit, puree vegetables (not starches)	Mashed potatoes, puree scrambled eggs, puree meat	Ground meat, regular scrambled eggs, canned fruit, soft cooked carrots, beets, bread Chopped meat, sandwiches (tuna, egg, bologna) Unrestricted diet
Properties	Easily deformed, moves very readily in response to gravity and compression	Less easily deformed than thin liquids, moves fairly readily in response to gravity or compression.	Less easily deformed, so may obstruct a narrow passage. Slides in response to gravity or compression.	Less easily deformed, thus can obstruct narrow passage. Transferred mostly by compression.	As the bolus becomes more viscous, it is less and less easily deformed, less likely to move in response to gravity, more reliant on dental and lingual competence for mastication and transit, sensory competence and judgment of bolus characteristics, adequate salivation, and healthy mucosa.
Transit	Thin liquids are most likely to move through the upper digestive tract quickly and completely.	Variably likely (depending on the degree of thickness) to move through the digestive tract easily without falling into the airway and to pass fairly well through narrow sites such as strictures.	Slippery purees are more likely to stop at obstacles such as webs and strictures, but may be less likely to "stick."	Purees are likely to stop at obstacles and may not slide easily along dry mucosa. Purees will not move through the pharynx without adequate compression/constriction. Complete transit requires adequate salivary and mucosal health.	Adequate oral and pharyngeal patency and strength of compression/ constriction is requisite for safe swallow of high-viscosity foods once mastication has transformed the solid into a puree. Adequate transfer requires adequate salivary and mucosal health.

continues

Table 10–5. continued

	Thin Liquids	Thick Liquids	Slippery Puree	Puree	Foods Requiring Mastication (in order of descending difficulty)
Airway	Agility of laryngeal airway closure for swallow is a prerequisite for ingestion of thin liquids.	Swallow of thick liquids requires less laryngeal agility because thick liquids are less easily deformed and move more slowly (speed varies with thickness) in response to gravity or compression.	Slippery purees require less laryngeal agility but more competent oral and pharyngeal constriction. If the bolus is not adequately transferred, residue may fall into the airway after the swallow. The properties of purees present a greater risk of obstructing the airway than liquids.	Because they do not move readily in response to gravity, purees are less likely to fall into the airway quickly. However, if oral and pharyngeal clearing is incomplete because of poor constriction or xerostomia, pharyngeal residue presents a risk to the airway after the swallow has been completed. The properties of purees present a greater risk of obstructing the airway than liquids.	Adequate airway protection during swallow of solids is reliant on adequately complete oral and pharyngeal transit. The airway can be obstructed if penetrated by solid bolus residue, even if mastication is fairly adequate. The properties of solids present a greater risk of obstructing the airway than liquids.
Patients	Patients with prolonged or incomplete oral, pharyngeal, or esophageal transit because of poor muscular constriction or narrowing (eg, stricture), but who are alert and enjoy good laryngeal function are most likely to achieve adequate intake with liquid consistencies.	Patients with prolonged or incomplete oral, pharyngeal, or esophageal transit because of poor muscular constriction or narrowing (eg, stricture) are most likely to achieve adequate intake with liquid consistencies. Patients with mild cognitive deficits or who show poor oral bolus control or impaired initiation of swallow gestures may require thickened liquids.	Patients who are slow to initiate swallow gestures, including airway closure, but who are able to apply some compression to accomplish oral and pharyngeal bolus transfer would tolerate slippery purees.	Patients who are able to apply adequate pressures to transfer the bolus through the oral and pharyngeal cavities completely will tolerate puree consistencies.	The goal of mastication is to produce a "swallow safe" bolus, probably one approximating a puree. The ability to tolerate degrees of viscosity in the solid range is dependent on lingual agility and ROM, judgment re: bolus readiness, salivary flow, and dentition.

Source: Modified from Mackenzie S, Lorens B. In: Leonard R, Kendall K, eds. *Dysphagia Assessment and Treatment Planning.* San Diego, CA: Plural; 2008

Table 10–6. The Relationship Between Solid Textures and Swallowing Severity

	NPO	Pureed	Mechanically Altered	Advanced	Regular
Function Impairment Level	Severe Impairment: All nourishment via alternate feeding method (NPO); trial oral intake with SLP only.	Moderately Severe Impairment: Alternate feeding method is primary source of nourishment. Limited, inconsistent success with oral intake. Requires constant supervision; some assistance required in feeding but SLP introduces new items or techniques.	Mild–Moderate Impairment: Fairly reliable swallowing of prescribed diet but may have difficulty with clear liquids or solids; requires supervision.	Mild Impairment: Intake of regular diet with some food restrictions; may require specific techniques or procedures to achieve successful swallowing. Does not require close supervision.	Minimal Impairment: Efficient chewing and swallowing of all food consistencies with occasional episodes of coughing and/or requires additional time for adequate intake. Normal: safe and efficient chewing and swallowing of all food consistencies.
Dysphagia Severity Rating: Parkinson Disease	Severe Dysphagia: More than 10% aspiration for all consistencies. "Nothing by mouth" recommended.	Moderate to Severe Dysphagia: Patient aspirates 5–10% on one or more consistencies, with potential for aspiration minimized by use of specific swallowing instructions. Cough reflex absent or nonprotective. Alternative mode of feeding required to maintain patient's nutritional need. If pulmonary status is compromised, "NPO" may be indicated.	Mild–Moderate Dysphagia: Potential for aspiration exists but is diminished by specific swallowing techniques and a modified diet. Time required for eating is significantly increased, and supplemental nutrition may be indicated.	Mild Dysphagia: Oral pharyngeal dysphagia is present but can be managed by specific swallowing suggestions. light modification in consistency of diet may be indicated.	Minimal Dysphagia: Videofluoroscopy shows slight deviance from a normal swallow. Patient may report a change in sensation during swallow. No change in diet is required. Normal swallowing mechanism.
Severity Scale Primarily Related to ALS	Aspiration of Secretions: Secretions cannot be managed noninvasively. Patient rarely swallows. Secretions are managed with suction/medication; patient cannot safely manage PO intake. Patient usually swallows reflexively.	Tube Feeding With Occasional PO Nutrition: Primary nutrition and hydration are accomplished by tube. Patient receives less than 50% of nutrition. PO intake alone is no longer adequate. Patient uses or needs a tube to supplement intake. Patient continues to take significant (less than 50%) PO. Liquified diet: oral PO intake is adequate. Nutrition is limited primarily to liquefied diet. Adequate thin liquid intake usually a problem. Patient may force self to eat.	Soft Diet: Diet is limited primarily to soft foods. Requires some special meal preparation. Prolonged time or small bite size: meal time has significantly lengthened and smaller bite sizes are necessary. Patient must concentrate on swallowing liquids.	Minor Swallowing Problems: Complains of some swallowing difficulties. Maintains an essentially regular diet. Isolated chocking episodes. Normal abnormalities: only patient notices slight indicator such as food lodging in the recesses of the moth or sticking in the throat.	Normal Swallowing: Patient denies any difficulty chewing or swallowing. Examination demonstrates no abnormality.

Source: Adapted from Cherney LR, Pannell JJ, Cantieri CA. Clinical evaluation of dysphagia in adults. In: Cherney LR, ed. *Clinical Management of Dysphagia in Adults and Children.* Gaithersburg, MD: Aspen Publishers; 1994.

ORAL NUTRITION AND DYSPHAGIA DIETS

Oral nutrition is the goal for most patients with dysphagia due to stroke or for those who have undergone head and neck cancer surgery. Conversely, for patients with progressive neuromuscular diseases, oral nutrition may be the starting level of intervention, with progression to an enteral feeding stage due to the progress of the disease.

Oral nutrition diets are organized on the basis of viscosity of the foods and liquids. Safe swallowing requires temporal management of the neuromuscular behaviors at each stage of the swallow.

National Dysphagia Diet

Dysphagia diets vary considerably from facility to facility. Although many hospitals, clinics, and nursing homes are beginning to adopt many of the recommendations and features of the National Dysphagia Diet,[11] considerable variation for specific patients remains. The NDD requires both the specification of food consistency and its viscosity.

> All dysphagia diets should adjust food/liquid intake for: (a) amount, (b) viscosity, (c) consistency, and (d) timing of the meal to achieve maximal nutrition and maintenance of the desired viscosity over the course of the feeding period.

Traditional oral dysphagia diets are typically a stepwise progression to the normal diet and grouped into liquids and 4 levels of viscosity/consistency boluses. According to the NDD, these are:

Liquid Consistency: Thin, nonaltered liquids such as coffee, tea, frozen desserts, and soft drinks.

Level 1: Pureed food and thickened liquids, the most conservative level. This diet is used for patients with severe oral preparatory, oral phase, and pharyngeal dysphagia. It includes homogeneous consistencies such as pudding and blenderized mashed potatoes. It avoids "lumpy" consistencies such as oatmeal and cottage cheese.

Level 2: Pureed and mechanically altered foods, plus thick or thickened liquids and very soft foods that require minimal chewing (eg, cottage cheese, macaroni, pancake with syrup). A Level 2 diet can also include those foods that are soft and easily formed into a bolus, such as cooked fruit and bananas. This diet avoids dry foods, or foods with skins. It is used with deficits of the oral phase or decreased pharyngeal peristalsis. It is also the most common diet for those suspected or identified with aspiration. It is first used under therapeutic control, and then the patient is advanced to it on her or his own when the clinician deems it safe to do so.

Level 3: Advanced soft and solid foods with nearly regular textures. This level will still avoid foods that are hard, foods with skins, and seeds or nuts. It allows breads, cakes, and tender whole meats with liquids, if they are allowed and tolerated. This diet is advised for individuals who are beginning to chew and to rehabilitate chewing and bolus propulsion.

Level 4: Regular soft foods and all liquids, avoiding rough or coarse foods. This diet usually precedes advancement to a regular diet. It is usually undertaken under supervision at first.

American Dietetic Association Diet

Although somewhat similar to the traditional levels noted above, the American Dietetic Association lists 4 levels of semisolids and solids in their recommendations for a dysphagia diet. These are:

Level 1: Dysphagia pureed—homogeneous, very cohesive puddinglike consistency; requiring bolus control, no chewing required.

Level 2: Dysphagia mechanically altered—consisting of cohesive, moist semisolid foods requiring chewing ability.

Level 3: Dysphagia advanced—consisting of soft foods that require more chewing ability.

Level 4: Regular—consisting of all foods allowed.

Diets and Consistencies

Liquids

Recently, terms have been proposed for liquids based on their viscosity ranges. The results were summarized recently by McCullough et al[12] and include the following 4 terms:

Thin

Nectarlike

Honeylike

Spoon-thick

Consistency Modifications

Liquid modification: Used to increase or decrease the viscosity of the liquid in order to achieve bolus control.

Thin: Clear liquids, milk, coffee and tea, and broth-based soups.

Thick: Milkshakes, strained cream soups, and nectars.

Thickened: Thin or thick liquids may require thickening agents to modify the consistency. It should be remembered that these thickeners may also alter other aspects of the bolus, as reviewed above in the section on viscosity. A number of food thickeners are now available in supermarkets, pharmacies, and health food stores. Table 10–7 lists commercial thickening agents that may be used. The recent literature suggests that not all are of equal consistency and therefore do not provide a stable viscosity. Because new products are being developed and marketed constantly, it is not the purpose of this chapter to recommend one manufacturer over another. Rather, clinicians will have to keep up with new materials and with the modifications that companies offer as rheological testing becomes more common. The amounts to be mixed will vary

Table 10–7. Commercial Thickening Agents

Company	Brand Name	Product Basis
Nestle Nutrition http://www.nestlenutritionstore.com	Thicken Up	Modified cornstarch
Woodbury Products http://www.woodburyproducts.com	Thick-It	Modified starch
	Thick-It 2	Modified starch
Simply Thick http://www.simplythick.com	Simply Thick	Starch base
Gillco Ingredients http://www.gillcoingredients.com	Pectin Gel	Polymeric carbohydrate
Hormel Health Labs http://www.hormelhealthlabs.com	Thick and Easy	Modified food starch
	Nutra Thick	Modified food starch
Total Care Home Medical http://www.tchomemedical.com	Variety of Products	Several
Bernard Foods http://www.edietshop.com	Ultra Thixx	Cornstarch
Links Medical Products http://www.linsmed.com	Hydra Aid	Starch with other materials added

substantially and the clinician may resort to "trial and error" mixture consistency for each individual. However, as pointed out above, this could lead to vastly different consistencies and affect the safety of oral nutrition.

Solid food modification: A means to advancing the diet in steps consistent with patient progress.

Pureed/liquefied: Regular food may be blenderized with added liquid as needed to form a smooth consistency. The consistency may vary from a thick liquid consistency to a pastelike consistency. The consistency of baby food is often best tolerated; however, it should be adjusted to meet the individual's needs.

Mechanically altered: Chopped and ground foods, very soft foods such as pasta and casseroles, and foods that easily form a cohesive bolus.

Soft: Naturally soft foods that require a minimal amount of chewing. Meat may need to be cut in small pieces and rough food such as nuts, popcorn, raw vegetables, and salads are avoided. Avoid foods that crumble or are of mixed consistency. Table 10–8 presents 3 categories of foods that are not well tolerated by individuals with swallowing problems.

Table 10–8. Three Categories of Foods That Are Not Well Tolerated by Individuals With Swallowing Problems

Crumbly and Noncohesive Foods	
Plain ground meat, chicken, or fish	Peas, corn, or legumes
	Cornbread
Scrambled eggs	Cottage cheese
Rice	Coconut
Jello	Nuts and seeds
Crackers	

Mixed Consistency Foods	
Vegetable soup	Salad with dressing
Soup with large pieces or chunks of food	Canned fruit
	Gelatin with fruit
Cold cereal with milk	Yogurt with fruit
Citrus fruit	

Sticky Foods
Dry mashed potatoes
Peanut butter
Fresh white or refined wheat bread
Fudge or butterscotch sauce/caramel
Bagels or soft rolls

NONORAL DIETS

Introduction

A large number of patients are unable to take adequate nutrition orally. This may be temporarily in patients who have had surgery for oral pharyngeal or laryngeal disease or patients who are acutely recovering from a stroke or those patients with a neuromuscular degenerative disorder who no longer can manage oral nutrition.

Enteral feeding is the type of feeding that occurs by way of the intestine. In patients who are unable to take adequate nutrition by mouth but otherwise have a functioning gastrointestinal (GI) tract, this type of feeding can be used. The enteral approach may reach the stomach, duodenum, or jejunum via a feeding tube placed through the nose. Table 10–9 summarizes the common feeding tubes, with their advantages and disadvantages.

Nasogastric, Nasoduodenal, and Nasojejunal Tubes

Nasogastric tubes (NG) are the most commonly placed tubes. Their use is typically short term (3 to 21 days) and they are placed with the expectation that swallow rehabilitation will be aggressive and fast paced. In some cases, the NG tube must be replaced by a more permanent nonoral feeding tube, but these cases are usually the result of additional morbidity that was not expected at the time of NG

Table 10–9. Common Feeding Tubes With Their Advantages and Disadvantages

Access Site	Advantages	Disadvantages
Nasogastric	Minimally invasive, easy placement; suitable for short-term use; transitional to bolus feeding; radiographic confirmation not necessarily required but recommended for liability issues	Cosmetic: feeding tube visible unless patient self-inserts each feeding; risk of sinusitis; lack of intact gag reflex may (not necessarily) indicate increased aspiration risk; stomach must be uninvolved with primary disease
Nasoduodenal	Minimally invasive, easy placement; suitable for short-term use; reduced risk of pulmonary aspiration; useful in conditions of gastroparesis or impaired stomach emptying; useful if esophageal reflux present; allows for feeding when bowel sounds are diminished or absent	Requires radiographic confirmation of placement; Cosmetic: feeding tube is visible; requires 43" length feeding tube; may not remain placed in duodenum due to tube migration; typically, smaller diameter tube than NG, more prone to plugging if not properly maintained
Nasojejunal	Same advantages as nasoduodenal; placement of tip further down GI tract minimizes dislocation to stomach; 60" length tubes available offering even greater placement security	Similar disadvantages as nasoduodenal, except placement of tip more secure
Cervical Esophagostomy	Improved cosmetic appeal as end of tube more easily concealed; ease of feeding over gastrostomy as do not need to undress; more suitable for long-term feeding	Although more suitable for long-term feeding, the lower esophageal sphincter is stented open and same concerns for gastric and esophageal reflux with possible pulmonary aspiration are present as with the NG feeding tube
Gastrostomy	Suitable for long-term feeding; Cosmetically more appealing than a nasally placed tube; minimizes risk of tube migration and aspiration due to voluntary or accidental dislocation of nasoenteric tube by patient; percutaneous placement available (PEG); some GT have large bore tubes, which minimize occlusion from medications and high-viscosity formulas; most suitable of all tubes for use of homemade formula, provided tip is placed in stomach and it is a large bore tube; bolus feeding option available if tip of tube in stomach	Potential risk of pulmonary aspiration; lack of intact gag reflex and/or presence of esophageal reflux may indicate increased risk or aspiration; insertion site care needed; potential skin excoriation at stoma site from leakage of gastric secretion; potential fistula at insertion site after FT removal; If GT feeding tip port is placed in duodenum, usually a smaller bore tube is used and it is subject to more occlusion risk

placement. Figure 10–1 shows a typical NG feeding tube that may be used for both short-term or long-term nutritional support. The tube is placed by the physician, and usually an x-ray is taken to validate the final location of the tube. Nasogastric tubes have their termination in the stomach.

Nasoduodenal tubes are also used for short-term dysphagia. They are useful when there is a strong suspicion of **esophageal reflux** or **gastroparesis** (inability to empty the stomach due either to bilateral vagotomy or neural damage to the vagus nerve).

Nasojejunal tubes terminate in the jejunum, which is the midsection of the small intestine. In the jejunum are small fingerlike outgrowths that allow for digested food or liquid to be absorbed, thus providing the needed nutrition even when the stomach cannot tolerate food or liquids.

Gastrostomy Tubes

A gastrostomy tube is surgically placed directly into the stomach. Feedings via gastrostomy tube can be

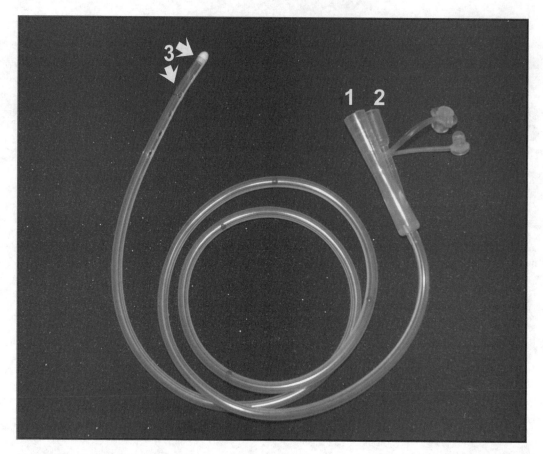

Figure 10–1. Kendall Argyle silicone Salem Sump tube, 16-Fr., 48" length (Tyco/Healthcare). Dual Lumen. Y-connector with (1) suction drainage lumen/feeding port, (2) suction vent lumen, and (3) closed-end tip with multiple exit ports. **Source:** *From Leonard R, Kendall K. Dysphagia* **Assessment and Treatment Planning: A Team Approach** *(2nd ed.), San Diego, CA: Plural, 151 (Figure 10–2).*

administered by continuous feeding or by bolus feeding. Gastrostomy tubes are preferred for long-term nonoral feeding because they are less likely to become dislodged than nasal tubes. For the patient who is ambulatory, gastrostomy tubes are easily hidden, avoiding less social embarrassment. In addition, medications are more easily administered due to the size of the gastrostomy tube. Gastrostomy tubes are less likely to clog than NG tubes and they do not irritate the interarytenoid area.

A gastrostomy can be created through a percutaneous endoscopic route (PEG), by surgical (ie, laparotomy or laparoscopic) placement of a tube, or creation of a stoma. The PEG has become the procedure of choice, because it can be done in the intensive

care unit or the procedure room under local anesthesia. In general, the PEG takes less time and costs less than laparoscopic-assisted or open gastrostomies. Figure 10–2 shows a typical gastrostomy tube.

From an anatomical standpoint, the gastrostomy can be classified into 2 categories: those that are lined with serosa (temporary) and those lined with mucosa (permanent). Functionally, this relates to not only the care of the gastrostomy site, but what is required for reversal when it is no longer needed. Serosa-lined gastrostomies include PEG, laparoscopic-assisted gastrostomy, and open (Stamm) gastrostomy. They are in fact serosa-lined gastrocutaneous fistulas. The lining of the tract is granulation tissue, which will quickly close if the tube is removed for any reason.

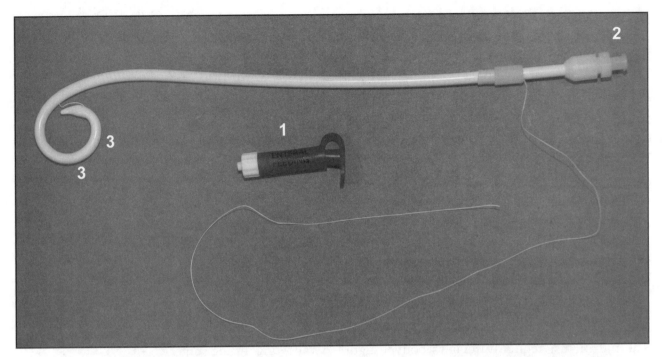

Figure 10–2. Deutsch Gastrostomy Catheter with AQ Hydrophilic Coating, 16-Fr., 25 cm long with Cook-Cope type locking loop. (1) Enteral feeding adapter with male Luer lock fitting, (2) Luer lock tube opening, and (3) exits ports. Source: *From Leonard R, Kendall K.* Dysphagia Assessment and Treatment Planning: A Team Approach *(2nd ed.), San Diego, CA: Plural, 153 (Figure 10–6).*

Therefore, if this type of gastric tube is displaced, it must be replaced within 4 to 6 hours if the tract is to stay open.

The "permanent" or mucosa-lined gastrostomy (Janeway gastrostomy) requires a laparotomy in the operating room and is constructed by creating a tube of stomach, which is brought out through the anterior abdominal wall. The mucosa-lined gastrocutaneous fistula, as opposed to the serosa-lined fistula, will not close if the feeding tube is removed.

The following problems are the most commonly associated with placement of a gastrostomy tube:

- Excoriated skin around gastrostomy site
- Cellulitis around gastrostomy site
- Abscess at gastrostomy site (rare)
- Catheter clogging
- Gastrostomy tube extrusion

The decision to opt for nonoral feeding is often a critical one for the patient and family.

> Instrumental testing provides the basis for the decision to opt for nonoral feeding, but the decision is not based solely on radiographic, manometric, or endoscopic assessment.

Other factors used to decide in favor of nonoral feeding include: (1) time required to swallow; (2) energy level of patient; (3) need for alternative route for medications; (4) repeated episodes of dehydration; (5) history of pneumonia; and (6) unexplained weight loss or signs of malnutrition. All of the issues, those related to diagnostic finding as well as the clinical observations, must be discussed with the patient and family members when the option for nonoral feeding is part of the treatment plan.

It is equally important to present to the patient a strong rationale to elect nonoral feeding when there is a progressive neuromuscular disease such as amyotrophic lateral sclerosis (ALS). Logemann[13] has pointed out that the time to complete one swallow has diagnostic significance. This factor, along with those noted above, should be considered when a feeding tube is planned.

> The patient with ALS and other patients with neuromuscular degeneration will benefit from a feeding tube when they still have the energy and desire to maintain their nutrition.

Waiting until the patient is at or near the end of life denies him or her the quality of life that might otherwise remain if nutrition was maintained.

MALNUTRITION AND DEHYDRATION

Patients with swallowing disorders should be monitored for signs of malnutrition and dehydration. The nutritionist regularly reviews body weight, caloric intake, liquid intake, feeding schedules (oral and nonoral), medication/nutrition interactions, and biochemical data. However, it is up to the entire dysphagia team to be alert for those factors that lead to dehydration and malnutrition.

Stroke

Stroke patients may be the largest group of individuals with dysphagia to be at risk for malnutrition and dehydration. Cognitive defects, hemiparesis, spatial neglect, and motor disabilities all contribute to the risk of malnutrition in stroke patients. Malnutrition in stroke patients may be as high as 56% at some point during a 3-week hospital stay.[14]

Malnutrition occurs as a result of poor or inadequate oral or nonoral intake. **Protein-calorie malnutrition (PCM)** is one of the most common types of malnutrition. PCM has the power to fatigue muscles, alter the neuromuscular function of the swallow muscles, and contribute to increasing the severity of dysphagia.

> Other factors such as increased stress reaction, higher incidence of respiratory and urinary infections, and bedsores come into play once malnutrition is present.

Given these comorbidity factors, one might expect longer hospital stays, poorer outcome, and greater risk of further illness with the presence of malnutrition.

In a systematic review of nutritional status during the acute and rehabilitation periods, Foley et al[15] found malnutrition ranging from a low of 8% to a high of 52.6%. Interestingly, the findings of malnutrition were increased during the rehabilitation period compared to the acute stroke period (0 to 7 days postonset). Others have found that malnutrition in the stroke patient is also related to the severity of the stroke[16] and to the lack of swallowing therapy during the poststroke period.[17]

Head and Neck Cancer

The problems with nutrition following head and neck cancer relate primarily to the loss of organs for swallowing during surgery.

> Patients with cancers in the head and neck often have significant swallowing problems prior to surgery.

They may already be suffering from malnutrition due to their inability to tolerate foods and liquids either due to the pain, the inability to move foods through the mouth, or the blockage of food by tumors in the pharynx or esophagus. Following surgery, the pathway to swallowing may be significantly altered. If radiation therapy is prescribed, further difficulties occur with mucositis, pain, or simply fatigue. A greater incidence of tracheostomy dependence and increased incidence of aspiration are noted when structures that have previously contributed to valving have been removed (eg, supraglottic laryngectomy, partial laryngectomy).[18]

Long-term effects of head and neck cancer also contribute to malnutrition due to the changing and fibrosing structures associated with radiation. PEG dependency rates increase due to the inability of the postradiation patient to manage bolus transfer due to tissue fibrosis and achalasia.[19]

When there is a concern about malnutrition, weight, or weight history, serum albumin and prealbumin are capable of identifying the majority of patients requiring nutritional attention. In the acute and rehabilitation settings, weight should be checked every 2 days. For home health care, weight should be checked at every visit. For patients undergoing longer treatments such as radiation therapy or chemotherapy, weight should be checked weekly and nutritional reviews should be done if a weight change is noted from one period to the next. Patients should understand that a feeding tube need not be a permanent nutritional route but rather a part of the rehabilitation from the underlying condition, whether it be a stroke or treatment for head and neck cancer. Whenever signs of malnutrition and dehydration are observed, a dietitian should be consulted.

NUTRITION IN THE AGING POPULATION

Swallowing problems with advancing age are a major health problem in the elderly but otherwise well individuals, as well as in hospitalized individuals and nursing home residents.

> An estimated 40% to 60% of nursing home residents have signs of swallowing disorders.[20]

It is in this group and the elderly patients in general that nutrition and eating play an important part of life, whether to maintain health or to aid in recovery from disease or sickness.[21] Because of the importance of eating, no diet should be recommended simply on the basis of a diagnosis or on the basis of an instrumental test. There are many factors that go into the nutritional needs of patients with dysphagia, as we have reviewed above. This is especially true in elderly patients, including those restricted to nursing or those otherwise healthy elderly individuals with other comorbidities. In both groups, the diet should be as liberal as swallowing safety allows. The elderly dysphagic population may face many problems affecting nutrition, such as poor eyesight, eating alone, and limited hand mobility. All of these problems have a bearing not only on what the patient may or may not eat but also on the patient's

quality of life. The importance of qualified dietitians to oversee the content of meals for the elderly should not be overlooked in the rehabilitation process. However, the dietitian should not undertake the management of nutrition in the elderly as their responsibility solely.

> Especially in elderly patients, the dietitian must work with the SLP, the physical therapist, and the attending physician to make sure that the nutrition needs are met within the framework of the medical conditions present, the physical abilities and limitations of the patient, and the quality of life needs that apply to each particular patient.

In some patients, this may mean a more liberalized diet to enhance quality of life; in others, it may mean restrictions in certain food groups or viscosities.[22]

Table 10–10 summarizes the major considerations that must be considered when preparing diets for elderly individuals. The dietitian must take all of these into consideration, along with the nutrition requirements of each individual. These considerations

Table 10–10. Considerations When Planning a Nutritional Rehabilitation Program for the Elderly Patient

Living situation
Dentition
Physical disabilities and limitations
Participation in physical activities
Social interactions at mealtime
Nutritional needs — weight maintenance, weight gain, weight reduction
Mental function
Emotional function
Religious preferences
Ethnic food preferences
Swallow security
Available community diet services
Meal delivery systems

are important because it is not always possible to do the proper tests or complete tests in elderly individuals. Thus, the choice of food consistencies and the viscosities and combinations of viscosities may be more subjective than objective. There is a need to talk to the families if available, other caregivers such as nurses and attendants, and roommates or neighbors to get a feel for what the elderly patient's needs are when the patient himself or herself cannot or does not express those needs. In all elderly patients, no diet should be so restrictive that it discourages oral intake. The American Dietetic Association favors a liberalized policy when considering diets for the elderly.[23]

> It is the position of the American Dietetic Association (ADA) that the quality of life and nutritional status of older residents in long-term care facilities may be enhanced by a liberalized diet. The ADA advocates the use of qualified dietetic professionals to assess and evaluate the need for medical nutritional therapy according to each person's individual medical condition, needs, desires, and rights.
>
> Although this statement addresses elderly in long-term care facilities, it is appropriate in treating all elderly individuals. Food and liquid, although primarily for nutrition and health maintenance, also play a role in one's social life. It is up to the members of the swallowing and feeding team to keep the broad-based role of nutrition in mind when managing dysphagia in the elderly.

SUMMARY

This chapter discussed the importance of integrating the work of the nutritionist with that of the SLP to avoid such problems as dehydration and malnutrition that can occur with patients following stroke, head and neck cancer, or other diseases leading to dysphagia. The SLP who treats swallowing disorders must not only use behavioral techniques to improve oral nutrition, but must also maintain knowledge of the properties of the foods and liquids that are being swallowed.

> Bolus size, consistency, and viscosity all affect the ultimate success of the patient's ability to achieve oral nutrition that results in adequate protein-calorie intake.

The study of rheology characterizes fluids according to their properties, but it is only in its infancy as it relates to dysphagia. Rheological advances have provided the basis for understanding why some viscosities are managed better than others. Proper viscosity allows the patient to control the speed of fluid transit and ultimately reduce the probability of penetration and/or aspiration. Diets for patients with dysphagia are organized on the basis of rheological properties and protein-calorie balance. Safe swallowing requires a combination of the proper consistency and viscosity along with the management of neuromuscular behaviors at each stage of the swallow. Viscosity modifications, either by changing the foods themselves or by modifying liquids and foods with thickening or thinning agents, provide the clinician with a range of options that can be used with various postures and techniques to achieve a safe swallow and advance the patient closer to a regular diet.

If oral nutrition is not possible, other means of nutrition must be invoked. The SLP who understands the basis of nonoral feeding, whether though a PEG or other means, can monitor the progress of the patient, along with the nutritionist. At the same time, oral motor exercises can be included in the treatment process to prepare the patient for the time when oral feeding may be tried.

STUDY QUESTIONS

1. The prime variable for studying the properties of liquids is:
   A. Density

B. Flow

C. Viscosity

D. Shear rate

2. Viscosity represents a characteristic of a liquid that can be described more simply as:

   A. Thickness

   B. Resistance to flow

   C. Degree of elasticity

   D. Type of texture

3. The National Dysphagia Diet is:

   A. A diet to be followed in nursing homes

   B. A proposed diet to allow comparisons of nutrition from facility to facility

   C. A research diet used to assess changes in swallowing function

   D. A diet that provides for recovery of dysphagia in patients with strokes

4. Chewing provides an opportunity for a food texture to be:

   A. Equally dense

   B. Equally homogeneous

   C. Equally cohesive

   D. All of the above

5. Total parenteral nutrition differs from percutaneous endoscopic gastrostomy feeding in that:

   A. It is continuous throughout the day

   B. It delivers nutrition directly to the bloodstream

   C. It can lead to dehydration

   D. It can only be managed in hospitalized patients

DISCUSSION QUESTION

Diabetic patients are a special group when it comes to nutrition requirements and limitations. Review additional literature to discuss the nutritional requirements and limitations for adult diabetes (usually Type 2 diabetes) as well as for childhood diabetes (usually Type 1 diabetes). How will oral and nonoral nutritional needs have to be adjusted for these groups?

REFERENCES

1. Nutrition management in dysphagia. In: *Manual of Clinical Dietetics* (5th ed.). Chicago, IL: American Dietetic Association; 1996.

2. Lewis MM, Kidder JA. *Nutrition Practice Guidelines for Dysphagia.* Chicago, IL: American Dietetic Association; 1996.

3. Li M, Brasseur JG, Kern MK, Dodds WJ. Viscosity measurements of barium sulfate mixtures for use in motility studies of the pharynx and esophagus. *Dysphagia.* 1992; 7:17–30

4. Cichero JA, Hay G, Murdock BE, Halley M. Videofluoroscopic fluids versus mealtime fluids: differences in viscosity and density made clear. *J Med Speech Lang Path.* 1997;5:210

5. Strowd L, Kyzima J, Pillsbury D, Valley T, Rubin BR. Dysphagia dietary guidelines and the rheology of nutritional feeds and barium test feeds. *Chest.* 2008;133(6):1397–1401.

6. Payne C, Methven C, Fairfield C, Bell A. Consistently inconsistent: available starch-based dysphagia products. *Dysphagia.* 2011 Mar;26(1):27–33.

7. Garcia JM, Chambers E, Clark M, Helverson J, Matta Z. Quality of care issues for dysphagia: modifications involving oral fluids. *J Clin Nurs.* 2010 June;19(11–12):1618–1624.

8. Bourne MC. *Food Texture and Viscosity: Concept and Measurement.* San Diego, CA: Academic Press; 1982:9–10, 115–117.

9. Leonard R, Kendall K. *Dysphagia Assessment and Treatment Planning.* San Diego, CA: Singular; 1997:240–241, 250–251.

10. Cherney LR, Pannell JJ, Cantieri CA. Clinical evaluation of dysphagia in adults. In: Cherney LR, ed. *Clinical Management of Dysphagia in Adults and Children.* Gaithersburg, MD: Aspen Publishers; 1994:77.

11. National Dysphagia Diet Task Force. *National Dysphagia Diet: Standardization for Optimal Care.* Chicago, IL: American Dietetic Association; 2002:1–15.

12. McCullough G, Pelletier C, Steele C. National dysphagia diet: what to swallow? *ASHA Leader.* 2003;16:27.

13. Logemann JA. Factors affecting ability to resume oral nutrition in the oropharyngeal dysphagic individual. *Dysphagia.* 1990;4:202–208.

14. Axelsson K, Asplund K, Norberg A, Ericsson S. Eating problems and nutritional status during hospital stay of patients with severe stroke. *J Am Diet Assoc.* 1989;89: 1092–1096.

15. Foley NC, Martin RE, Salter BA, Teasell RW. A Review of the relationship between dysphagia and malnutrition following stroke. *J Rehabil Med.* 2009;41:707–713.

16. Crary MA, Carnaby-Mann GD, Miller L, Antonios N, Silliman S. Dysphagia and nutritional status at the time of hospital admission for ischemic stroke. *J Stroke Cardiovasc Dis.* 2006;15:164–171.

17. Lin LC, Wang SC, Chen SH, Wang TG, Chen MY, Wu SC. Efficacy of swallowing training for residents following stroke. *J Advanced Nurs.* 2003;44:469–478.

18. Wein RO, Weber RS. The current role of vertical partial laryngectomy and open supraglottic laryngectomy. *Curr Prob Cancer.* 2005;29(4):201–214.

19. Corry J. Feeding tubes and dysphagia: cause or effect in head and neck cancer patients. *J Med Imaging Radiat Onc.* 2009;53:431–432.

20. Smith TL, Sun MM, Pippin J. Research professional briefs: characterizing process control of fluid viscosities in nursing homes. *J Am Diet Assoc.* 2004;104(6):969–971.

21. Centers for Disease Control and Prevention. Healthy aging: preventing disease and improving quality of life among elder Americans. Retrieved from http//www.cdc .gov/nccdphp/aag-aging

22. Kuzmarski MF, Dweddle DO. Position paper of the American Dietetic Association: nutrition across the spectrum of aging. *J Am Diet Assoc.* 2005;105(4):616–633.

23. American Dietetic Association. Position statement of the American Dietetic Association: liberalized diets for older adults in long-term care. *J Ame Diet Assoc.* 2002;102: 1316–1323.

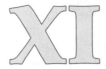

Patients With Voice and Swallowing Disorders

CHAPTER OUTLINE

  I. INTRODUCTION
  II. DIAGNOSIS
  III. INSTRUMENTATION
  IV. PERSONNEL
  V. FACILITIES
  VI. CASE STUDIES FROM VOICE AND SWALLOWING
     CENTERS
     A. Parkinson Disease
     B. Cough and Hoarseness
     C. Zenker Diverticulum
     D. Early Laryngeal Cancer
     E. Vocal Fold Paralysis
     F. Late Effects of Radiation Therapy in the Head and
       Neck Region
     G. Failure to Thrive in an Autistic Child
  VII. SUMMARY
  VIII. STUDY QUESTIONS
  IX. DISCUSSION QUESTION
  X. REFERENCES

INTRODUCTION

Speech and voice production and swallowing are overlaid functions of the organs in the head and neck. The lips, tongue, teeth, nasopharynx, velopharynx, oropharynx, and larynx are all involved in swallowing and speaking. Swallowing requires the manipulation of food in the oral cavity by the lips, tongue, and teeth, followed by transmission to the esophagus while protecting the airway by closing the vocal folds. Speech production requires air from the lungs, approximation and vibration of the vocal folds, and the modification of the tone and airstream by the lips, tongue, teeth, nasopharynx, and velopharynx, combined with neural integration of those structures. Anatomically, physiologically, and functionally, there is a significant overlap between the production of speech, voice, and swallowing functions. Clinicians who treat disorders of swallowing, speech, or voice should have specific knowledge of the structures and their functions as they relate to speech and swallowing.

From a practical point of view, there are many reasons for unifying the personnel who treat voice and swallowing disorders and the facilities where they are treated into a comprehensive center where patients can express their needs regarding both swallowing disorders and concerns about their speech or voice to individuals who have a keen interest and understanding of how disorders of speech, voice, and swallowing may interact. The development of a center that brings together those who have a special interest and expertise in the diagnosis and treatment of problems affecting the organs of voice and swallowing eliminates the need for a patient to travel from place to place to address these issues.

The management of speech, voice, and swallowing disorders in patients with head and neck cancer dates back over 100 years ago when the first laryngectomy was reported by Billroth and Gussenbauer in 1874, and reviewed by Fasching,[1] who also included a report of fitting a patient with a pneumatic artificial larynx. This device introduced sound into the pharynx through a surgically created fistula. Although the fistula aided the patient in communication, it also reduced the propelling force associated with swallowing and was eventually abandoned. However, since that time, the combined emphasis on postsurgical rehabilitation of swallowing and communication has been reflected in the advent of numerous surgical procedures designed to preserve voice and speech after head and neck cancer followed by rehabilitation by speech-language pathologists (SLPs), physical and occupational therapists, and dietitians. It is this group of specialists ho staff a comprehensive voice and swallowing center.

The modern era of team dysphagia management began with the publication of Logemann's text on the evaluation and treatment of swallowing disorders in 1983.[2] In that early work, clinicians were introduced to the importance of diagnosing and treating swallowing problems that arose from surgical sequelae, neurological events such as stroke, and degenerative neuromuscular diseases.

> Many of the current conservative surgical procedures, as well as the organ preservation protocols requiring radiation and chemoradiation to treat cancer of the head and neck, alter the natural swallowing patterns or compound the preexisting problems of speech and swallowing that exist in patients.

Logemann reported medical, surgical, and behavioral approaches for the management of swallowing disorders in patients with neurological disorders, as well as in patients following various surgical procedures.

Organ preservation procedures may also contribute to voice changes such as hoarseness and vocal weakness, disrupted resonance, and disorders of articulation. The comprehensive voice and swallowing center is composed of a team that understands the anatomy and physiology of the organs of the speech, voice, and swallowing mechanisms and brings together a unified program to maximize recovery of communication and swallowing functions.

In this chapter, the organization of a voice and swallowing center is described. The functional basis for a specialized voice and swallowing center will be shown with case studies of typical patients seen by the specialists in the center. In addition, the diagnostic equipment and space needed to maintain a functional voice and swallowing center are presented.

DIAGNOSIS

The oral cavity, pharynx, and larynx share the responsibility and burden of channeling expiratory airflow and voice upward and outward and propelling foods, liquids, and medications downward into the esophagus and stomach. Because of this shared passage, speech-language pathologists (SLPs) and otolaryngologists who are both uniquely trained in the anatomy, physiology, and neurology of the head, neck, and upper aerodigestive tract are uniquely qualified to develop and lead the team in the management of patients with voice, speech, and swallowing problems. The SLPs who treat voice and speech problems in head and neck cancer patients usually are trained to treat swallowing disorders in these patients. SLPs who treat language and speech disorders in the acute and long-term stroke and neurologically disordered populations are also involved in the treatment of swallowing disorders. The role of the SLP is to assess the patient's functional communication needs and safety of swallowing.

Once the assessment is made, the SLP and the otolaryngologist propose a plan of rehabilitation to the patient that may include pre- and postoperative treatments. The personnel of the swallowing center combine to work with the patient to achieve a safe and functional swallow and maximize communication.

The important elements for the SLP include the conditions at the onset of the problem, prior illnesses (including those related to birth or occurring at birth), genetic or inherited disorders and diseases, and the patient's family history of diseases related to the current condition. Currently prescribed and over-the-counter medications should also be noted. Also, during the speech and language history, the patient's prior level of function should be noted. Rehabilitation specialists should remember that treatment of swallowing requires a general level of cognition that allows the patient to follow commands, some of which may be complex.

The role of the otolaryngologist is to conduct a comprehensive head and neck examination, to recommend special tests, and to propose and manage medical or surgical intervention. The oral-motor examination, assessment of the sensory and motor functions of the cranial nerves involved in swallowing, and the ability of the vocal folds to function in voice production and swallowing along with specific tests of voice and swallowing are done by the otolaryngologist or by members of the voice and swallowing center. Special tests such as magnetic resonance imaging or pulmonary function tests to assess the respiratory control in these disorders are ordered by the otolaryngologist and reviewed by the swallowing team.

The otolaryngologist who treats swallowing disorders must have an understanding of the cranial nerve functions during voice production and swallowing. She or he must also recommend and conduct the proper tests to obtain a diagnosis and, along with the other members of the treatment team, offer a plan of rehabilitation. Table 11–1 summarizes major conditions and disorders routinely seen in a specialized voice and swallowing center. Some of these conditions are clearly more related to voice and speech disorders; others are primarily related to swallowing disorders. All these conditions are ideally seen by a coordinated treatment team whose members understand that speech and swallowing disorders may require specialized treatment.

> The members of a comprehensive voice and swallowing center determine the diagnosis and develop a plan of treatment using both patient complaints and documentation from the proper examinations, such as laryngeal imaging during swallowing or results of radiological studies of swallowing.

The medical diagnosis must be obtained prior to treatment for speech, voice, and swallowing disorders by the rehabilitation specialists. The diagnosis is made by the otolaryngologist, neurologist, or the pediatric otolaryngologist and they rely on the current test results and the patient's history.

Table 11–1. *Common Conditions, Disorders, and Diseases That May Have Components of Speech, Voice, and Swallowing Disorders*

Vocal fold paralysis	Laryngopharyngeal reflux
Vocal fold paresis	Gastroesophageal reflux
Superior laryngeal nerve paralysis	Dehydration
Vocal fold atrophy	Long-term intubation
Bilateral vocal fold paralysis	Tracheostomy
Chronic cough	Medications
Shortness of breath	Early postradiation dysphagia
Parkinson disease	Long-term radiation dysphagia
Cerebral vascular accident	Lingual, oral, and oropharyngeal cancers
Amyotrophic lateral sclerosis	Larynx preservation surgeries
Myasthenia gravis	Benign tumors of the head and neck
Vocal fold granuloma	Autism
Mental retardation	Autoimmune diseases

Prior to instrumental assessment or imaging of any type, the clinician will want to document the patient's problems using self-assessment tools whenever possible. Thus, diagnosis in the state of the art voice and swallowing center will include the use of patient self-assessment tools such as the Reflux Symptom Index (Appendix III), the SWAL-QOL, the Voice Handicap Index (VHI) and Voice Handicap Index-10 (Appendices IV-A and IV-B), and tests of motor speech functions.

INSTRUMENTATION

Special diagnostic and treatment equipment play an important role in the voice and swallowing center. Specifically, systems that allow the visualization of the upper aerodigestive tract structures under dynamic conditions guide clinicians in making the diagnosis and developing treatment plans. Transnasal flexible laryngoscopy (TFL) with a video camera attached to allow recording is used for the assessment of the nasopharynx, oropharynx, and larynx. The larynx and vocal folds may be observed during breathing, speaking, swallowing, and other vegeta-

tive activities during a TFL examination. TFL with video recording allows the clinician to perform and review FEES and FEESST examinations with the patient as well as to archive the exams for comparison after treatment.

Videostrobolaryngoscopy (VSL) with video recording is also a key instrument in the voice and swallowing center. VSL provides the clinician with a tool to observe the vocal folds under stroboscopic light for the purpose of assessing vocal fold closure patterns, motion, and symmetry. The use of high-speed digital imaging video is a relatively new tool for the diagnostician to examine details of vocal fold vibration. Recording at speeds of 2,000 frames per second and above, it captures the real-time motion of the vocal folds.

A typical scenario in a voice and swallowing center may begin with a patient coming with a complaint of "something sticking in my throat and occasional hoarseness." The FEES or FEESST examination may be the appropriate starting point. Likely, the patient will have significant laryngeal edema and erythema. If the remainder of the FEES or FEESST examination is normal, one possible initial treatment is medication for the edema and erythema. Following 3 to 6 weeks of medical treatment, the patient will return to the center. If hoarseness is still a complaint, a VSL examination will be done. The diagnosis may require treatment by the SLP as well as continued follow-up by the otolaryngologist.

Equally important to endoscopy and videostrobolaryngoscopy is an archiving system to maintain previous examinations for comparisons following various treatments. A video record that is maintained in an efficient archiving system allows the clinician to review patient progress and plan further treatment, if necessary, during subsequent visits.

Systems for the acoustic analysis of speech may also be used by swallowing specialists when there is a need to assess speech intelligibility, speech amplitude, or rate of speaking. Although these systems are used more commonly for primary complaints of voice and speech disorders, patients with many of the disorders listed in Table 11–1 may eventually require treatment for voice problems once they have achieved a safe swallow. These systems in the voice and swallowing center allow the clinician to obtain a baseline measure of all aspects related to the organs of swallowing.

Analysis of airflow and air pressure is reserved primarily for problems related to the voice; however, the same measures may also be important in assessing vocal fold closure, monitoring of breathing function during swallowing, and obtaining subsequent measurements of these parameters as the patient progresses in rehabilitation. Martin-Harris and colleagues[3] described a system for observing and recording apnea during swallowing. Observations of the respiratory patterns provide an understanding of the coordination of the respiratory and phonatory systems during swallowing. Other systems such as those described by Pitts et al[4] have been shown to be successful in improving glottic closure and thus improving the protective mechanism of the vocal folds as well as improving overall loudness of the patient.

Electromyography (EMG) is becoming more important in the diagnosis and treatment of swallowing and voice disorders. Although it is not critical to have EMG equipment available in the voice and swallowing center, its availability eliminates the need for a second trip to a specialist's office. With EMG in the office and a consulting neurologist available, information regarding nerve function can be obtained during the same visit, avoiding further delays to the start of treatment.

PERSONNEL

The development of a voice and swallowing center brings together specialists who have a special interest in the speech and swallowing organs and expertise in the diagnosis and treatment of problems affecting these organs. SLPs who are engaged in the diagnosis and treatment of voice and swallowing disorders should maintain contact with the American Speech-Language-Hearing Association's Special Interest Divisions 3 and 13. Each division offers special courses at the organization's annual convention as well as maintains websites with access to resources, special programs, and continuing education. In the United States, not all SLPs treat swallowing or voice disorders on a regular basis. In some countries, the SLP is considered the voice therapist, the voice clinician, or the dysphagia therapist, indicating special training or extensive expertise in these areas. The American Academy of Otolaryngology-Head and Neck Surgery has a speech and swallowing subcommittee to monitor regulations and propose standards to improve patient safety and clinical compliance with existing diagnostic and treatment codes.

> *Nothing is as valuable as shared real-time experience.*
> — Anonymous

In a comprehensive voice and swallowing center, communication between clinicians and patient and among clinicians is ongoing and direct. Using this clinical service delivery model, the key members are in close proximity and interact in the testing and treatment phases of patient care. The rationale for having all specialists in close proximity is that individuals with different professional backgrounds can see the same patient, conduct their tests and assessments within the same day, and communicate the results to each other without delay. The nonsurgical therapeutic aspects of swallowing disorders provide unparalleled continuity of care for the patient if all of the specialists are "in the loop." The digital or analog media of a particular swallowing examination allows all members of the therapeutic team to see the same examination but attend to different aspects as they relate to the presenting symptoms. Having the specialists in close proximity adds to efficient use of everyone's time, especially the patient's, and allows for shared real-time experiences during and after the examination.

Physicians and other health care professionals with specific areas of expertise in swallowing, in addition to an understanding of the neurophysiology of swallowing, are integral to the comprehensive care of patients seen in a voice and swallowing center. In particular, the following physician specialties are necessary: gastroenterology, pulmonology, neurology, psychiatry, and radiology. Nonphysician health care professionals are also vitally important to deliver complete care to patients with voice and swallowing disorders. They include nurses, registered dieticians, physical therapists, occupational therapists, and social workers.

FACILITIES

A defined space is necessary to house the medical and rehabilitation staff and the special equipment used by the individuals involved in the management of patients with swallowing and voice disorders. Treatment rooms should be well lit and have a decor that fits the mission of the center. The waiting area and treatment rooms should be designed for patient comfort. Reading materials or brochures that focus on voice, communication, and swallowing should be available in the waiting areas. These may be obtained from the American Speech-Language-Hearing Association and from the Academy of Otolaryngology-Head and Neck Surgery.

Rooms should be large enough to accommodate the specialists, the patients, and significant others as well as consultants who will come to participate in specific portions of the examinations. Although the voice and swallowing center is usually located in a medical setting, the need for patient comfort and convenience of a treatment center should not be overlooked.

CASE STUDIES FROM VOICE AND SWALLOWING CENTERS

It is not always obvious to a patient or to the referring internist if the patient's primary problem is a voice disorder (dysphonia) or a swallowing disorder (dysphagia). The value of a comprehensive voice and swallowing center to the referring physician is that she or he will know that, by referring the patient to a place where a group of individuals have expertise in both areas, the diagnostic workup will be comprehensive. The clinicians will evaluate both the voice and the swallowing complaints and suggest an orderly treatment approach. The internist will not have to find additional resources and will only need to maintain contact with one group. The following cases are common examples of the types of patients seen in a voice and swallowing center.

Parkinson Disease

There is probably no better example of the value of a voice and swallowing center than the needs of patients with **Parkinson disease**. These patients are usually referred by a neurologist because of either changes in the voice or difficulty swallowing certain food consistencies, usually solid foods. Their voices become noticeably weaker over a period of several months. The patient often reports a change in her or his voice coinciding with the diagnosis of Parkinson disease, but may not notice changes in swallowing other than an increase in throat clearing, excess mucus, globus sensation, and increased cough. However, on questioning, they may note that the cough is more pronounced after eating lunch and dinner. If the Reflux Symptom Index (RSI) is used, it is usually above normal and the Voice Handicap Index may also be above normal.[5,6] Weight loss may be reported.

Based on the patient's symptoms of voice change, dysphagia, and coughing after meals, a FEESST examination is appropriate. In some centers, this is done by the SLP; in others, it is done by the otolaryngologist. Once the endoscope is in place, velopharyngeal competency is assessed, the vocal folds are observed, and the general appearance of

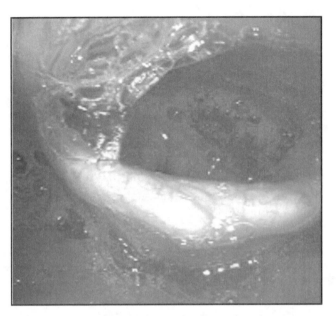

Figure 11–1. *Patient with diagnosis of Parkinson disease. The examination photo was taken after eating a small piece of cracker coated with food coloring. The patient noted that he swallowed it completely but coughed afterward.*

the larynx is viewed. Thick mucus in the piriform sinuses, epiglottis, and arytenoids is common in these patients.

Figure 11–1 was taken after swallowing a bolus consisting of a cracker. The patient is a 55-year-old male with a 2-year history of Parkinson disease. Evidence of the remaining bolus is present along with secretions, which the patient did not report feeling prior to the test.

Depending on the results of the sensory test, the laryngeal and vocal fold examination, and the FEES examination, the rehabilitation team prioritizes the treatment after reviewing the results with the patient. The otolaryngologist may elect to place the patient on a proton pump inhibitor (PPI) or other medication. The SLP may add a nutritional supplement to his daily diet. The SLP may also recommend following solids with a sip of water ("liquid washdown"). If there is a significant voice and speech disorder, the SLP may also recommend that the patient begin the Lee Silverman Voice Treatment, a special voice therapy for patients with Parkinson disease.[7]

In Chapter 6, we introduced expiratory muscle strength training (EMST). This exercise technique involves exhaling against a resistance, usually a small device containing some type of resistance. Although it has been used mostly for improving speech, several investigations have suggested that it has promise for improving swallowing as well. Rationale for the use of strength training was outlined by Burkhead et al[8] and suggests that strength training will increase functional muscle reserve, stimulate recruitment of additional motor units, and prepare the swallow organs for the rapid series of events that will follow. Given that the Parkinson patients have both a slow-acting neuromuscular system and weakness in that action, strength training may be a reasonable approach to improving both swallowing and voice in these patients. Work in this area will require not only effects on the practical outcomes of swallowing but also on the issues that underlie the functional gains using EMST.

The visit to a voice and swallowing center by a patient with Parkinson disease enables clinicians to maximize the value of the patient's visit. Specifically, clinicians are able to provide the patient with diagnoses and comprehensive treatments for the major problems of voice and swallowing in a single visit. The otolaryngologist and the SLP send one report back to the referring physician, which includes the results of the history, medical examination, test outcomes, and treatment plans.

The organization of voice and swallowing specialists under one roof facilitates a comprehensive diagnostic examination followed by a plan for the necessary treatments. There is no need for time-consuming referrals, loss of valuable examination data, or confusion about who is treating what aspect of the problem.

Cough and Hoarseness

Cough is a common complaint of patients seen in a voice and swallowing center. The patient may associate the cough with eating, talking, or no specific activity. The referring physician can feel assured that, by referring the patient to a comprehensive center, the issues related to voice and swallowing will be addressed.

Figure 11–2 shows the vocal folds of a 48-year-old male attorney who was referred by his internal

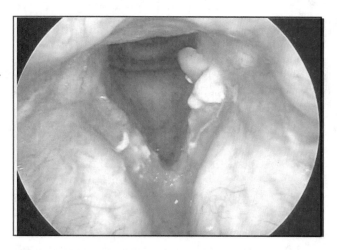

Figure 11–2. Vocal folds of a patient with left vocal fold granuloma. The white areas seen may be related to the extensive use of antibiotics, which were prescribed prior to his current examination.

medicine physician for examination following a complaint of increased cough and raspy voice that began about 4 months prior. The problem started about 2 weeks after he had surgery for gall bladder removal. At first, he noted simply a raspy voice, but then his cough increased. He noted the cough mostly when talking, although in the 3 to 4 weeks following surgery, the cough also occurred when he swallowed. His family physician prescribed an antacid, which did not improve the cough or the voice after 4 weeks. In fact, the patient noted that his voice had become "more raspy" in the past 2 weeks. His VHI was 16, above the normal value, and his RSI was 18, also above normal. Notable also was the rating of 5 for hoarseness on the RSI.

Given that his symptoms were related to his voice and also to his swallowing, a FEESST was selected as the diagnostic test of choice. The FEESST was administered by the ENT and SLP and revealed near-normal sensory response bilaterally. When given several consistencies of foods to swallow —applesauce, cracker, and apple—he showed no penetration, no aspiration, and no obvious delay or residual bolus in the piriform sinus or valleculae. The SLP reported normal swallow function. The otolaryngologist noted that he had a small lesion on the vocal process of the right arytenoid cartilage. This was diagnosed as a vocal fold granuloma and laryn-

gopharyngeal reflux (LPR) (see Figure 11–2). Appropriate results of the diagnosis and plan of treatment were sent to the referring physician. Interestingly, the white areas on his right vocal fold were previously diagnosed as an early vocal fold cancer and the reason that he was seen in the voice and swallowing center was for a second opinion of the treatment for the cancer. It was later determined that he had been using an inhaler and the white area was from the inhaler. As part of his treatment, he was given an antifungal medicine to start using and was told to stop the inhaler.

Based on the findings of the FEESST and the Reflux Finding Score (RFS) (Appendix II), the patient's antacid medicine was stopped and a proton pump inhibitor was prescribed twice daily, to be taken 30 to 60 minutes before breakfast and dinner. Because of his hoarseness, he was also referred to the SLP for vocal hygiene and voice therapy. The SLP saw him 4 times, working mostly on reducing the hard glottal onset in his speaking pattern and counseling him as to temporary diet and lifestyle changes necessary to treat the vocal fold granuloma. This included an increase in water consumption and reduction of caffeine, alcohol, chocolate, and mints, 4 foods/liquids that tend to produce increased episodes of acid reflux.

When he returned 2 months later, he noted that his coughing associated with talking was substantially reduced. His VHI rating was now a 7, slightly above normal. The vocal folds were examined via transnasal flexible laryngoscopy and the granuloma, although still present, was much smaller than it was 2 months earlier. There were no complaints of swallowing difficulty at this visit.

Four additional therapy sessions were agreed on with the SLP, the otolaryngologist, and the patient. Three months later, the patient reported no coughing when talking, a VHI score of 1, and no evidence of granuloma during flexible endoscopy.

Although this type of patient is often seen in a voice and swallowing center, the diagnosis and treatment may not always be obvious following the examinations. For example, a patient who initially seemed similar to the previous patient was concerned about his increasing hoarseness, which had been present for 8 to 10 months. His wife noted that he often coughed, but it was primarily after eating

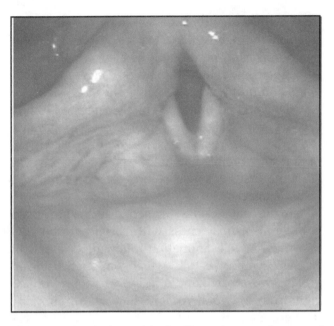

Figure 11–3. *Patient with significant laryngopharyngeal reflux, vocal fold edema, and right vocal fold paresis. Note the food coloring down to the level of the vocal folds, indicating penetration of colored water.*

or drinking or on waking up. An 8-pound weight loss over the past 6 months was reported. He was referred by his internist for evaluation of his voice. Sensation was examined initially. The sensory test revealed a high sensory threshold (8.5 mm Hg) on the right side and a near-normal (5.6 mm Hg) sensory threshold on the left side. The SLP noted the presence of a nasal quality in his speech. A complete FEESST was done. Figure 11–3 shows the result following a teaspoon of liquid of a nectar consistency. There was penetration to the level of the vocal folds. Based on the results of the SLP (nasal speech quality), the results of the sensory test (asymmetric sensation), and the swallowing examination (penetration), this patient was sent for a neurological consultation. He was ultimately diagnosed with amyotrophic lateral sclerosis (ALS).

In this case, the multiple findings obtained by the SLP and ENT combined to suggest a neurological disorder, specifically ALS. The diagnosis was confirmed by the neurologist, and the patient was referred back to the SLP for treatment of his swallowing and referred to the ALS self-help group located in the city.

Zenker Diverticulum

A 64-year-old man in otherwise good health complained to his primary physician of occasional hoarseness, occasional burping, and recently a "gurgling" sound in his throat. Following a cursory examination of the patient, the primary physician offered him a 4-week course of a popular proton pump inhibitor and dietary modifications. After 6 to 8 weeks, the problem had increased in severity, his hoarseness was more regular, and he indicated several episodes of regurgitation. The primary physician referred him to a voice and swallowing center, indicating in the referral letter that the patient was hoarse and not improving despite twice-daily proton pump inhibitor medication, a modest 3-pound weight loss, and discomfort due to the burping.

At the voice and swallowing center, the patient completed the Reflux Symptom Index, scoring 39, and the Voice Handicap Index, with a score of 17, both numbers above the normal values. Given the report from the family physician and the ratings of reflux and voice handicap indexes, it was decided to start the examination with a transnasal flexible laryngoscopy. On exposure of the larynx and vocal folds, there was clear evidence of regurgitation. Mucus was seen in the piriform sinus. A few sips of water were given to the patient. Although he swallowed all without penetration or aspiration, there were clear signs of regurgitation. At that point, the examination was ended and the patient was sent for a barium esophagram to determine if a Zenker diverticulum was present. Figure 11–4 shows the radiographic view of the Zenker diverticulum. His proton pump inhibitor medication was resumed and increased to twice daily, 30 minutes before breakfast and dinner. Because of his hoarse voice quality, he was referred to the SLP for a program of vocal hygiene and voice therapy. Voice therapy was an appropriate referral, as this was his original complaint to his internist and continued to be a complaint of his at the voice and swallowing center.

Ultimately, the patient was taken to surgery for a Zenker diverticulotomy and cricopharyngeal myotomy. His follow-up visit included a transnasal flexible laryngoscopy in which the piriform sinus areas were found to be clear of mucus. The noise associated with his swallow was also gone, and he

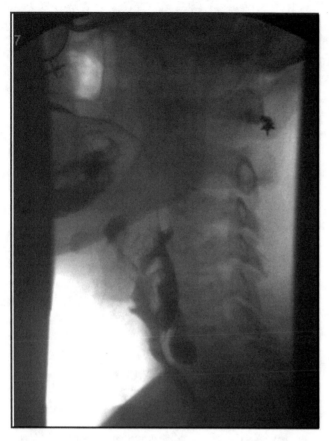

Figure 11–4. Radiographic image of Zenker diverticulum obtained during the barium esophagram.

no longer complained of regurgitation. His RSI was now 12. Because he remained somewhat hoarse, voice therapy was continued for 4 additional visits. At a 6-month follow-up visit, the patient was experiencing no swallowing problems and only occasional hoarseness. His VHI was a 3 and no further voice therapy was planned.

Early Laryngeal Cancer

A 49-year-old male accountant was sent to a voice and swallowing center by his family physician after a 4-month history of hoarseness, a 2-month history of throat pain while swallowing, and a 6-pound weight loss over the previous 3 months. He saw an otolaryngologist in his hometown who prescribed an antacid and suggested he see an SLP for the

hoarse voice quality. However, when the SLP conducted a thorough clinical history and review of his symptoms, she learned that he also complained of throat pain and that he had smoked cigarettes for 15 years and quit 7 years ago, and she suggested that he seek a second opinion. The SLP referred him to a voice and swallowing center. However, because the patient was very busy, he did not schedule the appointment immediately. In fact, it was 10 weeks after the first ENT visit before he was seen in the swallowing center.

In the center, it was decided to address the main complaint of hoarseness with a rigid strobovideolaryngoscopic examination following a review of his history and the VHI, which was 24. Significant edema was present and a lesion was found on the right true vocal fold. Vocal fold motion was normal, as were abduction and adduction. A direct laryngoscopy and biopsy was scheduled and a diagnosis of a T1 vocal fold cancer was made by the pathologist (Figure 11–5). The patient opted for radiation therapy. He was also referred to the SLP for vocal hygiene counseling during the radiation treatment. Three weeks following treatment, he remained hoarse, with a VHI of 11. He continued voice therapy sessions for 6 weeks. When he was seen in the voice and swallowing center 3 months after radiation treatment finished, the vocal folds were free of lesions and vibrating symmetrically. His VHI was 4. He noted that he could now return to full-time practice without vocal fatigue or significant hoarseness. Regular follow-up examinations were scheduled.

This case highlights the importance of the need for a comprehensive examination when a patient who is currently smoking or who has smoked in the past complains of hoarseness lasting more than 2 weeks. The SLP was correct in sending the patient back to his primary care doctor for a referral for a second opinion from a comprehensive voice and swallowing center. Small lesions on the vocal folds may not be apparent on direct observation. With the proper equipment to observe, record, and archive the examination, the otolaryngologist, the SLP, and the patient can all see the details of the examination and develop a plan of treatment without delay. In this case, there was considerable delay from the first visit to the internist followed by referral to an

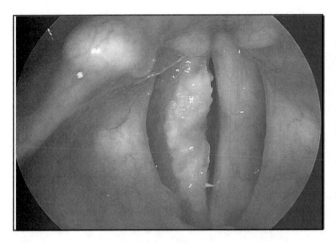

Figure 11–5. A 49-year-old male patient following biopsy of right true vocal fold. The diagnosis was T1 vocal fold cancer.

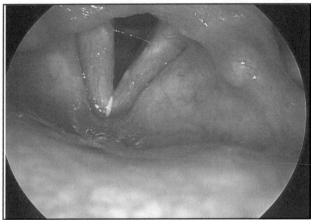

Figure 11–6. A 67-year-old male with a left vocal fold paralysis.

otolaryngologist, then the SLP, and finally the voice and swallowing center. Because of schedules and, to some extent, procrastination, it took nearly 3 months to obtain a definitive diagnosis.

Vocal Fold Paralysis

The onset of vocal fold paralysis may follow surgery or may develop along with multiple neuropathies. The patient may complain of weak voice, vocal fatigue, difficulty swallowing, or occasional cough after swallowing. Figure 11–6 shows the vocal folds of a 67-year-old male with a 14-month history of weak voice following coronary bypass surgery. Prior to his surgery, he spoke extensively as a trial lawyer. He reported an increase in coughing and occasional choking on liquids for 3 months. He was previously seen for 2 sessions of swallowing therapy in a rehabilitation center, which he noted had been helpful, especially when he used the supraglottic swallow. His voice was breathy and his maximum phonation time was 6.5 seconds. A modified barium swallow and a FEES test were done at previous examinations. Neither exam revealed penetration or aspiration, according to the written reports. He noted that when he was "careful," he could swallow small amounts of liquid without difficulty. During the current FEESST examination, the patient also swal-

lowed small amounts of liquid without difficulty; however, when challenged with repeated swallows, he began to cough. Trace amounts of liquid were seen at the level of the vocal folds. He indicated that on both previous tests, he was never challenged with repeated sips of liquid. Both previous tests were stopped after small amounts of liquid were swallowed successfully.

Because the patient had a weak voice and was experiencing aspiration, the recommended treatment for this patient was a thyroplasty, Type 1, followed by voice and swallowing therapy 1 week later. The goal was to increase his overall voice production and reduce penetration and aspiration through vocal fold approximation. Following his surgery, he reported improved swallowing and little or no coughing. He was seen for 4 sessions of voice therapy to improve his voice by reducing the associated strain that he developed following the vocal fold paralysis. Three months after surgery, his maximum phonation time increased to 14.5 seconds, and he was satisfied with his level of loudness. The SLP and otolaryngologist suggested no further treatment.

This case is an example of a team approach for both diagnosis and combined surgical and behavioral treatments. The SLP was part of the diagnosis process and realized that long-term voice or swallowing therapy would not be sufficient to treat the patient based on the findings of the voice and swallowing assessments. Following thyroplasty surgery, however, voice therapy was appropriate and helpful for increasing loudness and avoiding the strained voice quality.

Late Effects of Radiation Therapy in the Head and Neck Region

Radiation therapy (XRT) has been increasing in frequency for the treatment of cancer in the head and neck region. It is used as a single treatment in many cases, such as nasopharyngeal cancer, but it is more commonly used as a secondary treatment in other regions of the head and neck. During the course and for several weeks following radiation therapy, patients experience fatigue, mucositis, dysphagia, dysarthria, and dysphonia. This results in a decrease in quality of life following treatment. These changes are well-known, and with adequate care, proper nutrition, and rest, recovery from the XRT treatment regimen slowly occurs. Of course, depending on whether or not surgery preceded the XRT, some problems related to swallowing and speech may remain for a lifetime.

Recently, patients who have undergone XRT only for tumors of the oral cavity, larynx, and pharynx have been reporting increasing problems swallowing 3 to 5 years after successful treatment of their primary disease. Several studies have examined late effects of XRT. Suarez-Cunqueiro and colleagues[9] studied 851 patients and reported speech problems in 63.8%, and swallowing problems were reported by 75.4% of the group studied. The variables that presented a significant association with speech and swallowing impairment were gender, tumor location, stage of tumor, treatment modality, and reconstruction type. For patients who underwent XRT only, Langendijk[10] examined the later effects of patients who underwent XRT for various head and neck tumors and found that late radiation-induced toxicity, particularly in swallowing and xerostomia, have a significant impact on the more general dimensions of quality of life. These findings suggested that the development of new radiation-induced delivery techniques should not only focus on reduction of the dose to the salivary glands, but also to the anatomical structures that are involved in swallowing.

JW is a 51-year-old male who underwent radiation therapy for an early stage oral cancer tumor in 2006. He completed 30 sessions of radiation therapy over a 6-week period, a total of 70 Gy, considered a standard dose in the approximate period of time it usually takes for this amount of treatment. Over the course of treatment, he suffered minor mucositis and a 9-pound weight loss. His speech was only mildly distorted and gradually improved over the next 6 weeks. He maintained his nutrition on liquid supplements. Approximately 6 weeks following the completion of radiation therapy, he underwent a FEES examination that was reported to be normal, with no penetration or aspiration of liquids or foods. His medical record indicated normal laryngeal elevation and he was given the "OK" to swallow a normal diet. He reported only minor pain and moderate xerostomia initially. For this, he was prescribed medication to stimulate his saliva. Eventually, JW went back to work as an accountant. He maintained his regular visits with his oncologist and his otolaryngologist at 6-month intervals. At 3 years postradiation, he was seen for a regular visit with his oncologist, who noted a 5-pound weight loss since his last visit. Also noted was excessive throat clearing. The patient reported that he was having some difficulty swallowing foods even when he chewed carefully. He completed the RSI, with a rating 14, above the normal range and suggestive of laryngopharyngeal reflux. In addition, he was given the MDADI (see Chapter 5) and the results showed that his swallowing was having an impact on his quality of life. He subsequently was seen by his otolaryngologist and following a comprehensive head and neck examination, a FEES examination was ordered. It should be noted that during the head and neck examination, there was limited laryngeal elevation. When he was seen by theSLP for the FEES examination, there was mild dysarthria (distortions of /k, g, l, r/, and posterior vowels). His cough was strong and his voice was strong, but he remained with severe hoarseness and moderately severe breathiness. Figure 11–7 shows a still photo of the exam following a 10-cc bolus of honey-thickened liquid. The FEES examination was interpreted as penetration, minimal aspiration followed by a cough, and pooling of the material in the perform sinus and the vallecula. On 4 subsequent swallows, a chin tuck, a Mendelsohn maneuver, a

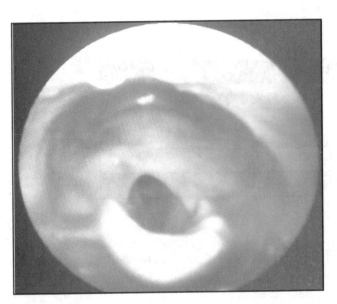

Figure 11–7. A 51-year-old male with late effects of radiation therapy toxicity.

head tilt backward, and a smaller bolus were tried. Only the Mendelsohn maneuver improved the swallow, showing less residual material in the piriform sinus with 2 swallows. A subsequent CT scan failed to identify additional cancer, and JW was told that he was experiencing late-stage toxicity from radiation that he completed 3 years before.

The swallowing problems that JW was now experiencing are due primarily to radionecrosis. There may also be loss of taste, continually decreasing salivary function, and dehydration.[11] Laryngeal radionecrosis is a difficult late complication of radiotherapy. It is associated with hoarseness, edema, pain, weight loss, and upper airway obstruction. The medical treatment options are limited, and in severe cases, the patient may require tracheostomy or laryngectomy. It is not uncommon for the patient to feel "better" 6 to 8 weeks after the completion of XRT and thus want to go on with his life away from day-to-day medical involvement; however, it is necessary to confront the issues of late toxicity and consider a long-term program of speech and swallow management. There is little data to suggest that a long-term program of speech and swallow exercises will help, but patients should be encouraged to continue to practice exercises that improve speech and swallowing. These exercises include tongue and jaw range of motion exercises and chewing exercises. A hygiene program of brushing teeth 3 times daily, maintaining hydration, avoiding drying foods and liquids, and of course avoiding cigarette smoking is recommended. The role of the SLP has not yet been fully outlined for these patients; however, as more and more patients with late effects of radiation are being seen, a greater awareness is building in the care of patients who have undergone XRT. We cannot say if JW would be speaking and swallowing better if he continued range of motion exercises and regular follow-up appointments with his SLP, but additional research may lead to evidence to support this type of treatment.

This case describes the late effects of XRT, which includes both severe speech and swallowing problems. It remains to be seen how these cases will be treated in the future, but based on general principles of muscle physiology and exercise, it might be expected that patients can experience less severe late complications of radiation therapy if an aggressive exercise program for speech and swallowing is undertaken shortly after recovery from the XRT treatment toxicity.

Failure to Thrive in an Autistic Child

A 3-year-old child (specifically, 31 months old) was seen by a pediatrician because the child was refusing to eat. An extensive history revealed that the child had a history of refusing to eat in the past but eventually began to eat. His mother described several interesting new behaviors. For approximately 6 months, he has pushed his food away from the table, spitting it out when he did eat it, and would run away from the table when his mother tried to place him in a high chair. He would often go to his room or another room in the house and start stacking books in a neat pile or taking his toys out of his toy box and lining them up on the floor and then replacing them in the toy box. The mother reported that recently, he would not answer her with yes or no responses. He would no longer smile when his father came home from work; he kept his head down and looked away from people when they talked to him. The pediatrician referred the child to the SLP because his language and speech also seemed inap-

Table 11–2. *Patient Characteristics of the Autistic Child Seen at the First Visit to the SLP Following Referral From the Pediatrician*

Age (months)	Weight (pounds)	Speech	Other Behavior Noted
18	22	Single-word responses	Occasional smile
24	24	Repeated singe-word responses	Rare two-word sentences
30	25	No two-word responses	No smiles
31	25	Single-word responses	Shrieks; no eye contact

propriate for his age. Table 11–2 reports the child's profile as reported by his parents.

The child was not cooperative when the SLP attempted to do an oral-motor examination. However, when the child was shown a series of pictures of animals, he began to stack the pictures in the corner of the room. The therapist then began to show him pictures of various parts of the body—face, hands, and so forth. When she showed him a picture that emphasized the stomach, the child turned the picture over and ran out of the room. A picture of a dog brought him back into the room. So the therapist began again to show him pictures and they made two stacks—animals on one side and pictures of faces on the other side. When she showed him the picture emphasizing the stomach, again the boy turned the picture over, but this time he went to the stack of animal pictures and lined them up in a row. The therapist engaged the boy to repeat the names of several pictures but when she showed him the picture that emphasized the stomach, he said "no" instead of repeating "belly."

This child was ultimately diagnosed as autistic by a pediatric psychologist. Because of the unusual behavior with the pictures reported by the SLP, the child was put on a mild medication for reflux disease. A plan for eating was developed by the SLP and the pediatric psychologist. One task that seemed to help in the feeding and eating program was to have the child use various pictures of food to feed his favorite pictures of animals. Ultimately, the group of foods that he selected to feed the dog and the horse were introduced into his diet.

The child began to gain weight. However, autism has many unusual behaviors and the child continued to have other autistic behaviors related to communication and socialization. He continued to receive treatment by the pediatrician, the pediatric psychologist, and the SLP. His parents were introduced to the problems of autism and joined a self-help group. After 6 months, the child maintained his weight and actually gained several pounds. Although still a problem because of food selection and distractions, eating substantially improved.

This case is unusual in that autism is often diagnosed earlier than 31 months of age. In addition, the fact that the lack of weight gain and growth was present diminished the other signs, although they were still present. The parents just associated the communication and socialization changes with the abnormal eating behaviors. Interestingly enough, once the SLP identified that eating was only a part of the problem, the child was diagnosed appropriately and the nutritional aspects of the autistic child could begin to be addressed.

SUMMARY

Having all specialists involved in diagnosis and treatment of speech, voice, and swallowing disorders available in a voice and swallowing center allows patients to receive diagnoses and treatment plans in a more timely manner than the multiple referrals necessary when specialists are in different facilities. In addition, it allows members of the team to review the same diagnostic tests and to consult, when necessary, to develop the most timely and optimal treatment plan for a patient.

1. In the assessment of a patient with a swallowing problem, the voice and communication needs of the patient should:
   A. Take precedence over the swallowing problem, because it is important for the patient to give a thorough case history
   B. Be equally important as the swallowing problem
   C. Be addressed after the safety of the swallowing problem is determined
   D. Be of little importance until a swallowing treatment program is begun

2. A swallowing team consisting of an otolaryngologist and an SLP should:
   A. Work in the same clinic so they can discuss the diagnosis and treatment of the patient
   B. Maintain regular communication and report changes in the patient's medical and swallowing status even if they do not work in the same center
   C. Maintain separate records of the patient's care, because there are patient privacy rules that must be maintained
   D. Each do an instrumental test of the patient's swallowing problem in order to compare results

3. Instrumental tests of swallowing are performed:
   A. On all patients seen in the swallowing clinic
   B. Only on adults, as children have problems with movement and the test may not be reliable
   C. On patients after the bedside assessment and trial swallows
   D. Only on patients that have not had the test in the past

4. Hoarseness for three weeks in a patient who comes to the swallowing clinic is a sign of:
   A. Voice disorder
   B. Reflux disease
   C. Dysphagia
   D. Possibly all three (A, B, and C)

5. If a patient swallows small amounts of a puree substance on 3 separate trials during the modified barium swallow examination without penetration or aspiration,
   A. The radiologist can make a diagnosis of no aspiration or penetration
   B. The SLP should ask to continue the examination
   C. The examination should be stopped and the patient put on a liquid diet
   D. The examination should be stopped and a diet should be prepared by the swallow team

Discuss the need for the swallowing team to be a virtual team rather than a team working together in one location. What are the advantages and disadvantages of the virtual team within a large medical center compared to the team being housed together in a specialized swallowing clinic?

1. Fasching W. The contribution made by the 2nd Department of Surgery, Vienna University, to the treatment of colorectal cancer (author's transl) [article in German]. *Wien Klin Wochenschr.* 1979 Feb 2;91(3):68–74.
2. Logemann JA. *Evaluation and Treatment of Swallowing Disorders.* San Diego, CA: College-Hill Press; 1983.
3. Martin-Harris B, Brodsky MB, Mickel Y, Ford CL, Walters B, Heffner J. Breathing and swallowing dynamics across the adult lifespan. *Arch Otolaryngol Head Neck Surg.* 2005:131(9):762–770.
4. Pitts T, Troche M, Mann G, Rosenbek J, Okun MS, Sapienza C. Using voluntary cough to detect penetration and aspiration during oropharyngeal swallowing in patients with Parkinson disease. *Chest.* 2010 Dec;138(6):1426–1431.
5. Belafsky PC, Postma GN, Koufman JA. Validity and reliability of the reflux symptom index (RSI). *J Voice.* 2002;16:274–277.
6. Rosen CA, Lee AS, Osborne J, Zullo T, Murry T. Development and validation of the Voice Handicap Index-10. *Laryngoscope.* 2004;114:1549–1556.

7. Ramig L, Gray S, Baker K, et al. The aging voice: a review: treatment data and familial and genetic perspectives. *Folia Phoniatr Logop.* 2001;53(5):252.

8. Burkhead LM, Sapienza CM, Rosenbek JC. Strength training exercise in dysphagia rehabilitation: principles, procedures and directions for future. *Dysphagia.* 2007; 22: 251–265.

9. Suarez-Cunqueiro MM, Schramm A, Schoen R, et al. Speech and swallowing impairment after treatment for oral and oropharyngeal cancer. *Arch Otolaryngol Head Neck Surg.* 2008 Dec;134(12):1299–1304.

10. Langendijk JA, Doornaert P, Verdonck-de Leeuw IM, Leemans CR, Aaronson NK, Slotman BJ. Impact of late treatment-related toxicity on quality of life among patients with head and neck cancer treated with radiotherapy. *J Clin Oncol.* 2008 Aug 1;26(22):3770–3776.

11. Givens DJ, Karnell LH, Gupta AK, et al. Adverse events associated with concurrent chemoradiation therapy in patients with head and neck cancer. *Arch Otolaryngol Head Neck Surg.* 2009 Dec;135(12):1209–1217.

Glossary

achalasia: A disorder of the esophagus that prevents normal swallowing. In achalasia, which means "failure to relax," the esophageal sphincter remains contracted. Achalasia affects the esophagus, the tube that carries swallowed food from the back of the throat down into the stomach. A ring of muscle called the lower esophageal sphincter encircles the esophagus just above the entrance to the stomach. Normal peristalsis is interrupted and food cannot enter the stomach. Achalasia is caused by degeneration of the nerve cells that normally signal the brain to relax the esophageal sphincter. The ultimate cause of this degeneration is unknown. Autoimmune disease or hidden infection is suspected.

akathisia: A movement disorder characterized by inner restlessness and the inability to sit or stand still. Akathisia may appear as a side effect of long-term use of antipsychotic medications, lithium, and other psychiatric drugs. Persons with akathisia typically have restless movements of the arms and legs such as tapping, marching in place, rocking, and crossing and uncrossing the legs. They may feel anxious at the thought of sitting down.

amyotrophic lateral sclerosis (ALS), often referred to as "Lou Gehrig's Disease," is a progressive neurodegenerative disease that affects nerve cells in the brain and the spinal cord. Motor neurons reach from the brain to the spinal cord and from the spinal cord to the muscles throughout the body. With voluntary muscle action progressively affected, patients in the later stages of the disease may become totally paralyzed. Dysphagia is progressive in ALS.

anaerobe: An organism that can live in the absence of free oxygen. Lactic acid and yeast are examples of anaerobes.

anterior faucial arches: The arches that separate the mouth from the pharynx.

aphasia: An acquired communication disorder that impairs a person's ability to process language, but does not affect intelligence. Aphasia impairs the ability to speak and understand others, and most people with aphasia experience difficulty reading and writing.

apnea: A period of time during which breathing stops or is markedly reduced. There are 3 forms of apnea: blockage of the airways, cessation of respiratory effort (usually brain related and referred to as "central") and a combination of airway blockage and central apnea. Apneas usually occur during sleep as well as briefly during a normal swallow.

apraxia: A disorder caused by damage to specific areas of the cerebrum. It is characterized by loss of the ability to execute or carry out learned movements despite the desire to do so. An example of an apraxia associated with swallowing is buccofacial apraxia, which may result in the ability to lick the lips or palate when food or liquid is there.

aspiration: The inhalation of either oropharyngeal or gastric contents into the airway below the vocal folds.

aspiration pneumonia: An inflammation of the lungs and airways to the lungs (bronchial tubes) from breathing in foreign material. Aspiration pneumonia is caused by breathing foreign materials (usually food, liquids, vomit, or fluids from the mouth) into the lungs. This may lead to:

- A collection of pus in the lungs (lung abscess)
- An inflammatory reaction
- A lung infection (pneumonia).

atrophy: Muscle atrophy is the wasting away or loss of muscle tissue. There are 2 types of muscle atrophy. Disuse atrophy occurs from a lack of physical exercise. In most people, muscle atrophy is caused by not using the muscles enough. The most severe type of muscle atrophy is neurogenic atrophy. It occurs when there is an injury to, or disease of, a nerve that connects to the muscle. This type of muscle atrophy tends to occur more suddenly than disuse atrophy.

Examples of diseases affecting the nerves that control muscles:

- Amyotrophic lateral sclerosis (ALS or Lou Gehrig's Disease)
- Guillain-Barré syndrome
- Polio (poliomyelitis)

autoimmune diseases: A varied group of more than 80 serious, chronic illnesses that involve almost every human organ system. It includes diseases of the nervous gastrointestinal and endocrine systems as well as skin and other connective tissues, eyes, blood, and blood vessels. In all of these diseases, the underlying problem is similar—the body's immune system becomes misdirected, attacking the very organs it was designed to protect.

autosomal dominant disorder: A disorder that is passed genetically from one abnormal gene from a family member. In many cases, one of the parents has the disease.

baclofen: A muscle relaxer and an antispastic agent. Baclofen is used to treat muscle symptoms caused by multiple sclerosis, including spasm, pain, and stiffness.

Beckwith-Wiedemann syndrome: A congenital growth disorder that causes large body size, large organs, and other symptoms. Symptoms include macroglossia (sometimes a protruding tongue), malocclusion (caused by macroglossia), and poor feeding skills

benzodiazepines are among the most commonly prescribed depressant medications in the United States today. More than 15 different types of benzodiazepine medications exist to treat a wide array of both psychological and physical maladies based on dosage and implications. Commonly prescribed benzodiazepines include Xanax (alprazolam), Librium (chlordiazepoxide), Valium (diazepam), and Ativan (lorazepam) and flunitrazepam, trade name Rohypnol. Many of these drugs slow down the motion of the esophagus.

beta-agonist: An agent, chemical, or chemical reaction that tends to null another.

bifid uvula: A bifid uvula is a uvula which is forked or split in appearance. The uvula is a structure in the rear middle of the mouth, located in front of the tonsils, which forms part of the soft palate.

bipolar electrocautery: An electrocautery in which both active and return electrodes are incorporated into a single handheld instrument, so that the current passes between the tips of the two electrodes and affects only a small amount of tissue.

bite reflex: A swift, involuntary biting action that may be triggered by stimulation of the oral cavity. The bite can be difficult to release in some cases, such as when a spoon or tongue depressor is placed in a patient's mouth.

bolus: A rounded mass that can be hard (pill) or soft (chewed food or liquids) that is given or taken and delivered to the swallowing organs of the body.

botulinum toxin (Botox): A neurotoxin made by *Clostridium botulinum*; it causes paralysis in high doses, but is used medically in small, localized doses to treat disorders associated with involuntary muscle contraction and spasms.

brachytherapy: An advanced cancer treatment. Radioactive seeds or sources are placed in or near the tumor itself, giving a high radiation dose to the tumor while reducing the radiation exposure in the surrounding healthy tissues.

brain stem stroke: A brain stem stroke is a stroke that originates in the brain stem. Because the brain stem handles many of the body's basic life support functions, such as swallowing, breathing, and heart rate, a brain stem stroke can be fatal. As with other strokes, early treatment is essential.

bruxism: The habit of clenching and grinding the teeth. It most often occurs at night during sleep, but it may also occur during the day. It is an unconscious behavior, perhaps performed to release anxiety, aggression, or anger.

Candida: A yeast infection of the esophagus caused by the same fungus that causes vaginal yeast infections. The infection develops in the esophagus when the body's immune system is weak (such as in people with diabetes or HIV). It is usually very treatable with antifungal drugs. Like *Candida*, HIV infection can develop in the esophagus when the body's immune system is weak. It is treatable with antiviral drugs.

celiac disease: A condition that damages the lining of the small intestine and prevents it from absorbing parts of food that are important for staying healthy. The damage is due to a reaction to eating gluten, which is found in wheat, barley, rye, and possibly oats.

The exact cause of celiac disease is unknown. The lining of the intestines contains areas called villi, which help absorb nutrients. When adults and children with celiac disease eat foods or use products that contain gluten, their immune system reacts by damaging these villi.

This damage affects the ability to absorb nutrients properly. A person becomes malnourished, no matter how much food he or she eats.

The disease can develop at any point in life, from infancy to late adulthood.

People with celiac disease are more likely to have:

- Autoimmune disorders such as rheumatoid arthritis, systemic lupus erythematosus, and Sjogren syndrome
- Addison disease
- Down syndrome

- Intestinal cancer
- Intestinal lymphoma
- Lactose intolerance
- Thyroid disease
- Type 1 diabetes

cervical osteophyte: A bony outgrowth or protuberance on the cervical vertebrae. Unless the osteophyte is exceptionally large, it will not interfere with swallowing even when it can be observed on radiological exams.

cervical spondylosis refers to common age-related changes in the area of the spine at the back of the neck. With age, the vertebrae (the component bones of the spine) gradually form bone spurs, and their shock-absorbing disks slowly shrink. These changes can alter the alignment and stability of the spine. They may go unnoticed, or they may produce problems related to pressure on the spine and associated nerves and blood vessels. This pressure can cause weakness, numbness, and pain in various areas of the body.

Chagas disease: Also called American or South American trypanosomiasis. An acute, subacute, or chronic form of trypanosomiasis seen widely in Central and South America, caused by *Trypanosoma cruzi*, and transmitted by the bites of reduviid bugs. The acute form, prevalent in children, is marked initially by an erythematous nodule (chagoma) at the site of inoculation; high fever; unilateral swelling of the face with edema of the eyelid (Romaña sign); regional lymphadenopathy; hepatosplenomegaly; and meningoencephalic irritation. The subacute form may last for several months or years and is characterized by mild fever, severe asthenia, and generalized lymphadenopathy. The chronic form, which may or may not be preceded by an acute episode, is characterized principally by cardiac manifestations (myocarditis) and gastrointestinal manifestations (including megaesophagus and megacolon).

Charcot-Marie-Tooth disease: A genetic disease of nerves characterized by progressively debilitating muscle weakness, particularly of the limbs. The foremost feature is marked wasting of the distal extremities, particularly the peroneal muscle groups in the calves, resulting in "stork legs." The disease usually weakens the legs before the arms. Charcot-Marie-Tooth is one of the more frequent genetic diseases and the most common genetic disease of peripheral nerves. Physical therapy can help to delay somewhat the wasting of limbs. The disease is genetically heterogeneous. It can be inherited as an autosomal dominant, autosomal recessive, or X-linked trait.

There are also sporadic cases with no family history of the disease that are due to new dominant mutations. Abbreviated CMT.

CHARGE syndrome: A recognizable (genetic) pattern of birth defects that occurs in about one in every 9,000 to 10,000 births worldwide. It is an extremely complex syndrome, involving extensive medical and physical difficulties that differ from child to child. The vast majority of the time, there is no history of CHARGE syndrome or any other similar conditions in the family. Babies with CHARGE syndrome are often born with life-threatening birth defects, including complex heart defects and breathing problems. Swallowing and breathing problems make life difficult even when they come home. All are likely to require special feeding arrangements. Despite these seemingly insurmountable obstacles, children with CHARGE syndrome often far surpass their medical, physical, educational, and social expectations.

chronic obstructive pulmonary disease (COPD): A disease of the lungs that makes breathing difficult. The air sacs in the lungs and the passageways to the lungs become flaccid and block air transport.

corticosteroids: Any of the class of drugs of steroid hormones made by the cortex or the adrenal gland. Used regularly in treating inflammation.

coughing: A cough is a forceful release of air from the lungs that can be heard. Coughing protects the respiratory system by clearing it of irritants and secretions.

craniotomy: A surgical operation in which an opening is made in the skull.

cricopharyngeal myotomy: A surgical operation that divides the cricopharyngeal muscle by cutting or slicing parts of the muscle to weaken or relax it. Thus, when an individual swallows, the small muscle is relaxed and does not prevent the flow of the bolus from passing into the esophagus. Prior to performing this operation, the surgeon may elect to dilate the muscle in the hope that dilation will achieve passage of the bolus.

decannulation: The removal of a cannula or tube that may have been inserted during a surgical procedure.

dehydration: Lack of proper fluids in the body. Dehydration is a dangerous condition that may cause tissue breakdown or even shock. Once diagnosed, the patient may require hospitalization and intravenous fluid support until stable.

dementia: Significant loss of intellectual abilities such as memory capacity, severe enough to interfere with social or occupational functioning. Criteria for the diagnosis of dementia include impairment of attention, orientation, memory, judgment, language, motor and spatial skills, and function. By definition, dementia is not due to major depression or schizophrenia. Dementia is reported in as many as 1% of adults 60 years of age. It has been estimated that the frequency of dementia doubles every 5 years after 60 years of age. Alzheimer disease is the most common cause of dementia. There are many other causes of dementia, including (in alphabetical order): AIDS (due to HIV infection), alcoholism (the dementia is due to thiamine deficiency), brain injury, brain tumors, Creutzfeldt-Jakob disease, dementia with Lewy bodies (tiny round structures made of proteins that develop within nerve cells in the brain), drug toxicity, encephalitis, meningitis, Pick disease (a slowly progressive deterioration of social skills and changes in personality leading to impairment of intellect, memory, and language), syphilis, thyroid disease (hypothyroidism), and vascular dementia (damage to the blood vessels leading to the brain).

diazepam: A benzodiazepine used as an antianxiety agent, sedative, antipanic agent, antitremor agent, skeletal muscle relaxant, anticonvulsant, and in the management of alcohol withdrawal symptoms.

diplopia: The perception of two images of a single object.

dopamine: A monoamine neurotransmitter formed in the brain by the decarboxylation of dopa and essential to the normal functioning of the central nervous system. Dopamine is classified as a catecholamine (a class of molecules that serve as neurotransmitters and hormones). Dopamine is formed by the decarboxylation (removal of a carboxyl group) from dopa. A reduction in its concentration within the brain is associated with Parkinson disease.

Down syndrome (see **trisomy 21 syndrome**)

dysgeusia: An unpleasant alteration of taste sensation, often with a metallic taste.

dystonia: A movement disorder characterized by sustained, irregular muscle contractions that result in writhing or twisting movements and unusual body postures.

Eaton-Lambert syndrome: A disease seen in patients with lung cancer; characterized by weakness and fatigue of hip and thigh muscles and an aching back; caused by antibodies directed against the neuromuscular junctions.

electrocautery: The cauterization of tissue by means of an electrode that consists of a red hot piece of metal, such as a wire, held in a holder, and that is heated by either direct or alternating current. The term *electrocautery* is used to refer to both the procedure and the instrument used in the procedure.

emphysema: A chronic respiratory disease where there is overinflation of the air sacs (alveoli) in the lungs, causing a decrease in lung function and often breathlessness.

enteral nutrition: A way to provide food through a tube placed in the nose, the stomach, or the small intestine. A tube in the nose is called a nasogastric tube or nasoenteral tube. A tube that goes through the skin into the stomach is called a gastrostomy or percutaneous endoscopic gastrostomy (PEG). A tube into the small intestine is called a jejunostomy or percutaneous endoscopic jejunostomy (PEJ) tube. Enteral nutrition is often called tube feeding.

epidemiology: *Classical*—The study of populations in order to determine the frequency and distribution of diseases and measurement of risks.

epiglottoplasty: Excision of redundant mucosa over the lateral edges of the epiglottis, aryepiglottic folds, arytenoids, and/or corniculate cartilages.

esophagectomy: A surgical procedure to remove a portion of the esophagus and then reconstruct it using part of another organ, usually the stomach or large intestine. Esophagectomy is a common treatment for esophageal cancer, and less common for Barrett esophagus and achalasia (a swallowing disorder).

esophagitis: An infection or irritation in the esophagus. An infection can be caused by bacteria, viruses, fungi, or diseases that weaken the immune system.

esophagoduodenoscopy: An endoscopic test of the esophagus and stomach usually done by a gastroenterologist. Now known as EGD.

esophagoglottal reflex (EGCR): The adduction of glottal folds upon esophageal provocation/stimulation.

esophagram: A series of x-rays of the esophagus. The x-ray pictures are taken after the patient drinks a solution that coats and outlines the walls of the esophagus. It is also called a *barium swallow*.

external beam radiation therapy (EBRT) uses high-energy rays (or particles) to destroy cancer cells or slow their rate of growth. A carefully focused beam of radiation is delivered from a machine outside the body. External beam radiation therapy usually involves treatments 5 days a week for about 6 weeks. The treatment itself is painless and much like getting a regular x-ray. Each treatment lasts only a few minutes, although the setup time—getting you into place for treatment—usually takes longer. EBRT has effects on swallowing, mainly related to inflammation.

fetal alcohol syndrome: The sum total of the damage done to the child before birth as a result of the mother drinking alcohol during pregnancy. Fetal alcohol syndrome (FAS) always involves brain damage, impaired growth, and head and face abnormalities.

Fetal alcohol syndrome is one of the leading causes of mental retardation in the US. FAS is an irreversible, lifelong condition that affects every aspect of a child's life and the lives of the child's family. However, FAS is 100% preventable—if a woman does not drink alcohol while she is pregnant.

There is no cure for FAS. Children born to mothers who drink alcohol demonstrate failure to thrive. As the child begins to mature, signs of mental retardation begin to appear. However, with early identification and diagnosis, children with FAS can receive services such as special feeding, modified diets, and ultimately special education that can help increase their potential.

fibrosis describes: (1) the formation of fine scarlike structures that cause tissues to harden and reduces the flow of fluids through these tissues; (2) the formation of fibrous tissue, as in repair or replacement of parenchymatous elements; or (3) tissue that has lost its normal elasticity due to scarring.

full-term newborn: Retained in the uterus for the normal period of gestation before birth (37 weeks).

gag reflex or pharyngeal reflex: A reflex contraction of the back of the throat, evoked by touching the soft palate. It prevents something from entering the throat except as part of normal swallowing and helps prevent choking. Different people have different sensitivities to the gag reflex.

gastroesophageal reflux: Return of stomach contents back up into the esophagus. This frequently causes heartburn because of irritation of the esophagus by stomach acid.

gastroparesis: A disorder in which the stomach takes too long to empty its contents. It is also called *delayed gastric emptying*. Normally, the stomach contracts to move food down into the small intestine for digestion. The vagus nerve controls the movement of food from the stomach through the digestive tract. Gastroparesis occurs when the vagus nerve is damaged and the muscles of the stomach and intestines do not work normally.

gastrostomy: A surgical procedure for inserting a tube through the abdomen wall and into the stomach. The tube, called a "g-tube," is used for feeding or drainage. Gastrostomy is performed because a patient temporarily or permanently needs to be fed directly through a tube in the stomach. Gastrostomy is also performed to provide drainage for the stomach when it is necessary to bypass a long-standing obstruction of the stomach outlet into the small intestine.

Gelfoam: A substance that is used to improve vocal fold bulk. Gelfoam is injected into paralyzed or partially paralyzed vocal folds to increase bulk and improve closure of the vocal folds.

globus: A word straight from the Latin, meaning (not unexpectedly) a globe or sphere. The word "globus" is used in a number of different contexts in medicine.

globus hystericus, sometimes just called globus, is the sensation of having a lump in the throat. This is a symptom of hysterical neurosis (conversion hysteria) as well as of diseases such as reflux laryngitis.

glossitis: A condition in which the tongue is swollen and changes color. Fingerlike projections on the surface of the tongue (called papillae) are lost, causing the tongue to appear smooth. Changes in the appearance of the tongue may be a primary condition or it may be a symptom of other disorders such as dehydration. Glossitis occurs when there is acute or chronic inflammation of the tongue.

glossodynia: A condition characterized by a burning or tingling sensation on the lips, tongue, or entire mouth. It is also called burning mouth syndrome (BMS), "burning tongue," or "orodynia"

glossopharyngeal nerve: The glossopharyngeal nerve is the ninth cranial nerve (CN IX). Problems with the glossopharyngeal nerve result in trouble tasting and swallowing.

Guillain-Barré syndrome: A disorder in which the body's immune system attacks nerves, resulting in weakness in various parts of the body. If the immune system attacks the respiratory or digestive system, the patient will experience shortness of breath and swallowing difficulty. Systemic attack may be sudden and may require medical emergency requiring hospitalization. The exact cause of Guillain-Barre syndrome is unknown, but it can be preceded by an infection such as an upper respiratory infection or stomach flu.

halitosis: The condition of having stale or foul-smelling breath.

hematoma: An abnormal localized collection of blood in which the blood is usually clotted or partially clotted and is usually situated within an organ or a soft tissue space, such as within a muscle; caused by a break in the wall of a blood vessel. The break may be spontaneous, as in the case of an aneurysm, or caused by trauma.

hemiparesis: A muscle weakness on only one side of the body. When hemiparesis happens as a result of a stroke, it commonly involves muscles in the face, arm, and leg. Swallowing is often seen being done in one side of the mouth.

hiatal hernia: An anatomical abnormality in which part of the stomach protrudes through the diaphragm and up into the chest. Hiatal hernia is a common abnormality, but symptoms, most often gastroesophageal reflux, only present in a small number of individuals.

Huntington disease: A hereditary disorder with mental and physical deterioration leading to death. Although characterized as an "adult-onset" disease, it can affect children as well.

Huntington disease describes an autosomal dominant pattern of inheritance with high penetrance (a high proportion of persons with the gene develop the disease). The characteristic findings of Huntington disease are caused by loss of neurons (nerve cells) in the brain.

The disease is due to a gene in chromosome band 4p16.3. The gene, called HD, contains an unstable repeating sequence of 3 nucleotide bases (CAG) in the DNA. Normal people have an average of 19 CAG repeats and at most 34 such repeats while virtually all patients with Huntington disease have more than 40.

The Huntington disease gene codes for a protein that has been named (confusingly) huntingtin, whose function is unknown. The elevated numbers of CAG repeats in the Huntington disease gene lead to the production of an elongated huntingtin protein, which appears to correlate with the loss of neurons in the disease.

Mood disturbance is usually the first symptom seen, with bipolar disorder–like mood swings that may include mania, depression, extreme irritability or angry outbursts, and psychosis. Other symptoms include dysphagia, chorea (restless, wiggling, turning movements), muscle stiffness and slowness of movement, and difficulties with memory and other cognitive processes. The HD gene is located on chromosome 4, and is an autosomal dominant gene. Only one copy needs to be inherited to cause the illness. Diagnosis is by genetic testing, and family members of people with Huntington disease may also want to know if they carry the HD gene. At this time, there is no cure for HD, although medication may be used to control symptoms of the illness, such as mood swings and chorea.

hypokinesia refers to slow or diminished movement of body musculature. It may be associated with basal ganglia diseases, mental disorders, and prolonged inactivity due to illness.

hypothyroid: A deficiency of the thyroid hormone, which is normally made by the thyroid gland located in the front of the neck.

hypoxia: A reduction of oxygen supply to a tissue below physiological levels despite adequate perfusion of the tissue by blood.

infant: A child in the earliest period of life, especially before he or she can walk. The term infant is typically applied to human children between the ages of 1 month and 12 months, although definitions vary between birth and 3 years of age.

insensate: (1) Lacking sensation or awareness; inanimate. (2) Lacking human feeling or sensitivity; brutal; cruel. (3) Lacking sense; stupid; foolish.

ischemia: Inadequate blood supply (circulation) to a local area due to blockage of the blood vessels to the area.

isokinetic neck exercises: Head exercises performed with a specialized apparatus that provides variable resistance to a movement, so that no matter how much effort is exerted, the movement takes place at a constant speed. Such exercise is used to improve muscular strength and endurance, especially after injury.

isometric neck exercises: Head exercises that only require your hands for strengthening your neck muscles. Isometric exercises are the very basic strengthening exercises to help build endurance to the muscle. Isometric exercises recruit muscles in order to strengthen without pain or movement.

jejunostomy tube: A feeding jejunostomy tube, also called a *J-tube*, is a tube inserted through the abdomen and into the jejunum (the second part of the small bowel) to assist with feeding and to provide nutrition.

Killian triangle: A triangular area in the wall of the pharynx between the oblique fibers of the inferior constrictor muscle, and the transverse fibers of the cricopharyngeus muscle, through which the Zenker diverticulum occurs.

laryngeal penetration: Material entering the laryngeal vestibule during the act of swallowing.

lipid: Sometimes used as a synonym for "fats," but may also include fatty acids and sterols, which contribute to cholesterol.

lower motor neuron: A nerve cell that goes from the spinal cord to a muscle. The cell body of a lower motor neuron is in the spinal cord and its termination is in a skeletal muscle. The loss of lower motor neurons leads to weakness, twitching of muscle (fasciculation), and loss of muscle mass (muscle atrophy).

Lyme disease: A bacterial illness caused by a bacterium called a "spirochete." Lyme disease is spread by ticks when they bite the skin. Lyme disease can cause abnormalities in the skin, joints, heart, and nervous system.

macroglossia: The abnormal enlargement of the tongue. In rare cases, macroglossia occurs as an isolated finding that is present at birth (congenital). In many cases, macroglossia may occur secondary to a primary disorder that may be either congenital (eg, Down syndrome or Beckwith-Wiedemann syndrome) or acquired (eg, as a result of trauma or malignancy).

magnetic resonance imaging (MRI): A special radiology technique designed to image internal structures of the body using magnetism, radio waves, and a computer to produce the images of body structures. In magnetic resonance imaging (MRI), the scanner is a tube surrounded by a giant circular magnet. The patient is placed on a movable bed that is inserted into the magnet. The magnet creates a strong magnetic field that aligns the protons of hydrogen atoms, which are then exposed to a beam of radio waves. This spins the various protons of the body, and they produce a faint signal that is detected by the receiver portion of the MRI scanner. A computer processes the receiver information, and an image is produced. The image and resolution is quite detailed and can detect tiny changes of structures within the body, particularly in the soft tissue, brain and spinal cord, abdomen, and joints.

malnutrition: Poor nourishment of the body often due to not eating healthy foods, improper digestion, poor absorption of nutrients, or a combination of these factors.

manometry: The measurement of pressure using a device called a manometer. Esophageal manometry is done to measure muscle pressure and movements in the esophagus in the evaluation of achalasia. Digital manometry is becoming more common in the evaluation of esophageal motility, often thought to contribute to regurgitation and reflux.

mastication: The act of chewing.

maxillectomy: A maxillectomy is a surgical procedure to remove all or part of the maxilla and is used to treat oral cavity cancer and cancers affecting the jaw and sinus cavity.

medialization laryngoplasty: A procedure that provides support to a vocal fold that lacks the bulk, the mobility or both, to achieve full adduction during vocalization and/or swallowing. A medialization laryngoplasty is done by inserting a Silastic shim or surgical Gore-Tex into the lateral portion of the vocal fold. It is also frequently called a thyroplasty since the procedure is performed through the thyroid cartilage.

motor apraxia: An inability to carry out, on command, a complex or skilled movement, though the purpose thereof is clear to the patient. Also known as kinesthetic apraxia and limb-kinetic apraxia.

myositis: An inflammation of muscle tissue. There are many causes of myositis, including injury, medications, and diseases.

myotomy: A myotomy is the dissection or cutting of a muscle, performed to gain access to underlying tissues or to relieve constriction in a sphincter, such as in severe esophagitis or pyloric stenosis. With the patient under general anesthesia, a longitudinal cut is made through the sphincter muscle to create a relaxed state in the muscle.

nasopharyngoscope: A nasopharyngoscope is a telescopic instrument, electrically lighted, for examination of the nasal passages and the nasopharynx.

Nd:YAG (neodymium-doped yttrium aluminum garnet; Nd:Y$_3$Al$_5$O$_1$) is a crystal that is used as a lasing medium for solid-state lasers.

neoplasia: New growth, usually refers to abnormal new growth and thus means the same as tumor, which may be benign or malignant. Unlike hyperplasia, neoplastic proliferation persists even in the absence of the original stimulus.

neoplasm: A neoplasm is an abnormal growth of tissue in animals or plants. Neoplasms can be benign or malignant. It is also called *tumor*.

neuroplasticity: The brain's ability to reorganize itself by forming new neural connections throughout life. Neuroplasticity allows the neurons (nerve cells) in the brain to compensate for injury and disease and to adjust their activities in response to new situations or to changes in their environment.

newborn: A human infant from the time of birth through the 28th day of life.

nonnutritive sucking: A natural reflex to satisfy a child's need for contact and may include unrestricted sucking on a breast, digit, pacifier, or other object like a blanket or toy. This nonnutritive sucking may make a child feel secure and relaxed, and allow the child to learn about the environment through mouthing objects.

nosocomial: Originating or taking place in a hospital, acquired in a hospital, especially in reference to an infection or pneumonia.

nosocomial pneumonia (NP; also known as hospital-acquired pneumonia [HAP] or health care-associated pneumonia [HCAP]): A pneumonia that occurs more than 48 hours after admission but that was not incubating at the time of admission.

nucleus ambiguus on each side is a motor nucleus within the medulla of the brain stem. It lies dorsomedial to the spinal lemniscus and ventral to the nucleus of tractus solitarius. It supplies skeletal muscle fibers via 3 cranial nerves:

- glossopharyngeal nerve: stylopharyngeus muscle
- superior laryngeal nerve to cricothryroid muscle
- recurrent laryngeal nerve to intrinsic muscles of the larynx

nucleus of the tractus solitarius is a brain stem nucleus on each side of the upper medulla. It lies lateral to the dorsal nucleus of the vagus, to which it has many connecting neurons, and medial to the spinal tract and the nucleus of the trigeminal nerve. The nucleus has afferent fibers that extend inferiorly within the upper medulla as the tract of solitarius. The superior part of the nucleus receives fibers from the:

- chorda tympani branch of the facial nerve, involved with taste sensation from the anterior two thirds of the tongue
- lingual branch of the glossopharyngeal nerve, involved with taste from the posterior third of the tongue
- internal laryngeal branch of vagus nerve, involved with taste in the region of the valleculae.

The inferior part of the nucleus receives fibers from the:

- vagus nerve
- glossopharyngeal nerve

Functionally, cells of the nucleus play a role in the:

- blood pressure regulation
- cough reflex
- gag reflex
- sneeze reflex
- vomiting
- inspiration

obturator: As related to dentistry, an obturator refers to a replacement prosthetic device that is used to replace upper teeth or associated structures (palate, gingiva, etc.) that may have been damaged in surgery, trauma, or altered development.

odynophagia: A severe sensation of burning, squeezing pain while swallowing caused by irritation of the mucosa or a muscular disorder of the esophagus, such as gastroesophageal reflux; bacterial or fungal infection; tumor; achalasia; or chemical irritation.

parenchyma: The tissue characteristic of an organ, as distinguished from associated connective or supporting tissues.

parenteral nutrition: Intravenous feeding. Also called parenteral alimentation

Passavant ridge: A prominence seen during swallowing on the nasopharyngeal wall by contraction of the superior pharyngeal constrictor; also called Passavant pad. When the palate is not optimally functioning during swallowing, this deficiency may be compensated for by a greater convergence of Passavant ridge.

pemphigus: One of a group of chronic, relapsing autoimmune skin diseases that cause blisters and erosions of the skin and mucous membranes. The immune system mistakenly regards the cells in the skin and mucous membranes as foreign and attacks them.

percutaneous endoscopic gastrostomy (PEG): An endoscopic medical procedure in which a tube (PEG tube) is passed into a patient's stomach through the abdominal wall, most commonly to provide a means of feeding when oral intake is not adequate. The procedure does not require a general anesthetic; mild sedation is typically used. PEG tubes may also be extended into the small intestine by passing a jejunal extension tube (PEG-J tube) through the PEG tube and into the jejunum via the pylorus.

peristalsis: A series of organized muscle contractions that occur throughout the digestive tract. Peristalsis is also seen in the tubular organs that connect the kidneys to the bladder. Peristalsis is an automatic and important process that moves food through the digestive system

pharyngoglottal reflex (PGCR): A protective reflex resulting in contraction of the pharynx and larynx upon stimulation.

photodynamic therapy (PDT): A treatment that uses special drugs, called *photosensitizing agents*, along with light to kill cancer cells. The drugs only work after they have been activated or "turned on" by certain kinds of light.

Pierre Robin sequence or complex: Pierre Robin was a French physician who first reported the combination of small lower jaw, cleft palate, and tongue displacement in 1923. Pierre Robin sequence or complex is the name given to a birth condition that involves the lower jaw being either small in size (micrognathia) or set back from the upper jaw (retrognathia). As a result, the tongue tends to be displaced back towards the throat, where it can fall back and obstruct the airway (glossoptosis). Most infants, but not all, will also have a cleft palate, but none will have a cleft lip. Almost all will have swallowing problems due to the anatomy of the oral cavity.

Pierre Robin sequence, like most birth defects, varies in severity from child to child. Problems in breathing and feeding in early infancy are the most common. Parents need to know how to position the infant in order to minimize problems (ie, not placing the infant on his or her back). For severely affected children, positioning alone may not be sufficient, and the pediatrician may recommend specially designed devices to protect the airway and facilitate feeding. Some children who have severe breathing problems may require a surgical procedure to make satisfactory breathing possible.

polymethylmethacrylate (PMMA): A suspension of microscopic synthetic polymer beads (microspheres) in a vehicle such as bovine collagen, hyaluronic acid, or some other colloidal suspending agent. Artecoll (PMMA suspended in bovine collagen) and Meta-Crill (PMMA suspended in a chemical colloid) are 2 brands of PMMA injectable augmentation products. The resin has long been used by orthopedic surgeons in bone cement for joint replacement or to replace a skull bone defect.

Pompe disease: A rare (estimated at 1 in every 40,000 births), inherited, and often fatal disorder that disables the heart and skeletal muscles. It is caused by mutations in a gene that makes an enzyme called acid alpha-glucosidase (GAA). Normally, the body uses GAA to break down glycogen, a stored form of sugar used for energy. Excessive amounts of lysosomal glycogen accumulate everywhere in the body, but the cells of the heart and skeletal muscles are the most seriously affected. Researchers have identified up to 300 different mutations in the GAA gene that cause the symptoms of Pompe disease, which can vary widely in terms of age of onset and severity. The severity of the disease and the age of onset are related to the degree of enzyme deficiency. The swallowing problems relate to muscle weakness and muscle fatigue.

postprandial: After eating.

Prader-Willi syndrome: A congenital disease. Newborns affected by this syndrome have problems sucking and swallowing and often do not gain weight. This medical condition also includes obesity and reduced muscle tone and mental ability.

progressive supranuclear palsy (PSP): A neurological disorder of unknown origin that gradually destroys cells in many areas of the brain, leading to serious and permanent problems with the control of gait and balance. The most obvious sign of the disease is an inability to aim the eyes properly, which occurs because of damage in the area of the brain that coordinates eye movements. Some patients describe this effect as a blurring. Another common visual problem is an inability to maintain eye contact during a conversation. This can give the mistaken impression that the patient is hostile or uninterested. Patients also often show alterations of mood and behavior, including depression and apathy as well as progressive mild dementia, lack of appetite, or dysphagia for solids.

The disease is "progressive" because it worsens over time; "supranuclear" because the main problem is not in the nuclei (clusters of cells in the brain stem) that directly control eye movements, but in higher centers that control the nuclei; and "palsy," which means weakness, in this case of eye movement.

PSP characteristically begins with loss of balance. Nearly all patients eventually develop the characteristic difficulty in moving the eyes up and down, the sign that often arouses a doctor's suspicion of the correct diagnosis. Although PSP gets progressively worse, no one dies from PSP itself. Difficulty swallowing can eventually permit aspiration of food into the trachea (windpipe). PSP may also be complicated by the effects of immobility, especially pneumonia, and by injuries from falls.

prosthodontist: A prosthodontist is a dentist with advanced specialty training including the design and fitting of prosthetic appliances, dental implants, dentures, veneers, crowns, and teeth whitening.

pseudobulbar palsy: Bilateral corticobulbar tract damage in which speech and swallowing disorders are common.

ptosis, also called drooping eyelid, is caused by weakness of the muscle responsible for raising the eyelid, damage to the nerves that control those muscles, or looseness of the skin of the upper eyelids.

pulse oximetry: A technique to measure the oxygen saturation of arterial blood by means of a photoelectric technique

pulsed dye laser (PDL): The pulsed dye laser uses a beam of light at a specific wavelength and is used for conditions or spots on the skin that are made up of blood and blood vessels.

regurgitation: A backward flowing, for example, of food, or the sloshing of blood back into the heart (or between chambers of the heart) when a heart valve is incompetent and does not close effectively.

Rett syndrome is a uniform and striking, progressive neurologic developmental disorder and one of the most common causes of mental retardation in females. It is an X-linked dominant neurological disorder that affects females only. Girls with the syndrome show normal development during the first 6 to 18 months of life followed first by a period of stagnation and then by rapid regression in motor and language skills. The hallmark of Rett syndrome is the loss of purposeful hand use and its replacement with stereotyped hand-wringing. Screaming fits and inconsolable crying are common. Because of these autistic-like behaviors, feeding is highly irregular.

Other key features include loss of speech, behavior reminiscent of autism, paniclike attacks, bruxism (grinding of teeth), rigid gait, tremors, intermittent hyperventilation, and microcephaly (small head).

rooting reflex: A reflex seen in newborn babies, who automatically turn their face toward the stimulus and make sucking (rooting) motions with the mouth. Elicited in a normal infant by gently stroking the side of the mouth or cheek. The rooting reflex helps to ensure breast-feeding.

sarcoidosis: An autoimmune disease of unknown origin that causes small lumps (granulomas) due to chronic inflammation to develop in a great range of body tissues. Sarcoidosis can appear in almost any body organ, but most often starts in the lungs or lymph nodes. It also affects the eyes, liver, and skin, and, less often, the spleen, bones, joints, skeletal muscles, heart, and central nervous system (brain and spinal cord).

In the majority of cases, the granulomas clear up with or without treatment. In cases where the granulomas do not heal and disappear, the tissues tend to remain inflamed and become scarred (fibrotic).

scleroderma: A disease of connective tissue with the formation of scar tissue (fibrosis) in the skin and sometimes also in other organs of the body. Scleroderma is classified into diffuse and limited forms. The CREST syndrome is a limited form of scleroderma. CREST stands for calcinosis (the formation of tiny deposits of calcium in the skin), Raynaud phenomenon (spasm of the tiny artery vessels supplying blood to the fingers, toes, nose, tongue, or ears), esophagus (esophageal involvement by the scleroderma), sclerodactyly (localized thickening and tightness of the skin of the fingers or toes), and telangiectasias (dilated capillaries that form tiny red areas, frequently on the face, hands, and in the mouth behind the lips).

silent aspiration describes aspiration without any obvious signs of swallowing difficulty, such as coughing or breathing difficulty. Silent aspiration is related to the loss of sensation in the vagus nerve.

slough: To separate dead tissue from surrounding living tissue.

squamous cell carcinoma: Cancer that begins in squamous cells—thin, flat cells that look under the microscope like fish scales. Squamous cells are found in the tissue that forms the surface of the skin, the lining of hollow organs of the body, and the passages of the respiratory and digestive tracts. Squamous cell carcinomas may arise in any of these tissues.

spasticity is stiff or rigid muscles with exaggerated, deep tendon reflexes (for example, a knee-jerk reflex). The condition can interfere with walking, movement, or speech.

stenosis: An abnormal narrowing in a blood vessel or other tubular organ or structure. It is also sometimes called a stricture.

stomatitis: An inflammation of the mucous lining of any of the structures in the mouth, which may involve the cheeks, gums, tongue, lips, and roof or floor of the mouth. The word "stomatitis" literally means inflammation of the mouth.

subluxation: Partial dislocation of a joint. A complete dislocation is a luxation.

sucking: To draw (liquid) into the mouth by contracting the muscles of the tongue and lips in an superior/inferior direction to create suction. To hold something in the mouth and draw at it by contracting the labial and cheek muscles.

suckling: To cause or allow to take milk at the breast with the tongue moving in an anterior/posterior direction.

tardive dyskinesia is a disorder that involves involuntary movements, especially of the lower face. Tardive means "delayed" and dyskinesia means "abnormal movement."

tonic contraction: Continuous contraction of a muscle.

torticollis: A muscle spasm in the neck causing the neck to twist often suddenly in one direction. Torticollis is triggered by a spasm in the spinal accessory nerve.

tracheostomy: A tracheostomy is a surgically created opening in the neck leading directly to the trachea (the breathing tube). It is maintained open with a hollow tube called a tracheostomy tube.

tracheotomy: A tracheotomy is a surgical procedure that opens up the windpipe (trachea). It is performed in emergency situations, in the operating room, or at the bedside of critically ill patients.

tractus solitarius: A tract composed of mostly sensory fibers that convey information from stretch receptors and chemoreceptors in the walls of the cardiovascular respiratory and intestinal tracts. Its fibers are distributed to the nucleus of the solitary tract.

transcutaneous: Through the skin.

transoral: By way of the mouth.

Treacher-Collins syndrome: An inherited condition that is passed down through families (hereditary) that leads to problems with the structure of the face. Symptoms include clefts in the face, cleft palate, a very large mouth, very small jaw, feeding and speaking difficulties.

trigeminal nerve: The trigeminal nerve (CN V) is responsible for sensation in the face. Sensory information from the face and body is processed by parallel pathways in the central nervous system. CN V is primarily a sensory nerve, but it also has certain motor functions (biting, chewing, and swallowing).

trismus: An inability to open the mouth fully. This may be due to spasm of the jaw muscles and be a symptom of tetanus (lockjaw) or it may be due to abnormally short jaw muscles, as in the trismus-pseudocamptodactyly syndrome.

trisomy 21 syndrome: A common chromosome disorder, often called Down syndrome, due to an extra chromosome number 21 (trisomy 21). The chromosome abnormality affects both the physical and intellectual development of the individual.

Trisomy 21 syndrome is associated with a major risk for heart malformations, a lesser risk of duodenal atresia (part of the small intestines is not developed), and a minor but still significant risk of acute leukemia. Children born with Down syndrome are often slow to acquire strong sucking ability, thus they may be slow to thrive if the swallowing problem is not detected early.

In Down syndrome, there are certain characteristic features in the appearance that may individually be quite subtle but together permit a clinical diagnosis of Down syndrome to be made at birth. These signs of Down syndrome include slight flattening of the face, minimal squaring off of the top of the ear, a low bridge of the nose (lower than the usually flat nasal bridge of the normal newborn), an epicanthic fold (a fold of skin over top of the inner corner of the eye, which can also be seen less frequently in normal babies), a ring of tiny harmless white spots around the iris, and a little narrowing of the palate.

upper motor neuron: A neuron that starts in the motor cortex of the brain and terminates within the medulla (another part of the brain) or within the spinal cord. Damage to upper motor neurons can result in spasticity and exaggerated reflexes.

vagus nerve (CN X): A remarkable nerve that supplies nerve fibers to the pharynx (throat), larynx (voice box), trachea (windpipe), lungs, heart, esophagus, and the intestinal tract as far as the transverse portion of the colon. The vagus nerve also brings sensory information back to the brain from the ear, tongue, pharynx, and larynx. It originates in the medulla oblongata, a part of the brain stem, and wanders all the way down from the brainstem to the colon.

velocardiofacial syndrome: A genetic condition characterized by abnormal pharyngeal arch development that results in defective development of the parathyroid glands, thymus, and conotruncal region of the heart. Medical problems include: cleft palate and other differences in the palate leading to speech and feeding difficulties.

verbal apraxia is a motor speech disorder. It is caused by damage to the parts of the brain related to speaking. Other terms include apraxia of speech, acquired speech apraxia, verbal apraxia, and dyspraxia.

vocal fold paresis: A condition of the vocal fold when it has lost partial neural innervation. Mobility of adduction and abduction is reduced and slower compared to normal function.

Wallenberg syndrome: A neurological condition caused by a stroke in the vertebral or posterior inferior cerebellar artery of the brain stem. It is also called lateral medullary syndrome. Symptoms include difficulties with swallowing, hoarseness, dizziness, nausea and vomiting, rapid involuntary movements of the eyes (nystagmus), and problems with balance and gait coordination. Some individuals will experience a lack of pain and temperature sensation on only one side of the face, or a pattern of symptoms on opposite sides of the body, such as paralysis or numbness in the right side of the face, with weak or numb limbs on the left side. Uncontrollable hiccups may also occur, and some individuals will lose their sense of taste on one side of the tongue, while preserving taste sensations on the other side.

xerophonia is a dry-sounding voice caused by diabetes medication.

xerostomia, more commonly known as dry mouth, is not a disease in itself. Rather, it is a symptom of many other diseases and conditions. These conditions cause saliva production to decrease or stop.

Zenker diverticulum, named in 1877 by German pathologist Friedrich Albert von Zenker, is a diverticulum of the mucosa of the pharynx, just above the cricopharyngeal muscle. It is also called *pharyngoesophageal diverticulum*.

Appendix I

Eating Assessment Tool (EAT-10)

Date: _____

Name: _____ MR#: _____

Height: _____ Weight: _____

Please briefly describe your swallowing problem.

_____

_____

Please list any swallowing tests you have had, including where, when, and the results.

_____

_____

To what extent are the following scenarios problematic for you?

Circle the appropriate response	0 = No problem; 4 = Severe problem				
1. My swallowing problem has caused me to lose weight	0	1	2	3	4
2. My swallowing problem interferes with my ability to go out for meals	0	1	2	3	4
3. Swallowing liquids takes extra effort	0	1	2	3	4
4. Swallowing solids takes extra effort	0	1	2	3	4
5. Swallowing pills takes extra effort	0	1	2	3	4
6. Swallowing is painful	0	1	2	3	4
7. The pleasure of eating is affected by my swallowing	0	1	2	3	4
8. When I swallow, food sticks in my throat.	0	1	2	3	4
9. I cough when I eat.	0	1	2	3	4
10. Swallowing is stressful.	0	1	2	3	4
				Total EAT-10:	

Appendix II

Reflux Finding Score (RFS)

A score of greater than 5 strongly suggests laryngopharyngeal reflux disease.

Findings	Scoring			
Subglottic edema (pseudosulcus vocalis)		2 if present		
Ventricular obliteration		2 if partial		4 if complete
Erythema/hyperemia		2 if arytenoid only		4 if diffuse
Vocal fold edema	1 Mild	2 Moderate	3 Severe	4 Polyp
Arytenoid/interarytenoid edema	1 Mild	2 Moderate	3 Severe	4 Obstruction
Posterior commissure hypertrophy	1 Mild	2 Moderate	3 Severe	4 Obstruction
Granuloma/granulation		2 if present		
Thick endolaryngeal mucus		2 if present		
			Total RFS:	

Appendix III

Reflux Symptom Index (RSI)

A score of greater than 10 strongly suggests that the patient has laryngopharyngeal reflux.

Within the last MONTH, how did the following problems affect you?	0 = No problem; 5 = Severe problem					
1. Hoarseness or problem with voice	0	1	2	3	4	5
2. Clearing your throat	0	1	2	3	4	5
3. Excess throat mucus or postnasal drip	0	1	2	3	4	5
4. Difficulty swallowing foods, liquids, or pills	0	1	2	3	4	5
5. Coughing after you ate or after lying down	0	1	2	3	4	5
6. Breathing difficulties or choking episodes	0	1	2	3	4	5
7. Troublesome or annoying cough	0	1	2	3	4	5
8. Something sticking in throat or lump in throat	0	1	2	3	4	5
9. Heartburn, chest pain, indigestion	0	1	2	3	4	5
					Total RSI:	

Appendix IV-A

Voice Handicap Index (VHI)

Instructions: These are statements that many people have used to describe their voices and the effects of their voices on their lives. Check the response that indicates how frequently you have the same experience.

(Never = 0 points; Almost Never = 1 point; Sometimes = 2 points; Almost Always = 3 points; Always = 4 points)

	Never	Almost Never	Sometimes	Almost Always	Always
F1. My voices makes it difficult for people to hear me.					
P2. I run out of air when I talk.					
F3. People have difficulty understanding me in a noisy room.					
P4. The sound of my voice varies throughout the day.					
F5. My family has difficulty hearing me when I call them throughout the house.					
F6. I use the phone less often than I would like.					
E7. I'm tense when talking with others because of my voice.					
F8. I tend to avoid groups of people because of my voice.					
E9. People seem irritated with my voice.					
P10. People ask, "What's wrong with your voice?"					
F11. I speak with friends, neighbors, or relatives less often because of my voice.					
F12. People ask me to repeat myself when speaking face-to-face.					

	Never	Almost Never	Sometimes	Almost Always	Always
P13. My voice sounds creaky and dry.					
P14. I feel as though I have to strain to produce voice.					
E15. I find other people don't understand me voice problem.					
F16. My voice difficulties restrict my personal and social life.					
P17. The clarity of my voice is unpredictable.					
P18. I try to change my voice to sound different.					
F19. I feel left out of conversations because of my voice.					
P20. I use a great deal of effort to speak.					
P21. My voice is worse in the evening.					
F22. My voice problem cases me to lose income.					
E23. My voice problem upsets me.					
E24. I am less out-going because of my voice problem.					
E25. My voice makes me feel handicapped.					
P26. My voice "gives out" on me in the middle of speaking.					
E27. I feel annoyed when people ask me to repeat.					
E28. I feel embarrassed when people ask me to repeat.					
E29. My voice makes me feel impotent.					
E30. I'm ashamed of my voice problem.					

Please circle the word that matches your voice today.

Normal   **Mild**   **Moderate**   **Severe**

P _____   **F** _____   **E** _____   **Total** _____

Appendix IV-B

Voice Handicap Index-10 (VHI-10)

Instructions: These are statements that many people have used to describe their voices and the effects of their voices on their lives. Circle the response that indicates **within the past month** how frequently you have the same experience.

0 = Never; 1 = Almost Never; 2 = Sometimes; 3 = Almost Always; 4 = = Always

1. My voice makes it difficult for people to hear me.	0	1	2	3	4
2. People have difficulty understanding me in a noisy room.	0	1	2	3	4
3. My voice difficulties restrict personal and social life.	0	1	2	3	4
4. I feel left out of conversations because of my voice.	0	1	2	3	4
5. My voice problem causes me to lose income.	0	1	2	3	4
6. I feel as though I have to strain to produce voice.	0	1	2	3	4
7. The clarity of my voice is unpredictable.	0	1	2	3	4
8. My voice problems upset me.	0	1	2	3	4
9. My voice makes me feel handicapped.	0	1	2	3	4
10. People ask, "What's wrong with your voice?"	0	1	2	3	4
				Total:	

Answers to Study Questions

CHAPTER I

1. **B**
2. **C**
3. **B**
4. **D**
5. **C**

CHAPTER II

1. **C**
2. Age   **T**
   Type of bolus   **T**
   Quality of dentition   **F**
3. **C**
4. **C**

CHAPTER III

1. **C**
2. **C**
3. **B**
4. **D**
5. **B**

CHAPTER IV

1. **D**
2. **E**
3. **D**
4. **C**
5. **A**

CHAPTER V

1. **C**
2. **B**
3. **C**
4. **C**

CHAPTER VI

1. **D**
2. **B**
3. **A**
4. **C**

CHAPTER VII

1. **A**
2. **D**
3. **C**
4. **D**

CHAPTER VIII

1. **C**
2. **E**
3. **E**
4. **E**
5. **E**

CHAPTER IX

1. **B**
2. **B**
3. **C**
4. **C**
5. **D**

CHAPTER X

1. **C**
2. **B**
3. **B**
4. **D**
5. **B**

CHAPTER XI

1. **C**
2. **B**
3. **C**
4. **D**
5. **B**

Index

A

abscesses, oral, 48
Acinetobacter lwoffi, 32
acquired immune deficiency syndrome (AIDS), 163
acyclovir, 49
ADA (American Dietetic Association)
 and aging population, 190
 and nutrition, 182–183
alpha adrenergic agonists, 46
alpha adrenergic antagonists, 46
ALS (amyotrophic lateral sclerosis), 139
 ALS swallowing severity scale (ALSSS), 35
 bulbar involvement, 34
 diagnosis, 34
 drooling, 36
 dysphagia, 35–36
 dysphagia etiology, 7
 fiberoptic endoscopic evaluation of swallowing
  (FEES) evaluation, 36
 food consistencies, 35
 malnutrition risk, 34
 nonoral feeding, 187–188
 nutritional deficiencies/dehydration, 35
 and oral content control, 34
 palatal lifts, 36
 PEG (percutaneous endoscopic gastrostomy) need, 34
 pulmonary aspiration, 34
 responses to aspiration, 34–35
 swallowing muscles weakness, 34
 velopharyngeal sphincter function enhancement, 36
Alzheimer disease, 34
 dysphagia etiology, 7
amantadine, 49
American Academy of Otolaryngology-Head and
  Neck surgery, 197
 speech and swallowing subcommittee, 197
aminoglycosides, 49
amyloidosis, 9, 43
analgesics, 49
anethole-trithione, 52
antacids, 46, 55
antibiotics, 48–50
anticholinergics, 49

anticonvulsants, 50
antidepressants, 49
antihistamines, 49–50
antihypertensives, 50
antineoplastic agents, 50
anti-Parkinson agents, 50–51
antipsychotics, 49, 51
antituberculous agents, 49
antivirals, 49
anxiolytics, 51
apnea, 23, 110, 127, 153, 197
Arnold-Chiari malformation, 34, 154, 163
artificial saliva, 55
ASHA (American Speech-Language-Hearing
  Association)
 special interest divisions, 197
aspiration
 defined, 29
 prandial aspiration, 29–30
 pulmonary syndromes related to aspiration
  ARDS (acute respiratory distress syndrome),
   30–31
  aspiration pneumonia, 31
  chronic pneumonia, 31
  risk factors, 32
aspiration pneumonia
 and altered mental status, 32–33
 anaerobic pneumonia, 30
 bacteriology of, 32
 defined, 30
 empyema, 30
 and GER (gastroesophageal reflux), 33
 lung abscess, 30
 and neuromuscular disorders, 33
 and prolonged mechanical ventilation, 33
 and upper aerodigestive tract tumors, 33
aspirin, 49
autism, 166, 205–206
autoimmune disorders, 9
 Crohn disease, 53–54
 dermatomyositis, 54
 epidermolysis bullosa, 54
 giant cell arteritis, 54
 MCTD (mixed connective-tissue disease), 54

autoimmune disorders *(continued)*
  myositis, 54
  ocular cicatricial pemphigoid, 54
  pemphigus vulgaris, 54
  polymyositis, 54
  Raynaud disease, 55
  rheumatoid arthritis (RA), 54–55
  sarcoidosis, 55
  Sjögren disease, 55
  systemic lupus erythematous, 55
  systemic sclerosis (scleroderma), 55
  Wegener granulomatosis, 55
azathioprine, 40

B

Bacteroides melaninogeniccus, 32
Bacteroides spp, 32
barbiturates, 46, 49
barium swallow studies, 41
Barrett esophagus, 48
bedside swallow evaluation (BSE)
  caregiver information acquisition, 73
  cost effectiveness, 4
  differential diagnosis, 79
  Mann Assessment of Swallowing Ability (MASA), 75
  Modified Mann Assessment of Swallowing Ability (MMASA), 75
  optimal protocols, 78
  physical examination, 78
  process, 74
  with pulse oximetry, 74–75
  and silent aspiration, 75–76
  trial swallows, 75
benzocaine, 49
benzodiazepines, 51
beta adrenergic agonists, 46
beta adrenergic antagonists, 46
beta antagonist medications, 36
botulinum toxin, 42, 45, 90, 137
botulism, 34
bromohexine, 52
bulbar palsy, 154
Burke Dysphagia Screening Test (BDST), 37

C

calcium channel blockers, 46
candidiasis, 48
carbamazepine, 50

case history, 73–74
  common clinical findings, 73
  critical components, 73
  questions to be answered by clinician in the process, 74
case studies
  autism, 205–206
  cough/hoarseness, 199–200
  laryngeal cancer, early, 202–203
  late effects of radiation therapy in head and neck region, 204–205
  Parkinson disease, 198–199
  vocal fold paralysis, 203–204
  Zenker diverticulum, 201–202
cerebral palsy, 6, 34, 154, 163
Chagas disease, 9, 48
chloroquine, 50
chlorpromazine, 51
cholinergic agonists, 46
cholinergic antagonists, 46
chronic intestinal pseudo-obstruction, 85
cisapride, 46, 50
cisplatin, 50
Citrobacter freundii, 32
Cogentin, 49
Compazine, 51
congenital conditions associated with swallowing disorders, 9
corticosteroids, 39, 54
cranial nerves
  clinical results following injury, 20
    glossopharyngeal nerve (CN IX), 22
    recurrent laryngeal nerve (RLN), 21
    superior laryngeal nerve (SLN), 21–22
    vagus nerve (CN X), 21
creep test, 175–176
cricopharyngeal achalasia, 90
critical care patients, swallowing sequelae, 41
Crohn disease, 53–54
curling (esophageal motility), 42
Cushing syndrome, 34
CVA (cerebrovascular accidents), 139
  brain stem strokes, 36
  Burke Dysphagia Screening Test (BDST), 37 (*See also* dysphagia screening)
  dysphagia following, 36–37
  early dysphagia screening value, 37
  lateral medullary syndrome (Wallenberg syndrome), 37
  left hemisphere strokes, 36
  multiple bilateral strokes/pseudobulbar palsy similarities, 37

posterior circulation strokes, 37
right hemisphere strokes, 36
site and size of lesions, 36
swallowing sequelae, 36
thrombosis of the posteroinferior cerebellar artery, 37
Wallenberg syndrome (lateral medullary syndrome), 37
cycloserine, 49

D

deep neck infections, 48
density, 175–178
dermatomyositis, 9, 54
diabetes mellitus, 4, 43, 85
diabetic neuropathy, 9
diazepam, 36, 46
dietitians
  elderly nutrition, 189
diets. *See* nutrition/diets
Dilantin, 50
diphtheria, 34
diuretics, 49
domeridone, 46
dopamine, 46
dopaminergics, 40
Duchenne dystrophy, 39
dysphagia lusoria, 9
dystonia/tardive dyskinesia, 34

E

Eating Assessment Tool (EAT-10), 71, 221
early intervention
  aspiration pneumonia in stroke, 5
  quality of life, 4–5
    SWAL-CARE, 5
    SWAL-QOL, 4–5
elavil, 49
elderly patients, 7
encephalitis, 9
endocrine conditions associated with swallowing disorders, 9
Enterobacteriaceae, 32
Enterococcus spp, 32
epidemiology
  comorbidities, 5
  etiologies, 5
    Alzheimer disease, 7
    amyotrophic lateral sclerosis, 7
    cardiac-related event, 6, 9

cerebral palsy, 6
cerebrovascular accident, 6–7
CNS involvement from AIDS, 6
craniotomy (aneurism repair), 6
degenerative neurologic disease, 6
dementia, 6
Huntington disease, 7
motor neuron disease, 7
multiple sclerosis, 7
neurological diseases, 6
Parkinson disease, 7
in patients exhibiting aspiration during videofluoroscopic examination/flexible endoscopic evaluation of swallowing, 6
progressive supranuclear palsy, 7
spinal cord injury, 6
vocal fold paralysis, adductor, 6
Zenker diverticulum, 6
epidermolysis bullosa, 54
epiglottitis, 48
erythromycin, 49
Escherichia coli, 32
esophageal cancer
  tumor treatments, 41–42
esophageal disorders, noncancerous
  achalasia, 42
esophageal diverticula, 43
esophageal inflammatory disorders, 43–48
esophageal phase of swallowing
  acid control/mucosal protection, 18
  bolus passage, 18
esophageal motility disorder, nonspecific, 43
esophageal spasm, diffuse, 42–43
esophageal webs/rings, 43
esophagitis, 48–49
ethambutol, 49
expiratory muscle strength training (EMST), 109, 111, 169

F

facioscapulohumeral muscular dystrophy, 39
fetal alcohol syndrome (FAS), 163
fiberoptic endoscopic examination of swallowing (FEES), 79–81
flexible endoscopic examination of swallowing with sensory testing (FEESST), 81–83
  and cardiac-related conditions, 9
  and PPIs (proton-pump inhibitors), 92
  reflux during, 92
Fusobacterium nucleatum, 32

G

gancyclovir, 49
gastroesophageal reflux disease (GERD), 9
   Barrett esophagus, 48
   defined, 43–44
   LPRD *versus* GERD symptoms, 48
   mechanisms leading to, 44–45
   substances influencing LES pressure, 46
   symptoms, 43–44
   24-hour esophageal pH monitoring, 92
   upper GI endoscopy/esophagogastroduodenoscopy (EGD), 90
   and Zenker diverticulum, 44–45
giant cell arteritis, 54
glossitis, 49
goiter, 9
Guillain-Barré syndrome, 34

H

H_1-receptor antagonists, 50
H_2 blockers, 55
Haemophilus influenzae, 32
Haldol, 49, 51
haloperidol, 51
head and neck oncology patients, 8
   radiation-associated xerostomia, 8
herpes simplex virus (HSV), 48
HIV (human immunodeficiency virus), 48
hospitalized patients
   assessment timing, 8
Huntington disease, 34
   dysphagia etiology, 7
Hurricaine mucosal anesthetic, 49
hypothyroid, 9

I

iatrogenic conditions associated with swallowing disorders, 9
Ig (immunoglobulin), 40
immunosuppressives, 39
inclusion body myositis, 39
infectious conditions associated with swallowing disorders, 9
infectious diseases/dysphagia, 48
inflammatory conditions associated with swallowing disorders, 9
instrumental assessment
   airway protection determination, 81

diagnostic tests of dysphagia and GERD, 89
   FEES (fiberoptic endoscopic evaluation of swallowing), 79–81
   FEESST (flexible endoscopic evaluation of swallowing with sensory testing), 81–83
      airway protection determination, 81
      and aspiration management, 82
      gathering information about withholding or allowing feeding, 82–83
   functional magnetic resonance imaging (fMRI), 88
   high-speed magnetic resonance imaging (MRI), 88
      MRI to identify lesion sites, 90
   manometry, 86
      esophageal manometry, 85
      pharyngeal manometry, 85–86
   modified barium swallow (MBS)
      8 steps of Penetration-Aspiration Scale (PAS), 84–85
      process, 83
      test observations, 84
   overview, 79
   positron emission tomography (PET), 88
   transnasal flexible laryngoscopy (TFL), 79, 93
   ultrasound, 87
      endoscopic ultrasound, 87–88
   videomanometry, 86–87
instrumental assessment and aspiration prediction
   FEES (fiberoptic endoscopic evaluation of swallowing, 85
   FEESST (flexible endoscopic evaluation of swallowing with sensory testing), 85
   MBS (modified barium swallow)
      MBS Measurement Tool for Swallowing Impairment (MBSImp), 85
instrumental tests associated with swallowing disorders
   CT (computed tomography) for defining bony anatomy, 90
   dual-probe 24-hour esophageal pH monitoring, 92
   EMG (electromyography), 93, 95
   esophogram (barium swallow)/UTIS (upper gastrointestinal series), 89–90
   LEMG (laryngeal electromyography), 93
   scintigraphy, 90–91
   sensory testing (ST)
      24-hour pH monitoring substitute, 92–93
   transnasal esophagoscopy, 90
   24-hour esophageal pH monitoring, 92
   upper GI endoscopy/esophagogastroduodenoscopy (EGD), 90
isoniazid, 49

K

Klebsiella spp, 32

L

laryngeal clefts, 9
laryngeal examinations
    breathing, 76
      laryngeal elevation, 78
      pitch control/range, 76
      saliva swallow, 78
      vocal quality/changes, 76
      volitional cough/throat clearing, 76, 78
laryngeal infections, 48
laryngopharyngeal reflux disease (LPRD)
    diagnosis, 46, 48
    dual-probe 24-hour esophageal pH monitoring, 92
    LPRD *versus* GERD symptoms, 48
    physical exam finding, 45–46
    Reflux Finding Score (RFS), 46 (*See also* dysphagia screening)
    RSI (Reflux Symptom Index), 45 (*See also* dysphagia screening)
    symptoms, 45
    TFL (transnasal flexible laryngoscopy), 93
Lasix, 49
lateral medullary syndrome (Wallenberg syndrome), 37
levodopa, 50–51
limb-girdle muscular dystrophy, 40
LPR (laryngopharyngeal reflux), 9
LSVT (Lee Silverman Voice Treatment), 103–104
Lyme disease, 9, 34

M

malnutrition/dehydration
    head and neck cancers, 188–189
    stroke, 188
MCTD (mixed connective-tissue disease), 54
medications
    acyclovir, 49
    alpha adrenergic agonists, 46
    alpha adrenergic antagonists, 46
    amantadine, 49
    aminoglycosides, 49
    anethole-trithione, 52
    antacids, 46, 55
    antibiotics, broad-spectrum, 48
    anticholinergics, 49

anticonvulsants, 50
antidepressants, 49
antihistamines, 49–50
antihypertensives, 50
antineoplastic agents, 50
anti-Parkinson agents, 50–51
antipsychotics, 49, 51
antituberculous agents, 49
antivirals, 49
anxiolytics, 51
artificial saliva, 55
aspirin, 49
azathioprine, 40
barbiturates, 46, 49
benzocaine, 49
benzodiazepines, 51
beta adrenergic agonists, 46
beta adrenergic antagonists, 46
beta antagonists, 36
botulinum toxin, 42, 45, 90, 137
bromohexine, 52
calcium channel blockers, 46
carbamazepine, 50
chloramphenicol, 49
chloroquine, 50
chlorpromazine, 51
cholinergic agonists, 46
cholinergic antagonists, 46
cisapride, 46, 50
cisplatin, 50
Cogentin, 49
Compazine, 51
corticosteroids, 39, 54
cycloserine, 49
diazepam, 36, 46
Dilantin, 50
diuretics, 49
domeridone, 46
dopamine, 46
dopaminergics, 40
elavil, 49
erythromycin, 49
ethambutol, 49
gancyclovir, 49
H_1-receptor antagonists, 50
H_2 blockers, 55
Haldol, 49, 51
haloperidol, 51
Hurricaine, 49
Ig (immunoglobulin), 40
immunoglobulins, 39

medications *(continued)*
  immunosuppressives, 39
  isoniazid, 49
  Lasix, 49
  levodopa, 50–51
  Mestinon, 39
  metoclopramide, 46, 50
  morphine, 46
  mucolytic agents, 50
  mucosal anesthetics, 49
  Nembutal, 49
  neuroleptics, 49
  nonsteroidal anti-inflammatory agents (NSAIDs), 49, 55
  parkinsonian weakness symptoms reaction, 49
  penicillin, 49
  phenobarbital, 49–50
  phenytoin, 50
  pilocarpine, 55
  pilocarpine hydrochloride, 52–53
  Plaquenil, 50
  PPIs (proton-pump inhibitors), 92
  prednisone, 40
  prochlorperazine, 51
  prokinetic agents, 46
  propulsid, 50
  Reglan, 50, 55
  rifampin, 49
  salicylates, 49
  sedatives, 49
  Stevens-Johnson syndrome-type reaction, 49
  sulfa, 49
  tamoxofen, 50
  tardive dyskinesia as negative side effect of antipsychotics, 51
  Tegretol, 50
  theophylline, 46
  thioridazine, 51
  Thorazine, 49, 51
  tricyclic amitriptyline, 36
  vidarabine, 49
  zidovudine (AZ17), 49–50
medications affecting swallowing
  analgesics, 49
  antibiotics, 49
  anticholinergics, 50
  anticonvulsants, 50
  antihistamines, 50
  antimuscarinics, 50
  antineoplastic agents, 50
  anti-Parkinson disease agents, 50–51
  antipsychotics, 51

  antispasmodics, 50
  anxiolytics, 51
  mucolytic agents, 50
  neurological agents, 50
  vitamins, 50
meningitis, 34
meningitis, chronic infectious, 34
Mestinon, 39
metoclopramide, 46, 50
Microaerophilic streptococci, 32
Mobius syndrome, 163
Moraxella catarrhalis, 32
morphine, 46
motor neuron disease, 34
mucolytic agents, 50
mucosal anesthetics, 49
multiple sclerosis, 34, 109, 111
  dysphagia etiology, 7
muscular dystrophy, 154
myasthenia gravis, 34, 102–103, 154
  botulism, 38
  compensatory training, 39
  Eaton-Lambert syndrome, 38
  meal timing, 39
  texture toleration, 38–39
  tongue weakness, 38
myasthenia gravis, adult-onset
  Eaton-Lambert syndrome, 38
  muscle fatigability, 38
myopathies
  dermatomyositis, 39
  Duchenne dystrophy, 39
  facioscapulohumeral muscular dystrophy, 39
  inclusion body myositis, 39
  inflammatory, 39
  limb-girdle muscular dystrophy, 40
  myotonic dystrophy, 40
  oculopharyngeal dystrophy, 40
  polymyositis, 39–40
  progressive supranuclear palsy (PSP), 40
  spinal muscular atrophies, 40
myositis, 54
myotonic dystrophy, 40
myotonic muscular dystrophy, 34

N

nasogastric tubes and GER (gastroesophageal reflux), 41
Nembutal, 49
neoplasias associated with swallowing disorders, 9
neoplasms and dysphagia
  exophytic tumor growth, 51

extrinsic tumor growth, 51
  infiltrating tumor growth, 51
neoplastic meningitis, 34
neuroleptics, 49
neurological disorders with dysphagic aspects, 34
newtonian fluid, 176–177
nonsteroidal anti-inflammatory agents (NSAIDs), 49, 55
nursing home residents, 8
nutrition/diets
  aging population
    ADA (American Dietetic Association), 190
    nutritional rehabilitation considerations, 189
    overview, 189
  dietitian nutritional assessment with comprehensive examination, 175
  nonoral diets, 184
    cervical esophagostomy, 185
    gastrostomy, 185–187
    nasogastric tubes (NG), 185
    nasojejunal tubes, 185

O

occupational therapists, 123, 169
ocular cicatricial pemphigoid, 54
oculopharyngeal dystrophy, 40
oculopharyngeal muscular dystrophy, 34
olivopontocerebellar atrophy, 34
oral examination
  articulation, 76
  reflexes/responses, 76
  resonance, 76
  secretions, 76
  sensation, 76
oral motor exercises (OME), 101–106
  enhancing control, agility, or neck rotation, extension, flexion, 105
  for absent tongue, 105
  for diminished labial opening, 105
  for incomplete glottic closure, 105
  for incomplete supraglottic closure, 106
  for missing palatal tissue, 105
  for pharyngeal constriction failure, 105
  for pharyngoesophageal segment (PES) opening inadequate for swallow, 106
  for trismus, 105
  for weakness or absence of mandibular support/control, 105
  increasing vocal fold closure/laryngeal elevation, 103–104
  Lee Silverman Voice Treatment (LSVT), 103–104

lip strength/bolus awareness in oral cavity, 101–102
TheraBite, 101, 103
tongue and mandible, 101–103
tongue strengthening, 103–104
oral nutrition/dysphagia diets
  commercial thickening agents, 183
  diets/consistencies
    consistency modifications, 183–184
    liquid thickness terms, 183
  NDD (National Dysphagia Diet)
    levels of viscosity/consistency of boluses
      liquid–level 4, 182
oral phase of swallowing
  bolus preparation/retention, 16
  fMRI studies, 17–18
  lips: bolus containment, 16
  tongue: food manipulation, 16
oral preparatory phase of swallowing, 2
  bolus formation/preparation, 16
  nerves involved, 16
  reduction phase, 16

P

Parkinson disease, 3, 34, 85, 109, 111
  case study, 198–199
  cricopharyngeal myotomy, 37
  dysphagia etiology, 7
  exercise value, 38
  and lingual function, 37
  oral swallow phase, 37
  pharyngoesophageal motor abnormalities, 37
  and pneumonia, 37
  prepharyngeal abnormalities, 37
pediatric swallowing/feeding disorders
  acquired immune deficiency syndrome (AIDS), 163
  anatomy, 151–152
  Arnold-Chiari malformation, 154, 163
  assessment of early reflexes
    gag reflex, 155
    oral infant reflexes, 155
    overview, 154–155
    suck reflex, 155
    swallow reflex, 155
  bulbar palsy, 154
  cerebral palsy, 154, 163
  CHARGE association, 169
  cleft of palate, lip, 154
  clinical examination, 153–154
  Down syndrome, 163, 169
  eating habits teaching charts, Web addresses, 166

pediatric swallowing/feeding disorders *(continued)*
  eating/swallowing treatment
    autism spectrum disorders, 166
    Beckwith-Wiedemann syndrome, 165–166
    cerebral palsy, 165
    Down syndrome, 165
    fetal alcohol syndrome (FAS), 166–167
    Pierre Robin syndrome, 165
    Rett syndrome, 167
    Treacher Collins syndrome, 165
    velocardiofacial syndrome, 165
  esophageal stricture, 154
  esophageal tumor, 154
  expiratory muscle strength training (EMST), 169
  feeding development, birth to 3 years, 156–158
  feeding programs, 169
  feeding/swallowing behaviors, 162
    and changes in respiratory patterns, 163
    and development delay, 163
    first feeding importance, 163
    hypotonia, 163
    nonnutritive sucking (NNS), 163
  feeding /swallowing factors
    human milk for premature infants, 168
    modified utensils and cups, 169
    special bottles, 169
    swallowing maneuver games, 169
  feeding/swallowing phases
    esophageal phase, 161
  fetal alcohol syndrome (FAS), 163
  foreign body sensation, 154
  incidence of, 148–151
  instrumental assessments, 155
    FEES (fiberoptic endoscopic evaluation of swallowing), 159–161
    FEESST (flexible endoscopic evaluation of swallowing with sensory testing, 159–161
    MBS (modified barium swallow), 159
    radiological, 159
  laryngomalacia, 154
  long-term gastrostomy, 163
  mental retardation, 163–164
  Mobius syndrome, 163
  muscular dystrophy, 154
  myasthenia gravis, 154
  normal coordinate feeding pattern, 163
  options in treatment
    oral motor interventions, 167–168
  oral motor examination, 154
  overview, 148
  physiology
    apnea/swallowing, 153
    neural development, 152–153
    reflexes, 153
  Pierre Robin syndrome, 154, 163
  poliomyelitis, 154
  Prader-Willi syndrome, 163
  psychological/behavioral systems of normal feeding, 162
  Rett syndrome, 163
  SOS (Sequential Oral Sensory) approach, 169
  sources for modified feeding and eating utensils and supplies, 168
  subglottic stenosis, 154
  tachypnea, 154
  tardive dyskinesia, 154
  tracheosophageal fistula, 154, 163
  treatment of feeding/swallowing disorders
    esophageal phase, 161
    preoral phase, 161
pemphigus vulgaris, 54
Penetration-Aspiration Scale (PAS), 84–85
penicillin, 49
Peptostreptococus spp, 32
pharyngeal examinations
  breathing, 76
  pitch control/range, 76
  saliva swallow, 78
  vocal quality/changes, 76
  volitional cough/throat clearing, 76, 78
pharyngeal phase of swallowing
  tongue, velopharyngeal, laryngeal interaction, 18
pharyngitis, 48
phenobarbital, 49–50
phenytoin, 50
physical therapists, 123
Pierre Robin syndrome, 163
pilocarpine, 55
pilocarpine hydrochloride, 52–53
Plaquenil, 50
poliomyelitiis, 154
polymyositis, 34, 39–40, 54
polymyositis/dermatomyositis, 34
polyneuropathies, 34
postsurgical swallowing disorders, 60
  anterior cervical spinal surgery (ACSS)
    airway edema, 60
    esophageal perforation, 61
    hypertonicity of upper esophageal sphincter (UES), 60–61
    prevertebral soft tissue swelling/epiglottis inversion, 60
    screw or plate displacement or extrusion following surgery, 61

size/positioning of bone graft and/or plate
suboptimal, 61
clinical manifestations of cranial nerve deficits, 65
etiological factors, 61
floor of mouth surgery, 63
glossectomy, partial, 63
head and neck surgery, 61
  abnormal oral phase swallowing, postsurgical, 62
  causes of abnormal oral phase swallowing,
    postsurgical, 62
  dysphagia after hypopharynx surgery, 62
  dysphagia after oropharyngeal resection, 62
hypopharyngeal surgery, 64
lip surgery, 63
mandibular surgery, 63
oropharyngeal surgery, 63
overview, 67
palate surgery, 63
reconstructive grafts/flaps can weaken laryngeal
    protection, 64
skull base surgery, 64
tracheotomy, 64
  airway pressure changes, 65
  expiratory speaking valves, 65
  glottic closure, 65–66
  laryngeal elevation, 65
  pharyngeal transit, 66
  physiological changes following, 65
Zenker diverticulum, 66
  surgical indications/contraindications, 67
  symptoms, 67
PPIs (proton-pump inhibitors), 92
prednisone, 40
prochlorperazine, 51
progressive muscular dystrophy, 34
progressive supranuclear palsy, 34
progressive supranuclear palsy (PSP), 40
prokinetic agents, 46
propulsid, 50
prosthetic management of swallowing disorders
  adjunctive swallowing treatments following partial
    glossectomy, 126
  IOPI (Iowa Performance Instrument) for pressure
    management, 122
  lingual prostheses, 125–126
  NSV (nasal speaking valve), 125
  oral prosthodontics/dentures, 122–124
  overview, 122
  palate lowering prostheses, 124
  physical/environmental adjustments for
    swallowing, 128
  rehabilitation goals after total glossectomy, 126

soft palate prostheses, 124–125
SWAL-QOL, 122
Pseudomonas aeruginosa, 32
PSS (progressive systemic sclerosis), 43

Q

quality of life
  aspiration, 2
  aspiration pneumonia, 2
  dehydration, 2–3
  and financial well-being, 4
  and general health, 3–4
  malnutrition, 3
  and pneumonia types
    CAP (community acquired pneumonia), 3
    nosocomial, 3, 8
  and psychological well-being, 4

R

rabies, 34
radiation therapy/swallowing disorders
  acute dysphasia from radiation, 52–53
  fractionated irradiation and salivary flow, 52
  irradiated salivary tissue degeneration, 52
  late effects complications, 52
  mucosal basal cell mitotic death, 52
  xerostomia, 52
Raynaud disease, 55
Reglan, 50, 55
Rett syndrome, 163
RFS (Reflux Finding Score), 46, 71, 222
rheology
  agents to alter viscosity, 177
  overview, 174–175
  terminology, 175–176
  viscosity, 176–178
  viscosity shear rate profiles/density measurements,
    177
rheumatoid arthritis (RA), 54–55
rifampin, 49
RSI (Reflux Symptom Index), 45, 71, 223

S

salicylates, 49
sarcoidosis, 9, 34, 55
scleroderma, 9, 85
screening for dysphagia
  Burke Dysphagia Screening Test (BDST), 71–72
  chest auscultation, 72
  dye test, 72

screening for dysphagia *(continued)*
    EAT-10, 71, 221
    MDADI (MD Anderson Dysphagia Inventory), 71
    RFS (Reflux Finding Score), 46, 71, 222
    RSI (Reflux Symptom Index), 45, 71, 223
    screening test limitations, 72–73
    screening tests, 71–73
    self-assessments, 70–71
    SWAL-CARE, 5, 70–71
    SWAL-QOL, 4–5, 70–71
sedatives, 49
sedentary elderly, 109
Sjögren disease, 9
speech-language pathologists (SLPs)
    and the BSE, 72
    collaboration in MBS administration, 83
    flexible endoscopic evaluation of swallowing with
        sensory testing (FEESST), 82
    physical examination, 78
    as primary member of the nonsurgical swallowing
        management team, 100
    voice and swallowing expertise, 197
sphincters, 19–20
    laryngeal, 21
    upper esophageal, 21
    upper esophageal (UES), 21
    velopharyngeal, 20
spinal muscular atrophies, 40
Staphylococcus aureus, 32
stomatitis, 49
Streptococcus pneumoniae, 32
Streptococcus viridans, 32
sulfa, 49
surgical treatment of swallowing disorders
    cricothyrotomy, 142
    decannulation, 142
    expiratory speaking valve, 141–142
    fenestrated tracheostomy tube, 142
    gastrostomy
        PEG (percutaneous endoscopic gastrostomy), 139
    laryngeal surgical closure
        laryngotracheal separation/Lindeman treatment,
          139–140
        proximal subglottic trachea closure as a blind
          pouch/a permanent stoma created from distal
          trachea, 140
    overview, 132
    palatopexy
        and VPI (velopalatine incompetence), 138
    pharyngoesophageal dilatation, 139
    tracheotomy for prolonged mechanical ventilation
        factors influencing recommendation for, 141–142

treating intractable aspiration schematic, 141
vocal fold medialization, 132–138 (*See also* vocal
    fold medialization *main entry*)
SWAL-CARE 15-item tool assessing quality of care/
    patient satisfaction, 5
swallowing, abnormal, 2, 28–29
    aspiration
        defined, 29
        risk factors, 32
    aspiration pneumonia
        and altered mental status, 32–33
        anaerobic pneumonia, 30
        bacteriology of, 32
        defined, 30
        empyema, 30
        and GER (gastroesophageal reflux), 33
        lung abscess, 30
        and neuromuscular disorders, 33
        and prolonged mechanical ventilation, 33
        and upper aerodigestive tract tumors, 33
    prandial aspiration
        classification, 29–30
    pulmonary syndromes related to aspiration
        ARDS (acute respiratory distress syndrome), 30–31
        aspiration pneumonia, 31
        chronic pneumonia, 31
swallowing, normal, 2, 56
    central neural control
        central pattern generator, 22
        cortical regulation, 22
        oral cavity receptor feedback, 23
        swallowing center, 22
        swallowing reflex, 22–23
    cranial nerves
        glossopharyngeal nerve (CN IX), 22
        recurrent laryngeal nerve (RLN), 21
        superior laryngeal nerve (SLN), 21–22
        vagus nerve (CN X), 21
    esophageal phase
        acid control/mucosal protection, 18
        bolus passage, 18
    oral phase
        bolus preparation/retention, 16
        fMRI studies, 17–18
        lips: bolus containment, 16
        tongue: food manipulation, 16
    oral preparatory phase, 2
        bolus formation/preparation, 16
        nerves involved, 16
        reduction phase, 16
    pharyngeal phase
        tongue, velopharyngeal, laryngeal interaction, 18

phase relationships
    variable bolus/timing, 18, 20
and respiration
    swallowing apnea, 23
sphincters, 19–20
    laryngeal, 21
    upper esophageal, 21
    upper esophageal (UES), 21
    velopharyngeal, 20
timely interaction of muscles and nerves, 28
swallowing following head and neck cancer
    early outcomes, 142–143
    late outcomes
        PEG feedings, 144
SWAL-QOL, validated assessment 44-item tool, 4–5,
    70–71, 122, 143
syndromes
    fetal alcohol syndrome (FAS), 166–167
    Rett syndrome, 167
    Pierre Robin syndrome, 165–166
    Down syndrome, 165
    Mobius syndrome, 163–164
syphilis, 34
syringobulbia, 34
systemic conditions associated with swallowing
    disorders, 9
systemic lupus erythematous, 55
systemic sclerosis (scleroderma), 55

T

tamoxofen, 50
tardive dyskinesia, 154
Tegretol, 50
textures
    characteristics, 178
    continuum of viscosities/textures, 179–180
    food categories not well tolerated by patients with
        swallowing disorders, 184
    solid textures/swallowing severity, 181
theophylline, 46
thioridazine, 51
Thorazine, 49, 51
tonsillitis, 48
torticollis, 34
tracheoesophageal fistula, 9
tracheosophageal fistula, 154, 163
traumatic brain injury, 34, 40–41
traumatic conditions associated with swallowing
    disorders, 9
treatment of swallowing disorders, nonsurgical, 100,
    118

compensatory swallowing therapy, 100–107
    expiratory muscle strength training (EMST), 109, 111
    Lee Silverman Voice Treatment (LSVT), 103–104
    neuromuscular electrical stimulation (NMES),
        109–111
    oral motor exercises (OME), 101–106
    Shaker exercise, 107–108
    thermal tactile oral stimulation (TTOS), 108–109
Lee Silverman Voice Treatment (LSVT), 103–104, 118
rehabilitative swallowing therapy, 115–116
    aspiration control, nonsurgical,
    chin down swallowing posture, 114–115
    effortful swallow, 112–114
    head back swallowing posture, 114–115
    head rotation swallowing posture, 114–115
    Mendelsohn maneuver, 112–114
    overview, 111–112
    postural techniques for aspiration or residue
        reduction or elimination, 115
    super-supraglottic swallow, 112–114
    supraglottic swallow, 112–114
    swallowing maneuvers for pharyngeal swallow
        bolus control, 112–114
    swallowing postures, 114–115
    swallowing therapy and aspiration, 115–116
    swallow-related disorders and possible
        interventions, 116–117
    tongue hold maneuver, 112–114
treatment of swallowing disorders, surgical
    cricothyrotomy, 142
    decannulation, 142
    expiratory speaking valve, 141–142
    fenestrated tracheostomy tube, 142
    gastrostomy
        PEG (percutaneous endoscopic gastrostomy), 139
    laryngeal surgical closure
        laryngotracheal separation/Lindeman treatment,
            139–140
        proximal subglottic trachea closure as a blind
            pouch/a permanent stoma created from distal
            trachea, 140
    overview, 132
    palatopexy
        and VPI (velopalatine incompetence), 138
    pharyngoesophageal dilatation, 139
    tracheotomy for prolonged mechanical ventilation
        factors influencing recommendation for, 141–142
    treating intractable aspiration schematic, 141
    vocal fold medialization, 132–138 (*See also* vocal
        fold medialization *main entry*)
tricyclic amitriptyline, 36
Trypanosoma cruzi, 48

V

vidarabine, 49
viral encephalitis, 34
viscosity, 176–178
vitamin A, 50
vitamin E, 50
vocal fold medialization
    laryngeal framework surgery, 134
    medialization laryngoplasty
        advantages/disadvantages, 135
        complications/limitations, 135
        cricopharyngeal myotomy, 137
        with Gore-Tex, 134, 136
        hypopharyngeal pharyngoplasty, 137
        with silicone, 134
    by vocal fold injection
        acellular dermis injection, 133
        advantages, 133
        autologous fat injection, 133
        calcium hydroxyapatite, 133–134
        complications, 133
        Gelfoam injection, 133
        hyaluronic acid injection, 133
        Teflon injection, 133–134
vocal fold paralysis, 34
voice and swallowing center model, 197
    case studies
        autistic child's failure to thrive, 205–206
        cough/hoarseness, 199–200
        laryngeal cancer, early, 202–203
        late effects of radiation therapy in head and neck
            region, 204–205
        Parkinson disease, 198–199
        vocal fold paralysis, 203–204

Zenker diverticulum, 201–202
    diagnostic considerations/tests, 195
        common conditions, disorders, diseases with
            elements of speech, voice, swallowing
            disorders, 196
    diagnostic considerations/tests/self-assessment
        tools, 195–196
    facilities, 198
    instrumentation (assessment/treatment
        verification), 196–197
        acoustic analysis systems, 197
        airflow/air pressure analysis, 197
        record keeping scheme, 197
        visualization, 196–197
    otolaryngologist/SLP shared roles, 195
    overview, 194–195
    personnel, 197–198
Voice Handicap Index-10 (VHI-10), 226
Voice Handicap Index (VHI), 196, 198, 201, 224–225

W

Wallenberg syndrome (lateral medullary syndrome),
    37
Wegener granulomatosis, 55
Wilson disease, 34

Z

Zenker diverticulum, 43–45, 66–67, 201–202
    case study, 201–202
    surgical indications/contraindications, 67
    symptoms, 67
zidovudine (AZ17), 49–50